W9-BSQ-323

Dian Shepperson Mills, CertEd (Nutrition), BA (Education and Psychology), DipION, MA (Health Education – Nutrition), is the Director of the Endometriosis and Fertility Clinic based at The Hale Clinic in London. As a clinical nutritionist, she holds clinics at The Institute for Optimum Nutrition (ION), in London and in Sussex, where she sees clients on a one-to-one basis for nutrition counselling. She can be contacted at www.endometriosis.co.uk, www.nutrition.us.com or www.makingbabies.com for consultations. In a link with the USA, she works with Total Wellness Inc. based in San Francisco. Her research interests include women's health issues, endometriosis, subfertility in both men and women, premenstrual syndrome, endocrine disorders, polycystic ovary syndrome and the menopause. She has published several papers, abstracts and book chapters, and has given lectures to scientific societies in Europe, the USA, Asia, Australia and South America.

A past trustee of the British Endometriosis Society, she is now a founder member of the SHE Trust (Simply Holistic Endometriosis), a charity that supports women with endometriosis who wish to use both orthodox and complementary therapies on their road to wellness. Dian has researched the relationship between endometriosis and diet, and works closely with doctors and consultants in the UK, USA and Europe. She is an active member of The European Society of Human Reproduction and Embryology (ESHRE), the American Society of Reproductive Medicine (ASRM), The She Trust (Simply Holistic Endometriosis) charity, founded to help women with endometriosis obtain unbiased information, and is an advisor to the International Endometriosis Association whose headquarters are in the USA.

As an advisor to the International Endometriosis Association, head-quartered in the USA, Dian has links to groups in the USA, Japan and Brazil, and the Nordic and other European countries, as well as to independent EA groups in Australia, New Zealand and Ireland. Dian holds nutrition clinics for one-to-one consultations in The Hale Clinic, London and at The Institute for Optimum Nutrition, London and in Sussex, England. Contact her via the web pages www.endometriosis.co.uk and www.makingbabies.com, and at dian@endometriosis.co.uk.

In addition to Dian's professional understanding of endometriosis, she has personal experience of the condition. During 1981–1982, she was bedridden for six months due to severe abdominal and leg pains that left her unable to walk. Endometriosis was written in her notes, but the gynaecologist did not believe that it could cause such pain and she was never told. She saw eight different specialists at this time and was even, for two weeks on a geriatric ward, placed on traction with a nine-pound weight hung from her left leg, and then fitted in a full-body plaster cast!

In the end, she was helped by herbs and homeopathy, and returned to fulltime teaching. In 1987 she was extremely ill again with ruptured ovarian cysts and excrutiating pain. The drug treatments given for pseudomenopause and pseudopregnancy made her even more ill. Laser surgery removed one cyst, but it returned within two weeks. The only treatment offered was a total hysterectomy with ovaries removed. Not wishing to have major surgery, Dian opted to look into complementary treatments. Her motto and philosophy has always been: 'Let's try the least harsh method first and work up.' The optimum nutrition route was a major part of her healing process. She consulted a clinical ecologist and closely followed his advice. By 1989, she began to be symptom-free and has remained so ever since. Having lectured in home economics and nutrition for 18 years, Dian has since retrained, for a further six years, in nutritional medicine, and has worked with thousands of women suffering from endometriosis and fertility problems worldwide.

Nutrition is not magical; it is logical. While following a healthy eating plan, women with endometriosis have seen a regression of their symptoms, and regained their energy and vitality. Improving quality of life is a key factor in regaining your health. There is no failure except in ceasing to try, as teachers say. Dian will go on researching to find the cause of endometriosis. Her quest is to eradicate period pain from the face of the planet. Dian now also works with Foresight – the Charity for Preconceptual Care – helping couples who have suffered miscarriage and fertility problems to conceive at The Endometriosis and Fertility Clinic, ION, London (tel: 020 8877 9993) and The Hale Clinic, London (tel: 020 7637 3377).

Michael W Vernon, PhD, HCLD is a reproductive physiologist and scientific director at the Woman's Hospital of Baton Rouge, Louisiana, USA. He previously held the post of Associate Professor at the University of Kentucky where he lectured on medical endocrinology. His research areas are uterine physiology, endometriosis and ART (assisted reproductive technology). He has published over 100 peer-reviewed papers, abstracts and book chapters, and has given plenary lectures to scientific societies in the USA, Europe, Asia and South America. Dr Vernon is an ad hoc member and past chair of the National Institute of Health (NIH), Washington, DC, in the field of reproductive biology.

He is an active member of several societies, including the American Society for Reproductive Medicine (ASRM), the Society for Gynecological Investigation (SGI), the Society for the Study of Reproduction (SSR) and the Endometriosis Association of the USA.

Dr Vernon has an extensive background in in-vitro fertilization treatment (IVF). He was part of the first research team at the Wisconsin Primate Center that successfully performed IVF in the rhesus monkey. He was the embryologist for the first babies born in Kentucky through IVF, GIFT, ZIFT, micromanipulation and cryopreservation.

Praise for

Endometriosis:

A Key to Healing and Fertility Through Nutrition

'Many women with endometriosis have found that nutrition can play a major role in overcoming some of the most debilitating effects of the disease. Dian Mills has studied the role of nutrition in treating endometriosis and, together with Michael Vernon, has made this information available in an understandable and compassionate way in this very helpful book.'

Mary Lou Ballweg, President

INTERNATIONAL ENDOMETRIOSIS ASSOCIATION

'The book is simple, easy to comprehend and will be embraced by a large majority, particularly those afflicted with endometriosis. It will be essential reading for scientists and the general public interested directly or indirectly in endometriosis.'

Dr O A Odukoya

DEPARTMENT OF OBSTETRICS AND
GYNAECOLOGY
JESSOP HOSPITAL FOR WOMEN
SHEFFIELD

'Endometriosis has an effect on all aspects of the life of a woman who suffers from this debilitating and perplexing condition. Modern medicine has made great strides in bringing help and relief to many women. Unfortunately, to date, there is still no known cure.

'During my years as Chair to the NES it became obvious that women are more than willing to help themselves. Regrettably, the tools to do this have been few and far between. With the publication of this book women will now have the opportunity to try to help themselves without resorting to powerful drugs and/or surgery, or to use the information as complementary alongside orthodox medicine. I welcome a book that will give women a choice.'

Diane Carlton, SRN, D/N Cert

SENIOR PRACTICE NURSE
CHAIR TO THE NATIONAL
ENDOMETRIOSIS SOCIETY 1983–97,
FOUNDER AND CHAIR OF
THE SHE TRUST

ENDOMETRIOSIS
A Key to Healing and Fertility Through Nutrition

Dian Shepperson Mills MA and
Michael Vernon PhD, HCLD

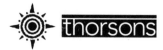

Thorsons
An Imprint of HarperCollins*Publishers*
77–85 Fulham Palace Road
Hammersmith, London W6 8JB

The website address is: www.thorsonselement.com

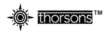

and *Thorsons* are trademarks of
HarperCollins*Publishers* Ltd

First published in Great Britain in 1999 by Element Books Limited
This edition published by Thorsons 2002

16 15 14 13

© Dian Shepperson Mills and Michael Vernon 1999

Dian Shepperson Mills and Michael Vernon assert the moral right to
be identified as the authors of this work

Text illustrations: Janice Sharp
Photography: R.S.A. Photography Ltd

A catalogue record for this book
is available from the British Library

ISBN-13 978-0-00-713310-9
ISBN-10 0-00-713310-3

Printed and bound in Great Britain by
Martins the Printers Ltd, Berwick-upon-Tweed

All rights reserved. No part of this publication may be
reproduced, stored in a retrieval system, or transmitted,
in any form or by any means, electronic, mechanical,
photocopying, recording or otherwise, without the prior
written permission of the publishers.

Note: the information contained in this book is true and
complete to the best of the authors' knowledge and is given
for the purpose of helping people who suspect or know that
they suffer from endometriosis. This book is not to be used as
a substitute for professional medical treatment. The ultimate
decision concerning care should be between you and your
doctor. The information in this book is general and is offered
with no guarantes on the part of the authors or Element
Books. The authors and Publisher disclaim all liability in
connection with the use of this book.

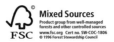
Mixed Sources
Product group from well-managed
forests and other controlled sources
www.fsc.org Cert no. SW-COC-1806
© 1996 Forest Stewardship Council
FSC

Contents

I would like to emphasize maternity as the frontier of human welfare and that the defence of mothers is the defence of nations. There is no place in the public health field that offers greater opportunity for service to mankind and the welfare of the human race than the application of newer and ever increasing knowledge of nutrition at the human frontier.

Ina May Hobbler, 1952

This human body, at peace with itself, is more precious than the rarest gem. Gherish your body, it is yours for this one time only. The human form is won with difficulty; it is easy to lose. All worldly things are brief, like lightning in the sky. This life you must know was the tiny splash of a raindrop. A thing of beauty that passes away even as it comes into being. Therefore set your goal, and make every day and night a time to obtain it.

Lama Tsong Khapa
14th century Tibetan scholar and yogi

Nuchi gusui – may your food and lifestyle heal.

The Okinawa Way Book

If you try, you might. If you don't, you won't.

W Pickles

Acknowledgements

To all those who believe and research into the power of sound nutrition principles in helping to strengthen new life, the words of Ina May Hobbler should echo around the world:

> I would like to emphasize maternity as the frontier of human welfare and that the defence of mothers is the defence of nations. There is no place in the public health field that offers greater opportunity for service to mankind and the welfare of the human race than the application of newer and ever increasing knowledge of nutrition at the human frontier.
>
> *Ina May Hobbler, Nutrition and*
> *Maternal Health, Proceedings of the First*
> *Conference on Human Nutrition, Ohio State*
> *Department of Health, Columbus, Ohio, 1952*

Thanks must go to those who have been supportive through the research and writing up of this book:

To Mike Vernon, for suggesting that we write this book together, and for all his encouragement and guidance throughout its inception. From a chance conversation on proteins in Houston in 1989, a book has grown, and its production has been tremendously rewarding and the greatest of fun, the happiest of times. We both wish to thank all the people who invented cyberspace and e-mail, which have made communication so easy.

To my husband, G J Mills, Mike's wife, Beverly Martin and his children, Tammy DiVito and Matthew for their support.

To my grandfather, who gave me an enquiring mind through all our childhood games with physics and chemistry experiments.

To my mother and father, who encouraged us to be caring of others.

To my friends and staff at the University of Brighton and at the Institute for Optimum Nutrition, for their guidance and encouragement.

To my ION students, who are always supportive and give great encouragement.

To Mary Lou Ballweg, of the International Endometriosis Association of America, for her inspiration, and to Mrs P Barnes of Foresight, whose dedication to endometriosis and infertility research made this book possible.

To Margaret and Arthur Wynn, in admiration, for their ongoing work in pulling together research from around the world on preconceptual care and nutrition, an inspiration to us all.

To all the women who have had faith enough to try the nutrition path, and especially to all those who have persevered and taken the time to write their story for inclusion in this book in the hope that they will inspire others to follow their lead.

To K Robinson, for her editing, support and friendship; to Rebecca Rose, for sheer delight and inspiration; to M Washington and Susan Wilson, for reading the book when it was in production and making all their suggestions; and to Sharyn Wong, for being the most supportive copy-editor who coached me through the process of completing this edition of the book.

To J Thomson, a fellow author, for her encouragement to write the book, and especially to Janice Sharp who, with her understanding of the subject, wove such beautiful drawings to adorn this book.

To Cassi Whiting, who has been an inspiration, whose support led me to develop all the fine detail about the ovaries and fertility.

To the gynaecologists who have aided our quest: Mr S Kennedy, of Oxford University, for taking the time to read this book in draft form, and for his support and belief in us; D Metzger, of Yale University and Mr O Odukoya, of Sheffield University, for their encouragement along the nutrition highway.

To Mike's former students and now new colleagues in endometriosis research, Drs Maria Bertero, Warren Nothnick and Kathy Sharpe-Timms.

To the Trustees of Lamberts Library Trust, because they understand the power of nutrition and have formed the largest nutrition library in Europe so that health professionals everywhere can tap this rich resource.

To all those women with endometriosis around the world who are suffering, whom we hope to give a path back to wellness.

Foreword

Women with endometriosis commonly complain that doctors do not take their symptoms seriously. There is a feeling that if doctors did listen and if only doctors knew more about endometriosis, women would not have to suffer years of pain without a definitive diagnosis. The frustration is justified as recent research has shown that it usually takes about ten years from the onset of symptoms for the diagnosis to be made.

I think that this apparent indifference to symptoms, such as painful periods and painful sex, merely reflects the lack of interest shown by society in general to health problems that are specific to women. I also think that sufferers themselves should be trying to raise awareness about endometriosis among both the medical profession and the general public. Endometriosis should be as well known as asthma or diabetes given how many women it affects and how much misery it creates.

The principal problem, however, is that not enough is known about the condition. Despite over 20 years of intensive research, we still do not understand what causes endometriosis; why there is such discrepancy between the intensity of symptoms and the severity of disease, or how best to treat patients. When doctors struggle in the dark because they do not comprehend a condition, it is inevitable that patients will receive care that they perceive to be unsatisfactory.

The other common complaint I hear is that sufferers feel restricted by the inability of many doctors to explain, using language that can be understood, the nature of the disease and the treatment options available. It is clear from recent research in Oxford that the failure to meet the information needs of sufferers leads to disillusion and a sense of disempowerment.

I believe that it is vital to provide women with high quality information, especially about treatment, to enable them to make the kind of important decisions that may potentially have a profound effect upon their lives. The reality, however, is that the treatment options are limited and the medications currently available rarely provide a cure. Therefore it is understandable that sufferers should seek complementary therapies that allow them to take control over their own bodies.

This book is unique because, for the first time, a highly respected scientist has teamed up with a nutritionist who uses complementary medicine, to give women a better understanding of the scientific basis for the use of nutritional therapies that many women around the world have found helpful. It should give encouragement to those in despair because conventional treatments have failed or produced unacceptable side effects. Eating healthily produces only good side effects.

The authors provide considerable evidence illustrating the role of basic nutrients in metabolic pathways involved in the normal menstrual cycle and pain-associated inflammation. Generally speaking, the medical profession has been slow to appreciate the importance of nutrients in the prevention and treatment of disease. For example, it has only recently been accepted that folic acid should be given to all women planning to conceive, so as to prevent neural tube defects. Much of what is said in this book, however, is common sense: eat well and your body will benefit. What is new is that Dian Mills and Michael Vernon provide the rationale for doing so in a condition that traditionally has been treated only with hormonal drugs and surgery. A holistic approach to endometriosis is vitally important because of the limitations of conventional medicine, and the authors are to be congratulated for providing the reader with a number of novel strategies for coping with this debilitating condition.

Stephen Kennedy
SENIOR FELLOW IN REPRODUCTIVE MEDICINE
UNIVERSITY OF OXFORD

1 What's happening to me?

The body has a miraculous capacity to heal itself.

Live and Learn and Pass it On,
quote from the Central Baptist Hospital
1997 calendar

You have a key to good health. Your body wants to be well, that is its natural state.

Endometriosis is a jigsaw puzzle of symptoms. You need to fit all the pieces together to provide clues as to what is happening within your body. This book will try to give you some of the pieces of the jigsaw, but you have to put them together yourself. This book will guide you to a truth. As you will read in the following chapters, some pioneering women have taken this path before and they share their success with you. Let them lead the way. They have found that, by giving the body the building blocks it needs, health can be regained.

That is the key, which you must always remember. Your body wants to be well. If you cut or burn your hand, you heal. If endometrial cells are growing in the wrong place, rest assured the body is trying to heal that area by whatever means it has available. Many women try drug and surgical treatments, and for some women they suppress some symptoms, but do not heal. Some people do get well, but many need other remedies or treatments.

Endometriosis is the second most common gynaecological complaint recognized by reproductive endocrinologists, affecting two out of every ten women. Endometriosis is everywhere and does not discriminate between women, race, colour, social status, body size, or colour of hair (although some women with red hair may have a greater incidence of endometriosis as they are more inclined to have allergies). It is possible that many women may have symptoms of endometriosis at some point in their lives, as every woman has the potential to develop endometriosis, but they do not always get a correct diagnosis. You are never alone with this disease – it is shared by many other women.

The term 'endometriosis' means that some of our body cells are growing in the wrong place, like weeds in a garden. Instead of staying inside the womb where they belong, to form the womb lining, these cells have spread outside the womb to infiltrate the ovaries and other areas of the body. If we knew exactly why these cells move around, it would be easier to find a cure. The endometrium normally grows only inside the womb. It is a nutrient-rich tissue designed to act as a food source and 'nest' for a fertilized egg. It also sets the stage for building the placenta which protects the baby as it develops in the womb.

For some unknown reason these endometrial cells migrate in endometriosis and seek other areas to grow. These areas are known as 'endometriotic implants' in medical terms, as they appear to seed themselves onto other organs in the peritoneal cavity (the abdominal area). Only cells from the spleen and endometrium in the human body are known to behave like this and migrate to other areas, and we need to understand why this happens in order to find a cure.

Women with endometriosis often ask 'Why me?' when they look around at their seemingly healthy friends. Endometriosis can be very distressing, and self-confidence may evaporate, but good health is not an impossible dream.

If you understand what is happening to you, it is easier to fight endometriosis and win. This book will look at how endometriosis manifests itself, how the body behaves, and how to approach drug and surgical treatments. It is important to look at how women as individuals can work with their bodies to help themselves heal, and to strengthen the immune and reproductive systems naturally using the nutrients which we ingest daily. The aim is to get the feel better factor!

We are all unique. No other person in the known universe is like you. People are meant to be different. Just look around in the street or your place of work at all the variables of face, hair colour, eyes, noses, height and weight. These differences are what make the strong gene pool of humankind. Orthodox medical and infertility treatments treat women as though they are all exactly the same. They take no account of your uniqueness. A 7-stone woman will be given the same dose tablet as a 14-stone woman. Treatments which work perfectly for you may not work as well for someone else because his/her body is slightly different. Moreover, many illnesses keep evolving, like the symptoms of ovarian/vaginal endometriosis, increasing levels of anxiety in those who suffer from them.

The purpose of this book is to outline the steps you can take to maximize your body's ability to fend off endometriosis. Although there is no known proven medical cure for endometriosis, nutrition may suppress the symptoms which are perceived as being due to endometriosis, and thus help to prevent them from interfering in your daily life. The book will review some of these options, especially the benefit of proper nutrition in the battle against endometriosis. Women who have tried these options and succeeded in combating endometriosis share their experiences.

Nutrition is not an alternative approach like herbal medicine or homeopathy. It is essential to life. *Eating is something we do every day. It sustains us and keeps us healthy, or it can make us unhealthy.* Unfortunately nutrition is no longer taught in schools. It is now assumed that we have a good choice of foods in the shops. But it is the quality of the foods you choose to eat which can make all the difference to your body's ability to heal itself. Nutrition is certainly very low on the list of doctors' priorities, many of whom may have had only a few hours of lessons in nutrition, and do not understand how nutrients relate to body biochemistry. It is a rare doctor who shows any interest in your food intake.

The 52 known nutrients in our foods are vital to all of us; they make our bodies work as nature intended. Vitamins, minerals and essential fatty acids and the actions of phytochemicals in plants are the body's building blocks to produce healthy new cells and to renew damaged tissue. For example, the mucous membrane which lines the digestive tract is renewed rapidly every 72 hours. New tissue can be formed very quickly on damaged organs, given the right building blocks of life. So the food you eat each day can help heal endometriosis.

Good quality, nutrient-rich food can improve the functioning of the body cells. This book will guide you through the selection of foods which will increase your intake of much-needed nutrients, especially those required by the reproductive and immune systems. It will give advice on which nutritional supplements may be helpful in the short term to boost body cells and correct hormone production, while you assess and improve your dietary intake.

The digestive system is the key to your healthy intake of nutrients, and improvement in this area can be a major factor in recovery from endometriosis. The gut flora and membranes must be healthy in order for all the nutrients from foods to be absorbed, so that they can reach the cells via the bloodstream. If your digestion is poor, it must be corrected before you can begin to get well. This is another key to your healing process. Once your digestion works efficiently, then the body can begin to heal itself.

Endometriosis can cause terrible pain, and adhesions which can stick organs together, possibly causing infertility in some women. The authors will inform you how the phytochemicals and nutrients in foods and herbs may work to reduce inflammation and pain. The known reasons for pain and infertility will be discussed, to help demystify endometriosis.

By understanding and improving the workings of your immune system, you can help to heal the reproductive system and improve fertility naturally, and the book looks at how assisted fertility works when endometriosis is present.

Gwenneth B of Sussex

The nutrition path was absolutely brilliant. I was so well while continuing it. Unfortunately I stopped. I have to go camping and go away with other groups from time to time. It then becomes impossible to follow the diet. I wish I had more self-control so that I could do it all over again. Any chance of a new start with some supplements again? Thank you for all your help in the past.

CASE STUDY

The incidence of endometriosis is high and many women may never even have heard of the condition, let alone be aware that their abdominal pain is due to it. Much of our society remains blissfully ignorant of endometriosis and of all its ramifications. All those with endometriosis need to teach everyone around them to understand this disease. The word endometriosis itself is disconcerting and cumbersome: 'endo-me-tree-osis'. This book will attempt to explain exactly what endometriosis is, and how you can try to reduce its symptoms by using the body's natural healing ability.

Furthering research is a main aim of the endometriosis groups all over the world, in America, Britain, Australia, New Zealand, Japan, India, Poland, Germany, Hong Kong, Singapore and Brazil. Women in the international endometriosis associations are pulling together around the globe to encourage governments to provide more funding for studying this disease, while also trying to raise money for research from their supporters. Research into endometriosis should continue apace to help improve diagnosis and treatment. Future research into how cells behave and how their basic physiology relies upon nutrients should lead to new ideas about endometriosis treatments. All women suffering from endometriosis should encourage new research in both orthodox and complementary fields to find a cure, and to prevent the next generation having to endure this disease and its traumatic treatments. We can all see hope for a future cure. Drugs and surgery are not the only answer, as we shall see. Healing from within is an important concept.

If you use this book wisely, it may help you to find the real you again – minus the symptoms of endometriosis. Feeling like a shadow of your former self is not a pleasant experience. Endometriosis leaves you with no energy to do anything. You feel so very tired from fighting the pain. You hope that the pain will just go away, but it doesn't. The body needs help in order to attempt to rid itself of the 'rogue' tissue of endometriosis. Seeking such help requires information and understanding, and in this book the authors hope that everyone will find the support they need to help them begin their healing process. Understanding is the key. Once you properly understand what you are fighting, it becomes easier. It helps to have all the information at your fingertips. If information is withheld from you, always be suspicious. Where your own body is involved you have a right to know what is being done and why. Always ask questions and only act when you feel satisfied with the answers. Truth is important to developing trust between practitioner and patient, so if information is withheld it prevents healing. When lies are told, trust is lost between the patient and expert.

Everyone wants to be happy and healthy and to enjoy life. Endometriosis hurts our lives. It stops us in our tracks. It prevents us living the life we want to lead. The pain associated with endometriosis can at times be so intense that women grow desperate to find a cure. When the body suddenly lets us down, the shock of feeling disabled is stunning and frightening. One feels out of control. Suggestions for treatments are made and you try them all. You just want to be well again; but fighting illness day in, day out causes despondency and great sadness for the lost time.

The medical profession has no absolute cure for endometriosis. It can support the patient and suppress the disease symptoms, but often the drug and surgical treatments do not get to the root of the problem and promote healing. Research shows that symptoms usually return within 18 months, after drug treatments are stopped. It is not uncommon for women to have taken five or six different drugs, one after another, and to have had several operations and still be in pain. Once all the reproductive organs have been removed, some members of the medical profession assume that endometriotic implants can no longer grow and women's symptoms can be dismissed and even ridiculed. Your local endometriosis group can advise you who is the right practitioner for you, and who is the most caring and compassionate.

Barbara B of Kent

The first benefit was the mental boost from feeling that I was actually taking control, doing something about my endometriosis. Within a very short time I had more energy and people stopped telling me how dreadful I looked! I also lost weight, which was great. I took the vitamin supplements and generally worked hard to improve my diet. My endometriosis was extremely severe and yet, even now, four years after a laparoscopy to remove cysts and reposition my womb, I remain totally free from endometriosis. My surgeon finds it unbelievable and constantly tells me how lucky I am. Thank you for all the support at the worst time in my life.

CASE STUDY

So what is this book going to do for you, the reader? Hopefully it will inspire you to know how magical your body can be. Both authors want to help you to find ways to let your body begin to heal itself. If you can give it the tools and the fuel it needs to fight the disease, that is a good start. Chapters 8, 9, 10 and 12 are a basic guide to the practical steps you can take as you attempt to heal yourself.

The keys to well-being are all around us. It is like a treasure hunt, but the treasure is not precious gems or gold; it is even more precious – health. For without that we can do nothing. Health is something which money cannot buy, but effort and willpower can take us a long way towards our goal. Strive to make it happen.

Feeling healthy and well is a right. Life without health can be intensely distressing. But it is important to fight to stay well, and one of the ways to help yourself heal is simply through eating good quality food. The word 'diet' is a misnomer. This is really just a Healthy Eating Life Plan – HELP – to bring you onto the road to recovery. It is an area of life over which you do have control. It is hoped that this book will inspire all women with endometriosis, and give you an insight into an area of self-help that is not difficult to follow. It will act to guide you, to choose food wisely, to enable you to absorb all the nutrients from your daily food intake, without making a meal of it.

> Don't count on anybody else coming along to relieve your stress.
> Put yourself in charge of managing the situation.
>
> *Ron Pound*

Take your health into your own hands and work with your body. Look after it. After all, it is designed to last almost a century, according to the latest research on ageing. At least a lifetime, and we all want that lifetime to be full to the brim.

Good luck on the road to recovery. There is light at the end of the tunnel. As Mary Lou Ballweg of the International Endometriosis Association, headquartered in the USA says 'Better to light one candle than to curse the darkness'.

It is up to you. There are many paths back to health – nutrition, gentle exercise and relaxation all have their part to play. Bring them together in your own life. Be gentle with yourself and learn to pace yourself. When the body has been ill for some time, it takes a while to get it back on track. There is a need to nurture yourself back to health. Take your life in both hands and let's go!

> Too much of a good thing can be wonderful.
>
> *Mae West, Actress*

SUMMARY

1 This book gives you the information about how endometriosis behaves and how nutrition may help you to combat the disease. Each chapter has a summary of all the key factors for you to follow, should you so wish.

2 Your body wants to be well. You are giving it a fighting chance to good health through choosing good quality food, fresh air, natural daylight and gentle exercise.

3 You are unique. Your body biochemistry is individual to you and needs treating as such. What works for one person may not work in the same way for you. Find out what suits you. Use your intuition. What feels right? Use this book wisely as a guide.

4 Your body cells use nutrients as building blocks to renew damaged tissues. These nutrients come from the freshest foods.

5 You can use your food choice to reduce inflammation and pain.

6 Arm yourself with a wide range of information which will enable you to choose wisely which treatments you feel are right for you. Never allow anyone to coerce you into having a treatment which feels wrong to you.

7 You can take control over what is happening to you by trying some self-help techniques, and working with your body, which is giving you signals that it needs help. Be gentle with yourself.

8 The medical profession has no cure for endometriosis and drugs and surgery can only suppress symptoms. Nutrition can help to speed up healing after surgery and, in some cases, can reduce the side effects of drug treatments.

9 Orthodox and complementary medicines can work alongside one another and enhance healing.

10 Develop your own Healthy Eating Life Plan – HELP yourself to heal.

www.endometriosis.co.uk
www.makingbabies.com
www.nutrition.us.com

2 How endometriosis affects your body

All is flux, nothing stays still.

Heraclitus, 540–480 BC

OH NO! MY PERIOD HAS STARTED AGAIN – SO SOON?

How many times have these words been uttered by women? The menstrual period has a way of appearing at the most awkward time and interfering with daily life. With endometriosis, menstruation may worsen, leading to severe, sometimes excruciating, pain and possible subfertility. It can interfere with normal daily activity, and we can shy away from learning about endometriosis when the cycle provokes such distress. When the monthly cycle includes pain or lack of a hoped-for pregnancy time after time, it becomes physically and emotionally draining. Other women seem to have no period pain and to fall pregnant so easily – it all seems so unfair. We stand aghast and become angry with our own body and its failings.

The reproductive system is the core of our feminine identity and its many subtleties and biological intricacies could be better understood. It should be celebrated as the focus of the origin of new life and menstruation should NEVER be painful. By understanding the reproductive system, you will be better able to understand endometriosis and how proper nutrition may help your body biochemistry to stay in balance and help you in your fight against this disease.

Our bodies are wondrous things, and understanding the amazing ways in which they work will help us to see more clearly what should be happening and just how endometriosis affects our whole body. Understanding can place us more in touch with the miracles going on within our cells each day. Endometriosis has the ability to mess up what should be a perfectly normal reproductive system, causing the wrong hormonal messages to be sent. The body always tries to get things right, so we have to enhance what it is attempting to do by natural means wherever possible.

THE REPRODUCTIVE SYSTEM

The menstrual or reproductive cycle of women is a complex process that involves many different endocrine glands and the hormones they secrete. These hormones all work together in a 28-day menstrual cycle that prepares the uterus for a possible pregnancy.

Women menstruate for about 40 years of their life. It is during this stage of their life that the symptoms of endometriosis will appear. The normal age for a girl's first period (menarche) occurs between 9.1 and 17.7 years with a median age of 12.8, while a woman's last period (menopause) occurs between 48 to 55 years with a median age of 51.4.

What is fascinating is that when women are assembled together, such as in schools, colleges and hospitals, their menstrual cycles align so that they all have a period at the same time. This is felt to be due to pheromones and an olfactory link to the pituitary gland.

The major organs of the reproductive system are the hypothalamus, pituitary gland, thyroid, ovary, uterus (womb), endometrium and Fallopian tubes. To understand how the menstrual cycle works, we need to look at where the various endocrine glands are located (figure 2.1). The glands control the whole reproductive cycle. People often assume that only the uterus and ovaries are involved. However, several endocrine glands control the system and they trigger the menstrual cycle. After we have familiarized ourselves with the reproductive system, this chapter will discuss how the glands and the hormones they produce interact during the reproductive cycle, and how endometriosis interferes with this cycle.

THE ENDOCRINE SYSTEM

It is the correct balance of hormones that controls this whole system. The endocrine system is scattered throughout the body and usually works perfectly, sending hormone messages from one gland to another via the bloodstream. Occasionally this system may go wrong and a polyendocrine disorder, where one or more glands are affected, can lead to illness. The thyroid, pancreas, adrenals and ovaries may all malfunction under stress.

HYPOTHALAMUS AND PITUITARY GLAND

The control centre for the reproductive cycle is the hypothalamus and the pituitary gland in the brain. The hypothalamus secretes hormones (chemical messengers) which control the timing and the amount of hormone produced by the pituitary gland in the brain (figure 2.1). The pituitary gland can be viewed as the 'master gland' of the endocrine system, since its hormones orchestrate the activity of most of the other endocrine glands of the body, including the ovaries in women and testes in men. Think of the pituitary gland as the conductor of the orchestra, wielding the baton, telling the other glands what to do and when.

The pea-sized pituitary gland nestles in a bony cavity at the base of the skull (figure 2.2). It has a rich blood supply that allows it to distribute its hormones rapidly throughout the body. The pituitary gland is divided into two parts: the anterior and posterior pituitary.

1 The anterior pituitary secretes several protein hormones which affect a variety of glands and tissues of the body. However, the two major hormones of the anterior

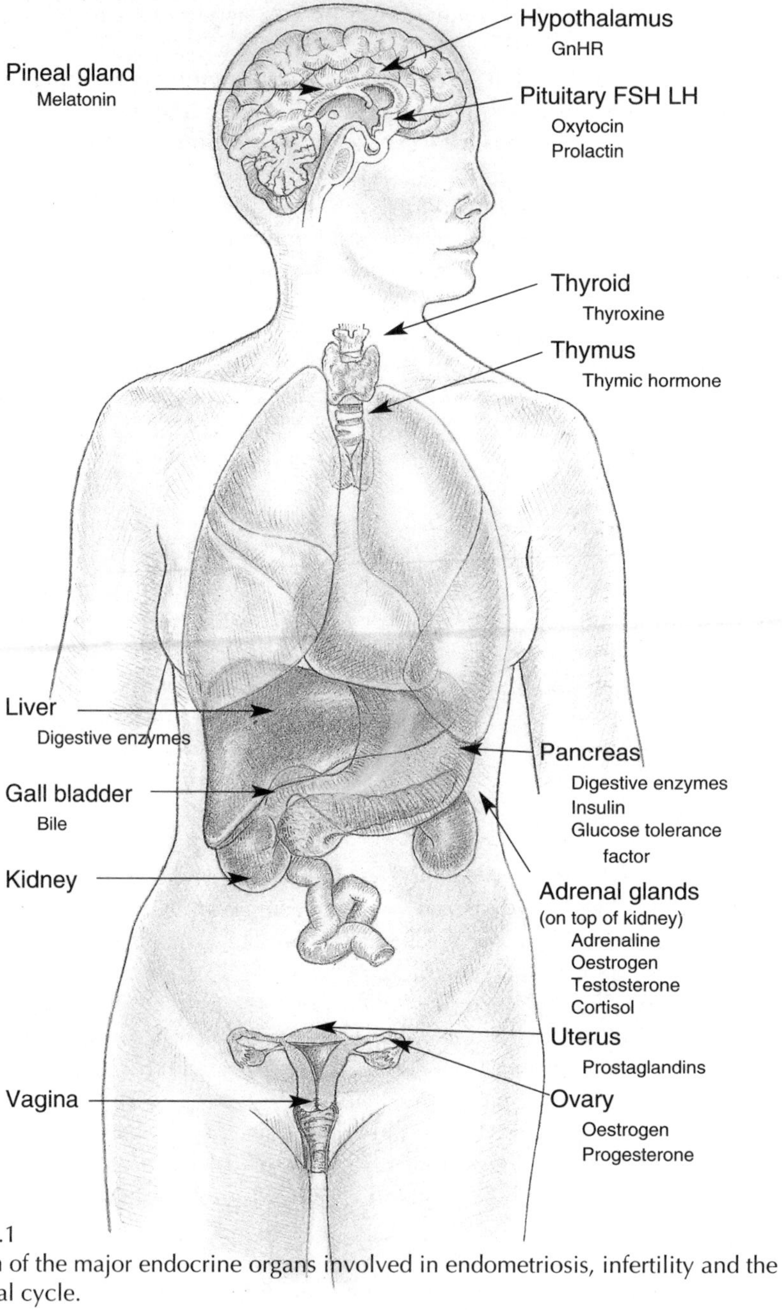

Hypothalamus
GnRH

Pineal gland
Melatonin

Pituitary FSH LH
Oxytocin
Prolactin

Thyroid
Thyroxine

Thymus
Thymic hormone

Liver
Digestive enzymes

Pancreas
Digestive enzymes
Insulin
Glucose tolerance
factor

Gall bladder
Bile

Kidney

Adrenal glands
(on top of kidney)
Adrenaline
Oestrogen
Testosterone
Cortisol

Uterus
Prostaglandins

Vagina

Ovary
Oestrogen
Progesterone

Figure 2.1
Diagram of the major endocrine organs involved in endometriosis, infertility and the menstrual cycle.

pituitary that affect the reproductive system are follicle-stimulating hormone (FSH) and luteinizing hormone (LH). These two hormones control the activity of the ovaries, and are very important controls for fertility.

2 The posterior pituitary also secretes several protein hormones. Oxytocin is the hormone that most directly affects the reproductive system. Oxytocin causes the smooth muscle of the uterus to contract during the birthing process. Oxytocin production is dependent on sufficient levels of the mineral manganese. It is thought to be important for bonding at birth and oxytocin levels are known to be increased in the brain when we fall in love.

THE THYROID GLAND

The thyroid is dealt with in detail in chapter 10. This gland can have an effect upon fertility; and lower than normal thyroid hormone levels (hypothyroid) cause infertility in both men and women. Indeed, auto-antibodies to the thyroid are used to predict which women are at risk from miscarriage.

Oestrogen acutely inhibits the rate of thyroid hormone release in adults.[1] In subclinical hypothyroidism, abnormal circadian TSH rhythm, elevated basal serum TSH concentrations and elevated titres of antithyroid antibodies are frequently seen.[2] Women with mild hypothyrodism have prolonged and heavy menstrual bleeding with a shorter menstrual cycle.[3] The thyroid enlarges in pregnancy and takes up more iodine as it makes more thyroxine.

THE OVARIES

The ovaries contain the female sex cells, also known as oocytes or eggs (*see* figures 2.2 and 2.3). All of the eggs that a woman has in her ovaries were produced while she was developing as a fetus in her mother's womb. The health of each egg inside a baby girl is therefore dependent upon the health of the mother. When a female fetus develops in her mother's uterus, her eggs increase in numbers until the seventh month of pregnancy, and then their numbers decline throughout the remainder of the pregnancy and throughout her life. As many as seven million eggs are present in a female fetus by the seventh month of pregnancy, but there are fewer than one million eggs at birth.[4]

From birth to puberty, the number of eggs declines further, from one million to about 400,000, which is the total number of eggs available to a woman during her reproductive years. During the reproductive years one egg is selected every month to develop to a stage that allows for ovulation, fertilization *and* conception. When a woman reaches 50 to 55 years of age, the supply of eggs is exhausted and the reproductive cycle stops. This is, of course, the time of natural menopause.

At any given time, two major structures, each about 1cm in diameter, can be seen within the ovary – the follicle and the corpus luteum (figures 2.2 and 2.3). Each follicle contains an egg surrounded by granulosa cells or 'nurse cells'. During the menstrual cycle the follicle becomes filled with follicular fluid and looks like a small cyst, about one centimetre in diameter. The granulosa cells of the follicle secrete the steroid hormone oestrogen; the corpus luteum produces the hormone progesterone.

Oestrogen has several roles:

1 It stimulates the endometrium to grow from day 1 to 14 of the cycle and replace the endometrial cells that were shed during menstruation. It is produced in the follicle of the ovary and in fat cells, and by the adrenal glands.
2 It enhances the contractions of the uterus and is required during the birthing process.
3 Too much oestrogen acts as an abortant. Too much produced very early in the pregnancy and not balanced by sufficient progesterone from the corpus luteum could trigger the loss of the pregnancy, as it is an abortive in high doses.
4 It increases the levels of neurotransmitters in the brain, improving mood and memory. If oestrogen is out of balance, it can trigger mood swings.
5 It is synthesized in the ovary from cholesterol, and secreted from the granulosa cells inside the follicles, the corpus luteum and the placenta.
6 It causes the liver to produce hormones.
7 It increases cholesterol production, produces weight gain and determines fat distribution.
8 It causes cell proliferation.
9 It deposits calcium into bones.
10 When its levels are high, women show greater verbal fluency.
11 When its levels are low, women use their hands more skilfully, and spatial ability is stronger.
12 Excess oestrogen may increase the level of antithrombin III, which increases the risk of blood clots.
13 Normal levels in the follicular phase are 30–150ng/ml. In menopause, oestrogen levels are 40–200ng/ml.

Progesterone, on the other hand, has different roles from oestrogen:

1 Stimulate the endometrium to become nutrient-rich in preparation for a pregnancy, from day 14 to 28 of the cycle.
2 Enhance relaxation of the uterus and prevent contractions of the uterine smooth muscle to prevent miscarriages.
3 Inhibit oestrogen from stimulating contractions of the uterus, maintain a pregnancy and prevent further ovulation.
4 Reduce the effect of the immune system to prevent the body from rejecting the embryo.
5 Raise the basal metabolic rate.
6 As a thermogenic, adjust body temperature, which rises from 97.8 degrees C to 98.3 degrees C just before ovulation.
7 It is synthesized from cholesterol in the corpus luteum and in the placenta from months three to nine during pregnancy.

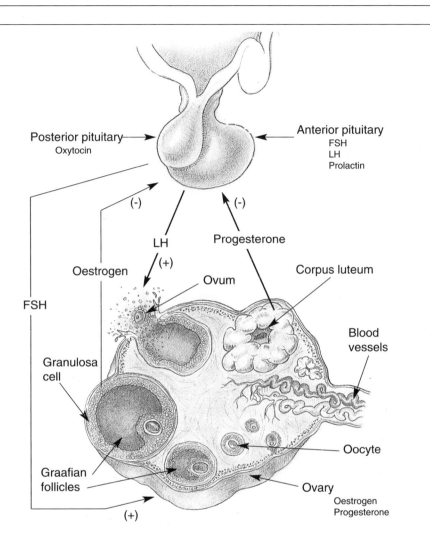

Posterior pituitary
Oxytocin

Anterior pituitary
FSH
LH
Prolactin

(-)   (-)

LH   Progesterone

Oestrogen   (+)

FSH   Ovum   Corpus luteum

Blood
vessels

Granulosa
cell

Graafian
follicles

Oocyte

Ovary
Oestrogen
Progesterone

(+)

Figure 2.2
Diagram of the endocrine (hormone) relationships between the anterior pituitary and
ovary. The pituitary secretes FSH (follicle-stimulating hormone) to stimulate the growth
of the follicle which contains the egg. When the egg is ripe and the follicle large, the
pituitary secretes LH (luteinizing hormone) and the egg is expelled (ovulated). After
ovulation, the follicle becomes the corpus luteum. The follicle produces oestrogen and
the corpus luteum progesterone [(+) means stimulates and (-) means inhibits].

8   Normal levels of progesterone are greater than 10ng/ml during the mid- to late luteal cycle.

The follicle granulosa cells produce oestrogen from day 1 to day 14 of the cycle; then the corpus luteum produces progesterone from day 15 to day 28 of the cycle. As these steroid hormones are both oil-based, the health of these hormones depends upon the quality of the oils you eat. Both are synthesized from cholesterol.

Androgens play a role in fertility:

1   They are precursors to oestrogen and come from the ovary and adrenal glands.
2   Testosterone is the male hormone produced in the testes, ovaries and adrenals. In women, excess may be produced if insulin levels are too high.
3   In women, testosterone levels are normally 35–50ng/ml. It is felt that there is a slight surge at the time of ovulation that increases the sex drive.

OVARIAN CYSTS

Often, women with endometriosis develop cysts on the ovaries. There are four main types of cyst:

1   Dermatoid cysts are rather bizarre and contain tissue that has developed into hair, nails and teeth. They are unusual.
2   Mucoid cysts are filled with a clear mucus and may grow to be very large.
3   Endometrial, or 'chocolate', cysts are related to endometriosis and appear to be unruptured follicles that fill with blood and become larger and larger. Size is usually given in terms of a fruit (tangerine-sized to grapefruit-sized), or up to the size of a five-month-old fetus in one case.
4   Polycystic ovaries, where six or more small cysts develop at the same time (see chapter 3).

The ovary is able to reabsorb cyst material and research suggests that a diet rich in B-complex vitamins aids this process. Cysts may grow within the ovary but, more often, they are attached to the ovary by a stalk. Pain ensues when this stalk becomes twisted or the ovary ruptures, spurting out hot stale, sticky blood onto the intestines. This pain is unbearable as the whole of the bowel muscles go into spasm and the body goes into shock. It is known that some cysts produce their own hormones, upsetting the hormonal balance. Small cysts can be reabsorbed, but those over 5cm in diameter are best removed surgically with a laser.

THE UTERUS

The uterus or womb is a little smaller than a woman's clenched fist, but during pregnancy, it can expand to over 45cm (18in) in length (see figures 2.1 and 2.3).

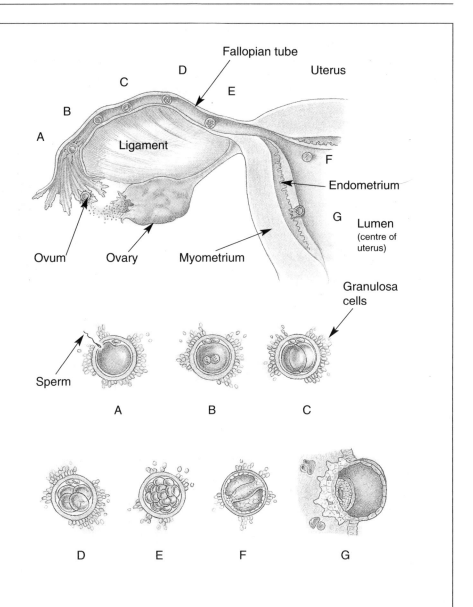

Figure 2.3
Cross-section of the uterus and Fallopian tube, and diagrams of the development of the egg to embryo. (A) Fertilization of ovum. (B) Fertilized egg with pronuclei. (C) Two-cell embryo. (D) Four-cell embryo. (E) Multicellular embryo (100 cells) – a morula. (F) Early blastocyst embryo. (G) Blastocyst invading the endometrium.

It consists of a well-developed muscular wall (the myometrium) and an inner mucus-like membrane (the endometrium). The smooth muscle wall of the myometrium expel the baby during the birthing process, and it is the contractions of these muscles that also cause menstrual cramps. These muscles require a balance of calcium and magnesium to help them function correctly. Calcium tenses muscles while magnesium allows them to relax. Magnesium-rich foods should be eaten when muscular cramps are a problem.

The uterus retains its full capacity to sustain implantation for up to 60 years of age. It clearly does not age in the same way as the ovary, as postmenopausal women can maintain a pregnancy after egg donation. 'The uterus is the main site for the production of the hormone prostacyclin, which protects women from heart disease and unwanted blood clotting. Since prostacyclin cannot be synthetically made in a laboratory, the removal of the uterus will ensure its production will cease forever.'[5] It also produces 60 different prostaglandins and enzymes.

THE ENDOMETRIUM

The endometrium (tissue lining the womb) plays a vital role in the reproductive process (*see* figures 2.3 and 2.4). The endometrium is brownish-red in colour with a fluffy appearance and slimy texture. The brownish-red colour is due to its nutrient-rich blood supply, and the slimy texture is due to the large amount of protein contained in its secretions. For a woman to conceive, the embryo must physically implant into this 'lush' endometrium. The endometrium is the sole source of nutrients and oxygen for the newly formed embryo. If nutrients are in poor supply, the womb lining will be unable to support the embryo's development. The growth of the embryo places a heavy nutrient demand on the endometrium, and this tissue needs to develop a rich blood supply. As we will see later, the quality of food eaten greatly influences the nutrients available to the endometrium. Pregnancy is rare if the endometrium thickness is less than 7mm. The chances of pregnancy are optimized if the endometrium is 9–14mm in thickness.[6]

The endometrium is also an important endocrine gland and secretes a family of hormones called prostaglandins (PG). Prostaglandin F (PGF) can stimulate strong uterine contractions (cramps) and prostaglandin E (PGE) can cause pain. These prostaglandins are the hormones directly responsible for most of the cramps and pain associated with endometriosis and menstruation. PGF also inhibits the development of the corpus luteum in the ovary and therefore reduces progesterone production. Therefore PGF has been used clinically to initiate abortions. If higher levels than normal of PGF are produced, miscarriages may occur.

As an endocrine gland, the endometrium is very responsive to the levels of hormones circulating in the blood. The balance of oestrogen and progesterone greatly affects the growth and activity of the endometrium. In chapter 11, the effects on the balance of what you eat will be clearly explained.

FALLOPIAN TUBES

The womb has two tube-like extensions called the oviducts or Fallopian tubes, which are the transport system (rather like a highway) for the sperm to reach the egg and for the embryo to reach the uterus (*see* figure 2.3). The process of fertilization takes place in the upper third of the Fallopian tubes, so the sperm have to be robust enough to be propelled from the uterus up two-thirds of the Fallopian tube to fertilize the egg. Contractions in the uterine muscle during orgasm are believed to assist this process.

The Fallopian tube enlarges at ovulation and secretes fluids as it responds to oestrogens. At midcycle, the fluid is copious, alkaline and contains nutrients, gases, proteins, electrolytes and steroids.[7]

ENDOCRINE COMMUNICATION

How does the body know when the embryo is entering the womb? The womb must have a precise line of communication to the ovary, where the eggs are manufactured and released. This is accomplished by endocrine communication. The pituitary and ovaries communicate with each other by sending 'chemical messengers' (hormones) through the blood system to tell each other what to do and when. Light hitting the retina of the eye stimulates the pituitary and hypothalamus, which releases GnRH, a hormone that triggers the release of LH from the pituitary. The LH surge causes the

Table 2.1
The major reproductive hormones of the menstrual cycle

ORGAN	HORMONE	ACTION
Hypothalamus	Gonadotrophin-releasing hormone (GnRH)	Stimulates the pituitary gland to produce FSH and LH
Anterior pituitary	Follicle-stimulating hormone (FSH)	Stimulates ovarian follicles
	Luteinizing hormone (LH)	Initiates ovulation
	Prolactin	Stimulates lactation
Posterior pituitary	Oxytocin	Stimulates uterine contraction
Ovary	Oestrogen	Stimulates endometrial growth and uterine contractions
	Progesterone	Maintains pregnancy
Uterus	Prostaglandins (PGE/PGF)	Stimulates uterine contractions, menstrual pain and birth

follicle membrane to rupture, releasing the egg. Ovulation occurs if the ovum meets a sperm in the Fallopian tube, and the follicle seals up to form a corpus luteum. This begins to produce progesterone to make the endometrium ready for implantation of the fertilized egg. Progesterone is produced by the corpus luteum until the third month of pregnancy, when the placenta is sufficiently mature to take over. If no fertilized embryo is implanted, the corpus luteum is reabsorbed into the ovary and the whole process begins all over again.[8] The major hormones involved in the reproductive system are listed in table 2.1.

Establishing the correct levels of these hormones is the key to getting the right message to the right place at the right time. When we say that the hormones are 'out of balance', the wrong messages are being sent and received, and things can begin to go awry.

FOLLICLE-STIMULATING HORMONE (FSH)

1 FSH is responsible for maturation of the ova in the follicle. Once a dominant follicle emerges with a diameter of 6.5–14mm, the rest will subside.
2 FSH production is inhibited by excess oestrogen and inhibin.
3 FSH causes granulosa cells to multiply rapidly and produce oestradiol.
4 Normal levels of FSH are 5–20mU/ml, depending on the day of the test.
5 When FSH levels are over 20mU/ml, menopause may be due within five years. Women with elevated FSH can still get pregnant as other factors, such as stress, can raise levels. After IVF treatments, where the ovaries have been hyperstimulated, many women find they have abnormal FSH levels for a time. Menopause is usually indicated with FSH levels of 40–200mU/ml.

LUTEINIZING HORMONE (LH)

1 LH secretion precedes ovulation and completes the maturation of the ovarian follicle.
2 LH stimulates androgen (testosterone) production.
3 LH is inhibited by oestrogen except just before ovulation, when it surges.
4 Progesterone may block LH secretion as it decreases the rate at which LH is pulsed from the pituitary gland.
5 LH receptors inside the granulosa cells develop as a result of FSH and oestrogen build up.
6 When LH surges, the dominant follicle grows between 1.4–2.2mm per day, reaching a maximum diameter of 18–22mm, and is ready for ovulation. It should be fully mature on day 14–16 of the menstrual cycle.
7 The interval between the LH surge and ovulation is 37–38 hours. Ovulation occurs randomly from left to right ovaries during natural cycles.
8 The Fallopian tubes enlarge at ovulation and secrete fluids as they respond to oestrogen and the LH surge.

9 Normal levels of LH are 7–14U/ml. While LH remains normal, ovulation is possible. FSH tests alone are not indicative of perimenopause as they can fluctuate wildly at this time. As LH levels rise abruptly at menopause, they should be tested with FSH.

PROLACTIN

1 This hormone inhibits ovulation.
2 Elevated prolactin can also be caused by high melatonin levels, resulting in decreased fertility (melatonin from the pineal gland increases when the eye registers darkness).
3 Excess prolactin can be caused by drugs such as tranquillisers, anti-ulcer drugs, high-dose oestrogen oral contraceptive pills, alcohol and street drugs.
4 Hypothyroidism and breast stimulation may also increase prolactin levels.
5 When prolactin is high, GnRH and LH are lowered. This can cause menstruation and ovulation to stop.

RELAXIN

1 This protein-based hormone, produced by the corpus luteum of the ovary, is similar to insulin and growth hormone.
2 It softens tissues and muscles, and may be responsible for morning sickness during pregnancy.

THE REPRODUCTIVE CYCLE

The bottom line of the reproductive system is to make a healthy bouncing baby through the processes of sexual intercourse, conception and pregnancy. One of the more formidable tasks of the female reproductive system is to prepare the lining of the womb (the endometrium) to feed and nurture the embryo. However, it is not possible for the body to maintain the endometrium in a continuous, heightened 'ready state' for pregnancy. Thus the body follows a monthly cycle of slowly building up the endometrium so that it will be in a nutrient-rich state only when a fertilized embryo may be around. Think of the endometrium as fresh food for the embryo; if it gets old (past its sell-by date) it is less nutritious and is less likely to sustain the pregnancy. This 'food for the fetus' is renewed each month, so the quality of food you eat is crucial to the health of this tissue. If a fertilized egg fails to appear, then the body flushes away the existing endometrium, and starts all over again. This flushing away of the endometrium is, of course, the menstrual period.

THE MENSTRUAL CYCLE

The menstrual cycle in most women lasts approximately 28 days, with the first day of blood flow (the menstrual period) usually designated as day 1 of the cycle (*see* figures

2.2 and 2.4). Around day 1 the hypothalamus secretes gonadotrophin-releasing hormone (GnRH) and, in response to this hormone, the pituitary gland secretes increasing amounts of FSH (follicle-stimulating hormone). FSH stimulates the granulosa cells (helper cells) in each follicle to ensure that each ova is 'fed' nutrients to help it produce oestrogen and to stimulate the egg to mature.[9] Oestrogen also sends a message to the womb to tell it to produce more endometrial cells, so that a healthy thickened endometrium will be present to accept the egg should it be fertilized by a sperm in the Fallopian tubes. Unfortunately, oestrogen also has some bad effects. It is responsible for the water retention between cells, which is why some women can feel bloated before a period, and for stimulating uterine contractions (menstrual cramps).

When the follicle reaches 15–17mm in diameter (around day 14–15 of the cycle), the pituitary produces a surge of luteinizing hormone (LH). This surge stimulates the egg to grow to 18–28mm in diameter and also signals the ovary to expel the mature egg (ovulate) out towards the Fallopian tubes. The mature egg is then sucked up by the Fallopian tube so that the sperm can fertilize it. Ovulation usually occurs on the 15th day of the cycle. If the body does not ovulate, then the LH surge may not be happening as it should, implying that the hypothalamus is not functioning efficiently. The hypothalamus requires vitamin B6 and zinc to produce GnRH. If it is not working efficiently, the right message is not passed to the pituitary gland for the LH release. All these hormones and the health of the egg are nutrient-dependent, and good blood flow is essential during this stage of growth.

After ovulation, the empty follicle undergoes a dramatic physical change. It turns a yellow colour (because of its oil-rich tissue) and is called the corpus luteum (which means 'yellow body'). The corpus luteum is very important as it secretes the hormones progesterone and relaxin, which send the message to the endometrium of the uterus to become receptive for a possible pregnancy (see figure 2.4). As its names implies, progesterone (which means 'for gestation') is required for the pregnancy to be maintained. In response to the progesterone, the endometrium starts to produce the nutrients the embryo will need for its development, and the myometrium (muscle) layer of the uterus relaxes. Without sufficient levels of progesterone, relaxin and magnesium, the uterus would start to contract and expel the developing embryo. Therefore, if the corpus luteum is poorly developed, a pregnancy may fail. Again, oils are implicated here. Studies show that 'Vitamin B6 (pyridoxine 5 phosphate) is necessary for the formation of the hormone progesterone' and the same source indicates that 'vitamin B6 is also required after ovulation when the body has a high level of oestrogen. B6 acts as a natural diuretic and helps alleviate some of the bloating associated with PMS. It is a precursor to progesterone'.[10] Moreover, 'the action of steroid hormones is balanced by B6 – it has an effect on endocrine diseases'.[11]

The fate of the egg is dependent upon whether or not it will meet up with a sperm in the Fallopian tube (see figure 2.3). If no sperm are present, both the unfertilized egg and the corpus luteum will degenerate (die) and be reabsorbed. The slow destruction of the corpus luteum leads to a decrease in progesterone and oestrogen secretion (see figure 2.4). Without these steroids, blood flow to the endometrium decreases and the

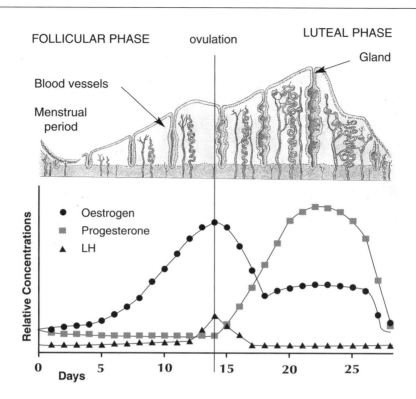

Figure 2.4
Graph of the day-to-day changes in the reproductive hormones during the menstrual cycle and the appearance of the endometrium during these changes. Note the endometrium becomes thick, and develops numerous blood vessels and glands because of the increase in oestrogen. The progesterone continues this build-up and makes the glands secretory, and prepares the endometrium for pregnancy. When the steroids decline at the end of the cycle, the endometrium sloughs off (menstrual period) and the cycle starts over again at day 1.

lush endometrium cannot be maintained. The endometrium starts to degenerate from a lack of oxygen and nutrients, and it begins to separate physically from the uterus and is shed. This withdrawal of oestrogen and progesterone is the cause of the menstrual period (blood flow). With the onset of the menstrual period, a new menstrual cycle starts all over again and a new lining of endometrium is made for another attempt at pregnancy.

Women often accept a very heavy menstrual flow as the norm because that is what they have come to expect. Dr Casmir Funk, the man who isolated vitamin B1 in 1912, described the effect of vitamin B-complex in reducing a woman's menstrual flow from five or six days to three or four days. He reported that menstruation came on 'completely without warning' (i.e. with no symptoms of premenstrual syndrome, or PMS) while these women were on B-complex vitamin therapy. He treated PMS successfully through nutrition, rather than drugs.[12] Large blood clots may be prevented when vitamins C and E are used together with evening primrose and fish oils as 'these all have oestrogenic properties, and certain oestrogens produce changes in blood clotting'.[13]

The amount of blood lost is usually about 60ml (2 fl oz).[14] At the beginning of the menstrual cycle, rich red blood should be the norm, whereas brown granular blood with chopped-liver-like clots implies poor nutrient uptake. The nutrients used to improve periods include iron EAP2, vitamin B6, B-complex vitamins, magnesium, chromium, vitamins C and E, and evening primrose and fish oils. If blood loss is excessive to the point of flooding, then a well-absorbed iron supplement such as EAP2 or citrate may be used for 1–2 months to normalize the flow.

• C A S E S T U D Y •

Gabi B of London

I'm 34, married with no children and live in London. I work as an IT consultant.

My periods were never a problem, more a slight inconvenience really. My story starts nine years ago, when I was around 25. My periods had become very heavy and painful. I thought this was how periods should be and that I'd been lucky up until then. So I put up with the pain, cramps, headaches and general grotty feeling for about a year. I then saw my GP, who referred me to a gynaecologist. My first visit was disappointing, to say the least. I was told that periods can be pretty unpleasant, and to come and see them again if the symptoms persisted. Well, after about two years, a laparoscopy confirmed that I had moderate endometriosis. I was put on a course of tablets to reduce the pain and inflammation. These tablets didn't really help with the symptoms, but added side effects to my list of complaints. After about a year, I was put on a course of Zoladex injections, very painful injections into the abdomen once a month. Now, at no time had I been told that there is no cure for endometriosis. The drug treatments can only ease the symptoms. Zoladex in effect makes you menopausal, thus stopping your periods. The lack of bleeding causes the endo-sites to decrease in size and shrivel up. This seemed to make sense to me and so I put up with the side effects – hot flushes, night sweats, headaches, nausea, exhaustion, mood swings and depression – because I genuinely thought this treatment would cure me. How naïve.

All was well for about a year, then the symptoms came back. So another laparoscopy confirmed endometriosis was still present. I was put on the pill to ease the bleeding and pain, and given Coproximal as needed, which I'm afraid I did.

About two years ago, I was finally given laser surgery to burn away the endo-sites. My condition was moderate-to-severe, my left ovary had become stuck to the cavity wall and there were a lot of adhesions. The surgery was a success, and I was skipping about with joy I felt so well. But then, nine months later, it was back with a vengeance.

I returned to my gynaecologist to discuss my options. I understood this was not going to go away, but wanted to know if there was anything I could do to help myself. I was told that surgery was not an option so soon, but they could prescribe a contraceptive pill which can be taken constantly, thus stopping my periods for six to nine months, which might decrease the size of the endo-sites. That sounded like good news to me. But when I read the booklet that came with the pills, the side effects sounded so severe that I decided to put up with the pain.

By this time I was a very unwell bunny. I felt ill for three weeks a month. Before my period, I felt like I was about to give birth to triplets. There were many different symptoms:

> constant severe ache in the abdomen
> shooting and throbbing pain on my left side
> shooting pains in my bottom
> headaches
> extreme bloating most of the time
> exhaustion
> nausea when the pain was really bad
> ovulation was like a full-blown period
> I couldn't use tampons and the pads just made me feel even bigger
> the blood was very dark and smelly, as if I was rotting from the inside out
> on top of these symptoms, my periods made me feel dirty.

I had managed to programme my periods to start on a Saturday, so I was able to spend the weekends in bed. Intercourse was impossible, and although my husband was very understanding, it was difficult not to be depressed. We had sex, but not intercourse. Sometimes I would demand intercourse, but would be in so much pain for days afterwards, it really wasn't worth it. I had a hot water bottle at work and used to spend a lot of time hanging onto the radiator in my office. I couldn't walk any distance and was exhausted all the time. We had to plan our life around my monthly cycle. I used to retire to bed most of the time. I think this was more depressing than anything. I hated having to cancel social events or even visiting my parents. People were very sympathetic, but I felt very pathetic. Life was not good.

I'd read a lot of books, many of which touched on nutrition, and I felt that maybe it was time to seek alternative help. I read Dian's book from cover to cover. It all made so much sense. I got her number from a friend of a friend, but I delayed making the call. I think I was afraid of another treatment not working, as what would I do then? I know this was the wrong attitude, but it wasn't until later that I realized that.

My life changed over a year ago. My period had come a day early and I had to take a day off work. As an IT manager, my work involved a lot of stress, running up and down stairs and humping heavy equipment from place to place. There is no way I could function with my period. It was like a battle and my endometriosis seemed to be winning. I finally made the call to the clinic from my bed. I was in tears and the receptionist was really sympathetic. I was amazed as, over the years, I have seen many medical people and I can't say that any of them were sympathetic. I wasn't expecting sympathy, but it would have been nice on occasions.

I saw Dian; we discussed my condition, lifestyle and diet. She prescribed multivitamins, minerals and fish oils. These were to give me a booster as I was so low. I was to give up *wheat, citrus, chocolate and coffee, and to reduce dairy, increase fruit, vegetables and oily fish, drink more water and generally avoid very processed foods. I decided to make a real effort and stick to the guidelines for a month to see what happened. I celebrated this with a cappuccino and a large piece of cheesecake followed by an orange.*

I kept a diary, recording what I ate and how I felt. It was a very useful process as I could refer back and see how well I was doing – or not. I thought about what I ate and ate regularly. I'd never had such exotic breakfasts! I knew that we ate food because our bodies needed it; I knew I should eat more fruit regularly, but just never fancied it.

After about three days, I felt fantastic, had loads of energy and didn't look so drawn. My husband said he could always tell the level of pain I was in by my eyes, and my eyes seemed bigger and brighter. I looked forward to food, and ENJOYED fruit. I had my period 10 days later. It was amazing. It hurt but was manageable. I almost enjoyed it (that was weird). The blood was bright red and, because of a major systems failure at work, I had to work on the weekend. I couldn't believe it. Not only was I standing up during my period, but I was working too.

It's been over a year now since I first met Dian and I am a different person. I wonder how much I have cost the NHS over the years in drugs, surgery and consultations, which weren't as successful as nutritional awareness has been.

It seems that wheat is my real problem, but because I now eat so well, my body can tolerate the occasional accidental wheat consumption. I am now very finely tuned so that if I do eat something that upsets me, I pretty much know immediately. I usually drink lots of water and cranberry juice, which seems to ease symptoms.

I had an amazing experience recently that confirmed my intolerance. I had a piece of chocolate cake – a real treat – which I was told was gluten-free. After a few mouthfuls, I found it physically hard to swallow. Within 10 minutes, I felt very tired and withdrawn. Later that afternoon, I had a pain in my left side and found it difficult to speak coherently. I knew something was wrong. I remembered I'd had some quiche at lunch and thought maybe the flour used was the problem. It turned out to be coeliac wheat flour but with the gluten removed. It is the wheat that affects me. I was very ill the next day and amazed by the severity of my reaction. I felt ill and tired the following week as well. It wasn't nice feeling ill again, but it confirmed to me how well I maintain my diet.

The point I want to get across is that I am an ordinary girl and lead an ordinary life. I sometimes stay out late and drink beer! But now I think about what I eat and I've got my life back. It isn't hard to change your diet because the rewards are immediate and your body takes control. Your body will let you know what vitamins and minerals you are lacking through cravings for different foods.

In a way I'm glad I was so ill when I first saw Dian because the change in me was immediate and immense. You don't have to live a miserable and painful life. There is help out there. I hope you are able to change your life like I have, and wish you a long good health.

FERTILIZATION

In women, the ovum lives for approximately 72 hours after it is expelled from the follicle. It may be fertile for less than half this time. Sperm survive in the female genital tract for 48 hours. Sperm have been seen to survive for one week after intercourse.[15] If sperm are present in the Fallopian tube, then the egg may be fertilized (*see* figure 2.3).

A fertilized egg, called a zygote, sends a hormonal message to the reproductive system that conception has occurred and the corpus luteum is prevented from degenerating. The corpus luteum of pregnancy continues to produce progesterone and the endometrium gets even more lush. As the zygote passes down the Fallopian tube its cells begin to divide to form the embryo. It keeps dividing, first into a two-cell embryo, then a four-cell embryo and then an eight-cell embryo, up to about 100 cells, at which point it is called a 'morula' (*see* figure 2.3).

At this stage of development, the cells of the embryo begin to develop into specific different types of body cells, and a fluid-filled area forms in the middle of the embryo. The embryo, now called a blastocyst, implants itself in the endometrium, a process dependent on enzymes rich in vitamin E and zinc. It takes about seven days for a fertilized egg to develop into a blastocyst and implant into the endometrium. Blastocysts may have 1,000 to 10,000 cells by day 8; by day 9 or 10, it should be firmly attached. On day 10, the placenta is formed when cells invade the maternal blood vessels. By day 19, the placenta has developed its own blood vessels.[16]

A woman is totally unaware of these important events. She will not know that she is pregnant for another week, when she misses her period.

Once the sperm has entered the egg, how does the body recognize that a conception has occurred? A message comes from the embryo that prevents the shedding of the endometrium. Within two weeks of conception the level of progesterone produced by the corpus luteum is maintained, and this protects the pregnancy. This progesterone enhances the ability of the endometrium to produce nutritious fluids that the embryo will need during its very early development.

Just imagine, from the tiny egg in the ovary and the minute sperm from the testes a whole new person can grow. The beauty of it is that each egg and sperm contain totally unique blueprints so that the baby developed from them will be a totally unique individual. We all began from this miracle of nature; we are indeed the stuff that stars are made of.

As complicated as the reproductive process is, it is easy to see that human procreation is a miracle. In fact, the incidence of subfertility in human beings is high, and as many as 15 to 20 per cent of all couples may be subfertile. Some of this subfertility may be the result of 'hiccups' in the reproductive process or a result of anatomical deformities in the reproductive system. As you will see in chapter 4, endometriosis may adversely affect many parts of the reproductive processes. What we have to do is make the body less tolerant of endometriosis, and get the right messages to the right place at the right time, to enhance the reproductive and immune systems. The correct choice of food will help our bodies to work efficiently as the nutrients help to trigger the correct hormonal messages.

CERVICAL MUCUS

The uterus is connected to the vagina through a small opening called the cervix, which acts as a physical barrier to protect the female reproductive organs from germs in the external environment. The state of the cervical mucus within the vagina is very important in achieving fertilization, and is also dependent on the correct hormonal messages.

Oestrogen makes the mucus runny and slippery, like egg white, making it easy for the sperm to swim through it and for conception to take place, rather like a super-highway for sperm. By watching for a clear mucus coming from the vagina, you will have a good indication as to when ovulation takes place. Mid-cycle (at ovulation) cervical fluid is copious and watery, and secreted at a rate of 600mg per day. It contains salts, amino acids, proteins, peptides and lipids.[17]

Progesterone, on the other hand, reduces the secretion rate to 20–60mg per day and thickens the mucus to stop sperm or bacteria from entering the womb during the second half of the cycle, when the uterus could contain a pregnancy that needs protection from the external environment. (*See* Appendix D, p. 350, for natural fertility guidance.)

ENDOMETRIOSIS

ENDOMETRIUM VERSUS ENDOMETRIOTIC IMPLANTS

The endometrium of the womb plays a vital role in the reproductive process. It is a dynamic tissue that undergoes continuous changes in the preparation for and maintenance of pregnancy. But although the endometrium is required for normal reproduction, it is also the major culprit in endometriosis. In this disease, pieces of endometrium grow and develop in areas outside the uterus. These rogue pieces of the normal endometrium are called 'endometriotic implants' by gynaecologists and scientists, and they can be found throughout the body. In general, however, endometriotic implants are usually found in the lower abdomen with the greatest number occurring in the base of the pelvis or the cul-de-sac/Pouch of Douglas and on the outer surface of the womb, ovary and the bowel, bladder and intestines (figure 2.5).

To a lesser extent endometriotic implants are found in the upper parts of the abdomen, including the small intestine, stomach, liver, gall bladder, kidney, pancreas and diaphragm, and also in the vagina and on the external genitalia. Implants have also been noted in lungs, skin spots, joints, the brain, gums and in the lining of the nose, but these locations are, thank goodness, fairly rare. They have even been observed in the scar tissue in women who have had hysterectomies or Caesarean sections. A bizarre location for endometriotic implants is in the joints of elderly men.[18] Three men in Australia were found to have endometriotic implants on their bladder as a result of taking oestrogenic drugs for cancer of the prostate.[19, 20] As men do not have a uterus, this is a true medical curiosity. Some scientists believe that we are born with a potential to develop endometriosis because, as a fetus develops, some of the endometrial cells migrate to the wrong place and are triggered by a hormonal message at some later date. Endometriosis is so curious and very difficult to live with, but fascinating in its bizarre behaviour.

WHAT CAUSES ENDOMETRIOSIS?

Although we do not have definitive proof of the true origin of this disease, several theories have been proposed as to what causes endometriosis. Dr Sampson in the early 1920s developed the theory of 'retrograde menstruation'.[21] He reported that endometrial tissues, in addition to flowing out of the vagina at the time of menstruation, also move up into the Fallopian tubes, from where they pour into the peritoneal cavity (abdomen). These backward-flowing fragments of endometrium then attach to the cells lining the abdomen and grow in a similar fashion to the uterine endometrium.

Sampson's theory has received the most support from the scientific community, since it agrees with the observation that the numbers of endometriotic implants increase with proximity to the opening of the Fallopian tube. As the endometriotic tissue flows out of the tubes, it would bathe the outer surface of the ovary and uterus, and large amounts would settle at the base of the pelvis in the cul-de-sac/Pouch of Douglas area. As mentioned above, these are the areas of highest occurrence of the disease. Recent research by Dr Jouko Halme of North Carolina University, USA, also supports Sampson's theory. Dr Halme examined the abdomen of his patients at the time of their menstrual flow. He observed the presence of endometrial fragments in the peritoneal (abdominal) fluid of 90 per cent of those who had normal, open tubes, compared with no endometrial fragments in the peritoneal cavity of the patients who had their tubes tied.[22]

These studies confirm that endometrial tissue can make its way through the tubes into the abdomen. Research performed by Dr Michael Vernon on monkeys has also shown that endometrial tissue placed on the surface of the cells lining the abdomen readily supports the growth and development of endometriotic implants.[23]

Thus it seems that Sampson's theory of retrograde menstruation provides a workable explanation of how endometriosis starts. However, it does not explain how endometriosis can develop in the bladder of men, so some additional theories have been suggested over the past 60 years. A second theory proposes that endometrial fragments work their way into the blood circulation or lymphatic system at the time of the menstrual period. The uterus has a rich supply of blood and lymphatic vessels (*see* figure 9.1, p. 166). As the endometrium is sloughed off, some pieces may enter open blood vessels or the lymphatic system and travel around the body. The lymphatic system is a part of the immune system and is explained in detail in chapter 9. It is similar to the blood circulation system, except that there is no heart to act as a pump. The body's movements aid the flow of the lymph, which is an oil-like fluid through which the white blood cells can flow. This theory offers an explanation for

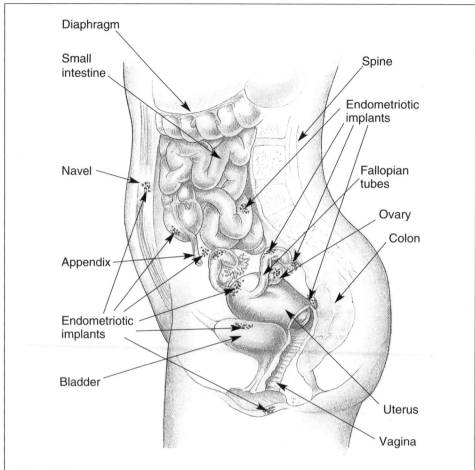

Figure 2.5
Cross-section of the female torso showing the areas of the body where endometriosis is most frequently found.

endometriosis in lungs, since endometrial fragments entering the circulatory system at the uterus would flow freely until they reach the small blood vessels in the lungs. It also may explain the presence of endometriosis in joints.

Another theory, noted by Meyer in 1927, proposed that epithelial tissue (the cells on the surface of most tissues) has the ability to transform into different types of epithelial tissue. Meyer proposed that some epithelial tissue (for example, joint epithelial cells) is converted into endometrial cells, thus explaining how men may develop endometriosis.[24] Quite perplexing, isn't it? The important question is 'Why does this happen in some women, but not in others?' Once we can find the answer to this, we will be nearer the cure. It is felt that a healthy immune system is the key to the removal of the endometriotic implants.

As the endometriotic implants are composed of a tissue very like that of the endometrium, the implants behave like the endometrium, and they respond to the same endocrine hormone messages. In fact, when Sampson first described the disease in the 1920s, endometriotic implants were sometimes referred to as 'mini-uteri'. Using microscopic observations, Dr Deborah Metzger of Yale University has closely examined the response of the endometriotic implant to ovarian hormones. She noted 'a correlation between morphological features (physical appearance) and the ability of endometriotic implants to respond to endogenous gonadal hormones (oestrogen and progesterone) in a manner similar to intrauterine endometrium'.[25] So the two tissues behave in an almost identical manner, one having a life-giving function and the other causing misery and pain.

Women with endometriosis in their noses actually have nosebleeds at the same time as their menstrual period. When the oestrogen of the ovary stimulates the cells of the uterine endometrium to proliferate, the cells of the endometriotic implant also increase. Therefore, endometriosis may 'spread' in response to the oestrogen produced during the menstrual cycle.

It has also been suggested that endometriotic implants may be fuelling their own growth by producing their own supply of oestrogen.[26] Such an 'intracellular' source of oestrogen could help to explain why some women's endometriosis does not respond to the standard drugs which reduce oestrogen production from the ovaries. It could be said that endometriotic tissue is very devious. It could be perpetuating its own growth by making its own home-grown supply of oestrogen.[27] Remember too that every fat cell as well as the adrenal glands and the ovaries also produce oestrogen. The key is how the digestive system excretes the oestrogen.

When the progesterone produced by the corpus luteum in the ovary stimulates the cells of the womb endometrium to become more secretory, the endometriotic implants also start to secrete large amounts of proteins, carbohydrates, fats and oils (lipids) and hormones. However, the big difference with endometriotic implants is that its secretions are not contained safely within the womb and excreted out of the vagina, but dumped into the abdomen or other areas of the body. The delicate organs and tissue inside the abdomen do not normally come in contact with these inflammatory secretions.

Some of these chemical secretions can be quite harmful to abdominal function and possibly to the ova and sperm. For instance, large amounts of prostaglandin E (PGE) and prostaglandin F (PGF) are produced by the endometrium and the endometriotic implant. PGE stimulates excruciating pain. Laboratory technicians who accidentally expose a cut or the mucous membrane of their nose to prostaglandin E feel severe pain for hours, and sometimes days, after the contact. Prostaglandin F can cause increased gut motility (causing irritable bowel syndrome) and stimulate diarrhoea. Prostaglandin F can also shut down the function of the corpus luteum and interfere with the reproductive cycle by reducing progesterone output. Thus, the pregnancy would fail. Balancing the anti-inflammatory and pro-inflammatory prostaglandins seems to be another of the keys on the road to reducing inflammation and pain. This balance is dependent on the quality of fats and oils which we take into our body, and on our absorption of zinc, magnesium, vitamin B6 and biotin, as these four nutrients are all involved in the metabolism of oils.

There is no medical cure for endometriosis. The primary reason for this is owing to the fact that the cells of the endometriotic implant respond to the same cues and chemical messengers as the uterine endometrium. If researchers developed a chemical or physical agent that destroyed the cells of the endometriotic implant, it would also destroy the endometrium lining the womb which would have very serious consequences for fertility. What we need to do is find the differences between womb endometrium and endometriotic implants so that we can destroy the endometriotic implants without harming the endometrium.

APPEARANCE OF ENDOMETRIOSIS

Not only does endometriosis appear in multiple sites within the body, it can also have a different physical appearance depending on its biochemical status. Several researchers have attempted to classify endometriosis by the appearance of the implant and some classification systems list over 30 types of endometriosis! Dr M W Vernon of the Woman's Hospital of Baton Rouge, Louisiana, USA, has developed a simplified classification system of endometriosis to explain the different physical appearance and biochemical status of the endometriotic implants.[28] In this system the implants are divided into three types:

1 *Red or petechial implants.* The first type owe their bright red appearance to a rich blood supply and look rather like a blood blister. These implants are the most biochemically active implants and may be the major culprit in the symptoms of endometriosis (i.e., pain and infertility), as they appear to secrete proinflammatory prostaglandins and the hormone oestrogen.
2 *Brown or intermediate implants.* These endometriotic implants look exactly like the fluffy, reddish-brown endometrium of the womb. They are less biochemically active than the red implants and are therefore called intermediate implants.
3 *Black or powder-burn implants.* These implants are virtually biochemically inactive. They have a poor capacity to secrete hormones, and they are associated with the formation of connective tissue that causes adjacent organs to become attached to each other (i.e., adhesion formation).

Adhesions can literally tie up organs, like the intestine, and cause serious gastrointestinal problems. Stretching these adhesions may also stimulate pain receptors on nerve endings. Adhesions are usually formed from sticky blood strands that set and harden between organs. The organs can then be pulled out of alignment. This tugging may cause sharp pain. The triggering of pain impulses and the production of the PGE proinflammatory series two prostaglandins directly by the implants may be the major cause of the pain associated with endometriosis, especially where the bowel may be attached to the ovary or uterus. Many women reading this book will understand exactly how excruciating that pain can be.

When a woman has endometriosis, the endometriotic implants are usually found in multiple locations in the body and all three types of endometriotic implants can be present at the same time. To help physicians determine the relative severity of the disease, the American Society for Reproductive Medicine (ASRM) has developed a classification system for endometriosis that has been used worldwide. This classification is based upon a scoring system that reflects the size, number and location of the endometriotic implants. Dependent upon the final score, the severity of a patient's disease is classified into one of four stages (*see* Appendix A, p. 341):

- Stage I or minimal disease
- Stage II or mild disease
- Stage III or moderate disease
- Stage IV or severe disease

The ASRM classification system has recently been revised by a group of international scientists, and the new revised system also incorporates the three types of endometriotic implants into disease assessment (*see* Appendix A, p. 341). It also records the percentage of the three types of implants, as well as the size, number and location of the implants.

In the future, most physicians who directly examine endometriosis through surgery will be able to classify the severity of the disease by ascertaining the stage of disease and the percentage of the incidence of the various types. Your gynaecologist should be able to tell you exactly what your implants look like. Ask about this! It is important that this information is in your notes if you change consultants.

The question arises as to how can such an important tissue as the endometrium turn into such a villain when it grows outside the womb and what can we do about it. The best way to elicit change is by helping the endocrine glands to send the right message, and to ensure that the immune system is working effectively to remove the rogue endometriotic implants and that the digestive system is excreting oestrogen correctly.

DIAGNOSING ENDOMETRIOSIS

The two major symptoms of endometriosis are pain and infertility. Unfortunately, to many doctors these symptoms sound vague and in themselves do not present definitive evidence of the presence of endometriosis. The pain that most women with endometriosis feel may be similar to the pain from a long list of medical problems, including extreme uterine cramps, gastrointestinal bloating (causing painful distention), childbirth contractions, stomach ulcers, pelvic inflammatory disease, kidney dysfunction, irritable bowel disease, diverticulitis, vulvadynia, cystitis and bladder infections and many others. Similarly, it is difficult to determine from a physical examination whether a patient is infertile due to endometriosis or some other reproductive problem (unless large lumps of endometriosis are palpable, but these could also be mistaken for fibroids or ovarian cysts). The only definitive proof of the presence of endometriosis is through direct observation, which means surgery.

To diagnose endometriosis, a doctor can look surgically for the disease via laparoscopy or laparotomy (*see also* chapter 6 for information on these procedures).

LAPAROTOMY

Laparotomy is a surgical procedure involving a 10–12cm (4–5in) abdominal incision and exposure of the peritoneal cavity. This is a very invasive procedure and is often unnecessary.

LAPAROSCOPY

Laparoscopy or 'belly-button surgery' is the second and preferred surgery (*see* figure 6.1, p. 110). In this procedure a fibre-optic device, called a laparoscope, is inserted through a small incision in the navel and the abdomen is examined and photographed or videoed. This procedure requires anaesthesia, but can be done in one day as an outpatient service. In the USA and Europe, some general practitioners can perform a mini-laparoscopy in their surgeries. As we will see in chapter 6, laparoscopy has the added advantage of allowing the consultant not only to diagnose the disease, but also to perform a simultaneous laser treatment, to 'burn' away visible endometriotic implants. If a woman consents to having a laparoscopic examination, she should confirm with the physician that in addition to diagnosing her disease, the endometriosis will be classified and photographed, and removed (by ablation, cauterization or laser). This spares her from a second operation and more anaesthetics, and the information will be very helpful in determining subsequent treatments. It would also prevent repeating the procedure if the patient changes doctors. Chapter 6 will discuss consent issues and medical ethics.

During laparoscopy, gases are pumped into the peritoneal cavity to increase the viewing area and to enable the consultant to move organs around in order to locate the endometriotic implants. Usually this form of surgery is successful in locating and ablating troublesome implants. The gases may dissipate to the four corners of the body, causing aching shoulders. Very occasionally the spine may need correcting by a chiropractitioner or osteopath as, when the body is tilted, unconscious, for several hours, the lumbar and cervical vertebrae may become misaligned. In order to speed up the healing of wounds after operations it has been shown that vitamin C and zinc supplements are helpful, as they are essential to the formation of collagen. Homeopathic *Arnica* 6X taken three days before and three days after an operation may reduce bruising. (Both Guy's and St Thomas's Hospitals in London, England, use this treatment for their patients after operations.)

CELLULAR BIOLOGY AND ENDOMETRIOSIS

Endometriosis happens at a cellular level; the implant attaches to the cell wall and hangs on for dear life. The important questions to ask are: Is something in the body weakening the cell membrane so that the endometriotic implants can take hold? How can we maintain the integrity of our cell membrane? If the cell membrane can remain strong, will it prevent the endometriotic implants from taking hold? Is a 'balanced' diet sufficient when we are so ill, or do we need nutritional supplements to help our bodies 'kick start' the healing process? Knowing how our cells work helps us understand why this may be essential in the short term.

Johannas Evers of Maastricht University in the Netherlands is 'looking at the behaviour of endometrium and peritoneum, and at how the endometrial fragments contact the peritoneal lining, how it apposes and attaches to cell membranes. How it subsequently invades organs remains enigmatic'. Somehow, it is felt that these fragments of rogue tissue are damaging the peritoneal membrane. Evers has shown that normal peritoneal tissue has 'Teflon'-like characteristics, which should be a defence against the endometriotic implants. But something secreted by the implants or immune cells may be disrupting this defence mechanism so that the peritoneal membrane behaves more like 'Velcro' and allows the endometriotic implants to stick fast to it.[29]

Research by Professor George Gray CBE has shown that cell membranes behave like liquid crystals. Liposomes (oils) give cell membranes integrity so that they act as a barrier to stop harmful chemicals from entering. Liquid crytals are rod-shaped molecules that are sensitive to light and heat. Local environmental conditions can affect the biology of these crytals. By increasing our knowledge of the dynamics involved, we can begin to understand why the cell membrane changes from 'Teflon' to 'Velcro'.

Nutritionally we know that magnesium and essential fatty acids enhance cell membrane integrity.

CELL STRUCTURE AND FUNCTION

There are many different types of cell in the human body – sperm cells in semen, bone-forming cells, red and white blood cells, cells forming connective tissue to hold us together, cells secreting acid in the stomach to help us digest food, cells storing fat in adipose tissue so that we are ready to survive a famine or drought, and the germ cells which form the ova. The list is endless. The basic structure is the same, but the function is very different for each cell. Together, cells make up the body in which we live. Each type of cell relies upon the nutrients in our diet to be fully functional. Low levels of essential nutrients cause cellular function to begin to fail.

Our bodies are about 70 per cent water. The cells also contain many minerals, trace elements and vitamins, often linked with sugars, fats or proteins. You are made up from what you eat.

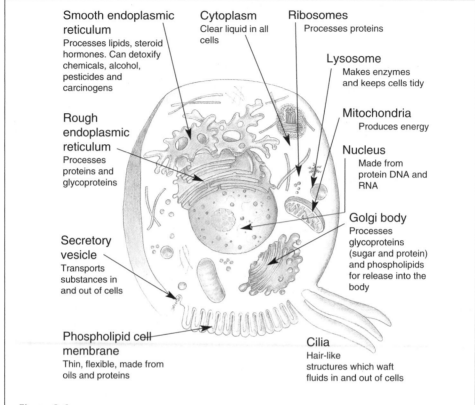

Smooth endoplasmic reticulum
Processes lipids, steroid hormones. Can detoxify chemicals, alcohol, pesticides and carcinogens

Cytoplasm
Clear liquid in all cells

Ribosomes
Processes proteins

Lysosome
Makes enzymes and keeps cells tidy

Rough endoplasmic reticulum
Processes proteins and glycoproteins

Mitochondria
Produces energy

Nucleus
Made from protein DNA and RNA

Secretory vesicle
Transports substances in and out of cells

Golgi body
Processes glycoproteins (sugar and protein) and phospholipids for release into the body

Phospholipid cell membrane
Thin, flexible, made from oils and proteins

Cilia
Hair-like structures which waft fluids in and out of cells

Figure 2.6
Cell diagram which shows all the major organelles within each cell. Rather like a small industrial centre, they take nutrients and process them to form new tissues and chemicals for our body to rebuild itself and stay healthy.

The basic cell structure (figure 2.6) consists of the outer layer or cell membrane, and the inner area which contains a fluid called cytoplasm. Within the latter are mini-organs rather like factories where proteins, fats, enzymes and hormones can be built. The centre of the cell contains the nucleus. This is the brain of the cell which controls how the cell behaves and how it will pass on its code to a new cell. The nucleus contains deoxyribonucleic acid (DNA), the genetically coded information that we have inherited from our parents. Cells chatter to one another and, if the message is disrupted, it becomes like a country trying to work without a postal service.

The cell membrane consists of phospholipids (compounds made up of cis-oils and phosphorus). In chapter 4, we look at the role of prostaglandins (which are oil-based hormones), and how the quality of the oils we eat is very important for fertility and pain reduction. The cis-fats found in natural oils can keep the cell membrane strong, whereas the trans-fats from manufactured or processed oils cannot lock into the membrane very well and leave the cell wall more likely to be breached by harmful substances. (Trans-fats may be made within the body or they could be from the environment.) The cell membrane is permeable, to allow nutrients and substances used for rebuilding the body cells to pass in and out.

A cell is rather like a little powerhouse, or production line. There are factories making proteins from amino acids, phospholipids from fats and oils, and glycoproteins from sugars and proteins. The structures called mitochondria take from your diet iron, vitamins C, B1, B2, B3 and B5, magnesium and coenzyme Q10, and with glucose, water and oxygen make all the energy the body needs. Magical stuff goes on in the twinkling of an eye.

We know that the amount of magnesium in the body is important for the integrity of the cell membrane. Research has shown that magnesium on the cell membrane can prevent the changes that cause cancer. Research shows that: 'Magnesium on the cell membrane helps cells stick together in a normal fashion. Magnesium is required in more than 30 enzyme systems that deal with cell growth and division, which are disordered in cancers.'[30] Endometriosis cells appear to mimic the way cancer cells grow and this may be important to understanding the disease. Endometriosis is thought to have nothing to do with cancer, but the way in which the endometrial cells can implant themselves in other tissues and travel all over the body has some resemblance to the attachment and movement of cancers. By understanding more about the mechanism of transport, it may help us understand better how we can prevent the disease from taking hold. As magnesium is required for DNA replication and is involved with the enzymes affecting cell growth and division, we know that this mineral could be vital for reproduction and possibly for prevention of endometriotic implants. More research is necessary to show how magnesium levels affect the ability of endometriosis implants to attach to the cell membrane.

Production of skin, mucous membranes, cell membranes and tissue renewal are dependent on vitamins A, C and E, zinc, manganese, choline and essential oils (fatty acids). The mitochondria are protected by manganese and choline. Deficiency of manganese leads to alterations in cell tissues. So our nutrient intake can make the skin, mucous membranes and cell membranes throughout our body much stronger. Our bodies can only use what we put into them. If we are stressed, take in too many anti-nutrients (such as coffee, chocolate, alcohol, refined sugars, fizzy pop and cigarettes), if we are surrounded by pollution (lead, cadmium, mercury, aluminium, food additives, pesticides and fungicides), or eat processed foods low in essential minerals (such as zinc, magnesium, manganese, chromium and selenium) and essential fatty acids, then it becomes more difficult for our poor bodies to cope.

FREE OXIDIZING RADICALS

Alex Comfort, the gerontologist, says 'FoRs are highly reactive chemical agents that will combine with anything that is around – like conference delegates.' To add insult to injury, 'free radical damage' to the cell membrane could be another problem. Free oxidizing radicals (FoRs) occur naturally in the body and are formed when glucose is burned to produce energy. Free oxidizing radical means that the molecules are incomplete; they have an electron missing, giving them an uneven, negative electric charge. As a result, the FoRs will rush around the body like mad things trying to steal an electron from an already complete molecule in order to make themselves whole.

However, changes in our diets and the environment have also caused an increase in the number of free radicals produced. FoRs are present in burnt food, fried food, sunshine, smog, industrial factory fumes, pesticides, tobacco smoke, upholstery and carpet treatments, barbecued food, and chemicals used in the building and paint trade. The high levels of FoRs can cause the body to become overwhelmed so that it can no longer make them all safe.

FoRs can cause injury, inflammation and mayhem to cell membranes, collagen (the building block of all human tissue) and to the DNA in the nucleus. Wherever they have been, they leave behind a compound which has been denatured and can no longer function as it should. For example, proteins are rather like tight curly hair; once they have been denatured, the proteins uncurl and lose their power. Protein-based hormones, such as oxytocin and prolactin, can be damaged in this way. The FoRs also damage the fats and oils in our bodies, including those oils making up the cell membrane, the steroid hormones, prostaglandins and the immune cells of the lymphatic system. All this thieving of electrons causes a domino effect, cascading through localized tissues and causing untold damage, as the cell loses control of its internal and external biochemistry.

FoRs cause damage in four main areas:

1 *Double bonds and DNA.* FoRs love the double bonds of DNA molecules and are attracted to them because of the electrons they contain. If DNA function is impaired it can no longer reproduce itself faithfully. Cellular mutations may occur, and the production of new enzymes, hormones and proteins can become faulty.

2 *Immune cells.* Because immune cells are so complex, they are susceptible to FoR damage. If the immune cells are damaged by FoRs they can no longer identify and attack invading 'aliens' effectively, thus leaving our body tissues open to more damage than would normally have taken place. This damage may lead cells to attack 'self' tissue as in auto-immune diseases, which could be the case in endometriosis.

3 *Cell membranes.* The cell membrane is made up of lipids (oils) and the FoRs attack the lipids' double bonds allowing harmful chemicals into the cell that may damage its working. Arachodonic acid from animal fats may trigger the cell walls to secrete prostaglandins which cause a proinflammatory reaction in the surrounding area, as happens with endometriotic implants.

4 *Proteins.* These are most susceptible to free radical damage. Once the electrons have been stolen from proteins they lose all their normal activity. This is very serious as all protein-based hormones, such as oxytocin, relaxin, inhibin and

prolactin, and enzymes suffer irreparable damage. Collagen (the substance which holds cells together) is affected and wrinkles in skin can result. Skin and internal mucous membranes age more rapidly.

The question is, therefore, how to reduce the amount of damage caused by FoRs? There are several enzymes in the body which exist in order to 'mop up' FoRs:

1   Super oxide dismutase (SOD) releases an electron to neutralize the FoR. For SOD to work, it needs regular supplies of copper, zinc and manganese from the diet. SOD forms part of a vital collection of genes which influence the repair of damaged DNA.
2   Glutathione peroxidase neutralizes FoRs by giving them an electron and stopping the damage before it begins. The amount of glutathione peroxidase present in the body is entirely dependent upon our absorption of selenium and vitamin B2 (riboflavin).
3   Catalase can only work when iron is present in sufficient quantity. It is an enzyme which plays an important role in the body's metabolism and it also neutralizes the effects of FoRs.

Antioxidants

Antioxidants are specific nutrients which can disarm the FoRs by adding an electron to the FoR and balancing the electric charge. The best-known antioxidants are vitamins A, C and E, and the mineral selenium. But coenzyme Q10, Quercetin (a flavinoid, *see* Glossary), and the amino acids taurine, glutathione and cysteine are also involved. Other substances which help support antioxidant activity are copper, manganese, iron, sodium and the vitamins B1, B2, B3, B5, B6, para-amino benzoic acid, choline and inositol. If our digestive systems are poor at absorbing these vital nutrients or our diets do not contain them in sufficient quantities, then we will sustain more FoR damage to our cells.

Does this mean that the damaged cell membranes may be prone to developing endometriosis? We don't know. More research is needed, but we can try to protect ourselves through our diet.

SUMMARY

1   The menstrual cycle is a complex mixture of interactions between the pituitary, the ovaries and the uterus.

2   The pituitary secretes the hormones FSH and LH which stimulate the ovary to produce mature eggs and steroid hormones (oestrogen and progesterone). The

ovarian steroids, in turn, prepare the uterus for a possible pregnancy by stimulating the uterine endometrium to become a lush tissue that secretes the nutrients required by a developing embryo.

3 Endometriosis is a disease that is characterized by the presence of uterine endometrium in areas outside of the uterus, primarily within the abdomen. These rogue patches of endometrial tissue are known as endometriotic implants.

4 Endometriotic implants interfere with the menstrual cycle in a subtle fashion that is not fully understood. But they can lead to pain and infertility in some women. The hormonal messages get mixed up in endometriosis.

5 Weakened cell membranes may make it easier for endometriotic implants to take hold.

6 Magnesium and natural cis-vegetable and fish oils are known to improve the integrity of cell membranes, which may prevent the endometriotic implants from sticking like 'Velcro'.

7 By reducing free radical damage the cell membrane may sustain less injury. Antioxidants such as selenium and vitamins A, C and E help to disarm free radicals. (A daily portion of fruit and vegetables will help to improve the dietary intake of these.)

8 Optimum nutrition and a healthy digestive system help to ensure that all cells work efficiently.

> You must be the change you wish to see in the world.
> *Mahatma Mohandas Karamchand Ghandi, 1869–1948*

3 Ovaries, ovarian cysts and syndrome X

To be surprised, to wonder, is to begin to understand.

Jose Ortega y Gasset

The ovary is a complex organ that works on a cyclic pattern to secrete hormones and mature existing ova, ripening them ready for release at ovulation. They react to the monthly hormone cycle that is dependent upon the release of hormones in the brain – from the hypothalamus and pituitary glands. In most women, this cycle just continues normally month in and month out, year in and year out, from teen years to the early 50s. Puberty usually begins at around the age of 13 to 14. In the 19th century, this was around the age of 17 years. In modern Western society, the onset is becoming earlier and earlier – many girls appear to begin their menstruation at age 11 or 12. Occasionally even children aged four to five years begin precocious puberty.

Research reported in the *Journal of Pediatrics* in 1999 noted that girls with the highest prenatal polychlorinated biphenyl (PCB) – oestrogenic pesticide – exposure tended to hit the first stages of puberty a bit earlier than others. In one study, 15 per cent of white girls were showing outward signs of puberty (breast buds and pubic hair growth) by the age of eight. Other research shows that overweight girls tend to mature earlier while very underweight girls mature later.

Early development may be caused by a protein hormone called leptin, produced by fat cells and known to be necessary for the progression of puberty. It functions in a lipostatic pathway and mediates energy production. The presence of leptin reduces appetite and increases energy production. It is possible that leptin and insulin work in a way to balance one another. Those girls who are overweight also have more insulin circulating in their blood, and high levels of insulin stimulates the production of sex hormones from the ovary and adrenal glands. No one has looked at the effects of growth hormones fed to beef and dairy cattle and their breakdown in the human body, so their effects in this area are unknown. But some research suggests that the chemicals used in plastics, like phthalates and bisphenol A – 'chemical cousins' to oestrogen – can affect the reproductive systems in animal experiments.[1]

Of course, such early development can bring endometriosis into the realm of adolescents. Already, one girl of 17 has reported to the author that she has undergone seven laser laparoscopies, and has been on the oral contraceptive pill once, and gonadotrophin-releasing hormone (GnRH) antagonists twice, to put her into a state of menopause, and had a Marina coil inserted – to no avail. A nine-year-old when operated on had her womb and ovaries stuck together with adhesions and active endometriotic implants, having begun her periods at the age of eight. We all have to find a less harsh approach than this for young girls.

> There are four kinds of people in the world:
> People who watch things happen,
> People to whom things happen,
> People who don't know what is happening,
> And people who make things happen.
>
> *Anon*

For some women and young girls, the normal hormone balance becomes disrupted, and ovarian tissue responds by developing abnormally; cysts and tumours may form. This may also be due to chemicals that pollute our world. Cysts appear and disappear all the time. Normal physiological cysts, such as follicular cysts and luteal cysts, are the only ones that are meant to be present and are discussed in chapter 2. The follicular cyst appears from day 1 to day 14 to ripen the ova and release it into the Fallopian tube. The luteal cyst (corpus luteum) appears from day 15 to day 28 and produces progesterone to maintain any possible pregnancy. They are usually 1cm in diameter, appear and are reabsorbed monthly.

When the follicular cyst bursts and releases the ova, it may spew out a small amount of blood, which gives rise to some short sharp pains and inflammation for a few minutes in some women midcycle (known as *Mittleschmertz*); this is normal. But if the pain is extreme, then something is wrong, and anti-inflammatory agents are needed to reduce the pain and immune support to clear away the debris. If a luteal cyst grows abnormally, it may cause hormonal problems. The excess progesterone may cause an irregularity of the menstrual cycle and stimulate the endometrium, thus altering blood loss.

ABNORMAL CYSTS

Endometrial cysts begin when the follicle does not burst and release an ova, or maybe a corpus luteum fills with blood and continues to grow and fill as the monthly bleed continues, trapping endometrium tissue inside. Endometriomas lie within the ovary or may grow from their surface. They have a wall around them not unlike moss on a stone. The term 'chocolate cyst' comes from the stale brown blood that they contain. They may be removed by laser or by aspiration (rupturing with a long needle), but they have been known to return within a few days unless their core has been removed by ovarian resection. Large ones up to 45cm diameter have been known, though most are 4–9cm in size. Strangely, gynaecologists always liken their sizes to fruits such as grapefruit, tangerine, orange or plum. These cysts produce oestrogen and, as such, can 'feed' the development of endometriosis. Ovulation can still occur with smaller cysts, though it may be erratic in the presence of excess oestrogen. It has been suggested that the presence of endometriomas alters the ova and may disrupt fertility.

Polycystic ovary cysts, on the other hand, produce more androgen hormones, such as testosterone, and do disrupt ovulation (see pp. 43–7).

Mucoid cysts are filled with clear mucus not unlike that of the nose, and can come and go within the ovary or be joined to it by a stalk. They are most often benign, but some can become malignant. They show up on scans as being full of dense matter and can grow alongside endometriomas.

Dermatoid cysts are bizarre, as they contain hair, nails and teeth. They can cause pain and need to be removed surgically. They are more unusual and develop if the cells that produce the ovum behave abnormally.[2]

When any of these cysts goes into torsion – where it twists on its stalk and cuts off the blood supply – great pain may be caused. Large cysts may also rupture, spewing out hot sticky blood or mucus all over the intestines. As bowel tissue is very sensitive and moves away if lightly touched during an operation, this shock of hot inflammatory blood causes the intestinal muscles to go into spasms.

The pain is so intense and terrifying that one wonders how the body can live through such pain. People who have not experienced this can have no idea of the severity of this pain. If we consider that most health professionals may have only ever experienced a severe toothache, it becomes understandable why they may have no idea of what we are talking about. Kidneystone pain may be the nearest agony the pelvic cavity can undergo. Often the body goes into shock and shakes violently, and there may be vomiting and cold sweats rather like standing under a waterfall. The immune system then has to work hard to clear up all the inflammatory debris that has been flung around the peritoneal cavity. Extra macrophages and polymorphs may be found in the fluid as they attempt to clear up the mess.

Some ovarian cysts are symptom-free and may only be found by chance on pelvic examination. Indeed, many women with endometriosis are asymptomatic and their cysts have only been discovered during an operation for sterilization. Sometimes women feel pain during intercourse, and the abdomen may become enlarged and uncomfortable if the cyst is large. The bladder may also be affected by the extra pressure, and urination may become more frequent. The vast majority of cysts are benign and the body is able to reabsorb those that are below 4–5cm in diameter (normal-sized). Larger cysts may require surgery to remove them, though they can recur within a few days in some cases.

New research suggests that cysts may be triggered by a variety of factors. Excess dairy foods, yoghurt and eggs are thought to be involved in cyst formation in some studies using Mormon women as controls. Another study found high copper levels when ovarian cysts are present. The latest research suggests an association with a high intake of refined carbohydrates and sugars. Research shows that B-complex vitamins aid the body in control of excess oestrogen, but excess sugars reduce their ability to work. Reduction of sugars and dairy foods, and an improved intake of B vitamin-rich foods, may help.

SYNDROME X OR INSULIN RESISTANCE

Syndrome X or insulin resistance is hidden and may be life-threatening. It affects body metabolism, and the evidence grows daily that many of us are inflicting it upon ourselves through chronic food intoxification. In the early stages it often goes unnoticed, the symptoms are silent and remain hidden – high blood pressure, raised levels of triglyceride fats in the blood, and insulin resistance (as the body struggles and acquires resistance to the insulin hormone, which normally enables the body to control glucose levels). Insulin is a hormone produced in the pancreas, an endocrine gland, and acts as a messenger between cells. It can affect the follicle of the ovary because it balances the effects of other hormones, including oestrogen, testosterone and glucose tolerance factor.

Insulin receptors are found in the ovaries, skin, brain, kidney and blood vessels. Insulin normally controls the enzymes involved in carbohydrate metabolism. It stimulates the storage of glucose in muscle and fat, and glycogen storage in the liver.

Insulin resistance is very complex. When extreme insulin reactions occur, it affects other steroid hormones. Too much insulin, and other hormones react badly; too little insulin, and hormones react poorly. The body always requires balance.

The liver holds the secret of syndrome X or insulin resistance. It deals with the products from digestion. Cell biochemistry research has shown that sugar can be as bad for the heart as saturated fats. The liver can flood the bloodstream with saturated fats as it deals with digestion. Since the 1960s, people have begun to shun the regular eating pattern of three meals a day and are now more likely to graze throughout the day. It is felt that this change in eating patterns may be why syndrome X is on the increase. Eating too frequently makes the liver continue to churn out digestive enzymes with no rest whereas eating three regular meals a day allows the liver a period of respite between each meal. Grazing or snacking all day long means that the overworked liver has to churn out fats, enzymes and hormones all the time. Every time we eat, the pancreas has to release insulin hormone into the bloodstream. Insulin encourages our body cells and organs to use up the glucose that surges through the bloodstream. Any glucose left in the blood for too long is dangerous as it sticks to proteins and leads to kidney damage or blindness. Insulin can also stop the liver from releasing excess fat. Excess fats in the bloodstream are dangerous as there they are altered biochemically and stick to the walls of the arteries, thus narrowing the blood channel. This can lead to heart attacks and strokes.[3]

Research suggests that when people munch on snacks – grazing throughout the day – instead of eating regular meals, the liver has to deal with insulin being around for long periods of time. This prevents the liver from withholding fats such as triglycerides and instead causes the opposite to happen. The liver releases an excess of triglycerides, which may lead to heart disease and other problems related to ovarian function. This excess of fatty triglycerides makes muscle cells insulin-resistant which, in turn, makes the liver secrete even more insulin. Even the fat cells, with all the extra triglycerides and glucose hurled at them to store, finally give in to insulin resistance. As the fat cells become overloaded, they push an excess of fatty acids into the bloodstream, and this overload kills off the important cells in the pancreas that produce insulin. What happens next is that insulin levels fall and glucose builds up in the blood to dangerous levels.[4]

As there is insufficient insulin left to maintain the normal balance of two teaspoons of glucose to eight pints of blood, type II adult-onset diabetes may then be diagnosed. (This may also be related to high dairy intake which, nutrition research suggests, may trigger an immune system reaction against cells in the pancreas.) If you eat a bar of chocolate containing eight teaspoons of sugar, the body has to react immediately to restore balance. The pancreas has to produce insulin and glucose tolerance factor in order to maintain normal blood sugar levels; doing this too often creates mayhem. The pancreas struggles to respond as sugar washes through the system. Eventually the pancreas cells reduce their response and are unable to cope with the demand, leaving these cells to die off.

How does this all relate to endometriosis and polycystic ovaries?

1   It affects liver function, and we need the liver to be extra efficient so that oestrogen is dealt with correctly and excreted from the body if in excess. If we eat too much sugar and saturated fats, we are tying up the liver to deal with sugar and triglycerides, leaving it too weary to balance oestrogen correctly.
2   Insulin affects ovarian function. The ovaries are very sensitive to insulin, as it has a steroidal action and makes the ovary produce an excess of the male hormone testosterone. This causes too many follicles to be stimulated, causing the ovary to have six or more follicles trying to ripen at any one time instead of the usual two or three. It may also have a relationship to the build up of ovarian 'chocolate' cysts.

POLYCYSTIC OVARY SYNDROME (PCOS)

Polycystic ovary syndrome is a common endocrine disorder affecting 5 to 10 per cent of women of reproductive age all around the world. Many women with endometriosis are also diagnosed with PCOS. Symptoms vary from irregular menstrual cycles with months in between, hirsutism, acne, frontal hair loss, skin tags and acanthosis nigrans (a velvet-like skin patch often found in the groin, neck, and under the breasts and arms). Weight accumulates on the stomach, thighs and hips. Though PCOS is independent of obesity, skinny and overweight women show signs of decreased insulin sensitivity. Obese women in general may exhibit insulin resistance. (Women with regular menstrual cycles do not show signs of insulin resistance.)[5]

In PCOS, hormone messengers from the pituitary gland to the ovary seem to be at abnormal levels, which in turn has a domino effect and creates havoc with the normal hormone balance. Lutenizing hormone (LH) levels are often abnormally raised, which stimulates the ovarian follicle, but the follicle is unable to mature fully as follicle-stimulating hormone (FSH) measurements are then at the wrong levels. High LH causes the ovarian follicle to produce more testosterone than is normal. This testosterone changes the oestrogen level and triggers menstrual dysfunction.[6]

These scrabbled hormones lead to the ovary's ending up with many small cysts – having between six to ten cysts constitutes a diagnosis of PCOS. Some contain eggs, others are dormant and the rest may secrete hormones. Unlike endometriotic (chocolate) cysts, which may grow as large as a five-month-old fetus, these PCOS cysts remain small and do not grow (8mm in diameter is maximum). They appear, are reabsorbed and others come to take their place, all due to receiving the wrong hormonal messages.[7]

Some women with endometriosis also appear to develop PCOS, but not every woman. PCOS tends to run in families, with evidence suggesting that there may be a genetic link.[8]

Lou C of Buenos Aires, Argentina

I would like to express my utmost gratitude to you for all your help and advice regarding my PCOS. After years of being pushed from doctor to doctor with no real answers being given, I decided to turn my back on conventional medicine and focus on dietary change. I am now a firm believer that 'you are what you eat'.

My symptoms started four years ago with hirsutism, weight gain, acne, severe mood swings, insomnia and depression, all of which pointed to PCOS. It took two years before I was diagnosed correctly. The only help offered was to go on the contraceptive pill Dianette. Purely by chance several years later, I saw a television programme on the Hale Clinic, offering alternative and complementary therapies. After my first consultation with you, it was clear that my condition could be greatly helped by dietary changes and food supplements. The main change in my diet was to reduce wheat products, avoid dairy products, eat less meat and drink less alcohol, and increase my intake of fish, vegetables and fruit.

The difference was amazing. Within two weeks, there was a noticeable 99 per cent improvement in all my symptoms. My husband said it was like having a new wife. My life has totally changed for the better and I feel like a totally new woman, full of energy and life. I am now nearly 99 per cent symptom-free – a change due completely to my new way of eating.

If you want something different for tomorrow, you have to do something different today! I cannot express my gratitude to you enough for all you have done for me. Many thanks!

• C A S E   S T U D Y •

PCOS AND ENDOMETRIOSIS

PCOS may or may not be found alongside endometriosis. With endometriosis, the link may be related to insulin resistance due to erratic hormone levels, liver dysfunction and poor food choice. When periods are erratic, and acne, hirsutism and weight gain are present, women may suffer from both conditions. Many sufferers of both PCOS and endometriosis may share the hyperinsulinism, high insulin secretion disorder. High insulin triggers the higher levels of testosterone and LH that give rise to these extra symptoms, and this can lead to anovulation, where the ovaries fail to produce a viable egg. It is the pituitary gland that produces growth hormone, stimulating the release of glucagons and insulin from the pancreas. This insulin acts on the outer layer of the ovary and stimulates the release of testosterone. The high testosterone then triggers high LH release from the pituitary. When the thyroid hormone thyroxine and the sex hormones oestrogen and progesterone do not work effectively, then blood sugar levels may rise. Severe shock may cause the pituitary and thyroid glands to function below par. Insulin is zinc dependent, and glucose tolerance factor (GTF), another hormone, depends upon chromium and vitamin B3. Both insulin and GTF are produced in the pancreas, an endocrine gland, and they work alongside other hormones in balancing the blood sugar levels in the body.

Insulin targets tissues to initiate the uptake of glucose and, of course, each cell requires glucose for energy production. Insulin binds to the cell's insulin receptors and this triggers a cascade of events. The amino acid tyrosine is involved in this process. Tyrosine is vital to the formation of thyroxine – the hormone from the thyroid gland in the neck that controls metabolism and temperature. How much everything in the body is interlinked! Once the target cells have received sufficient insulin, they can take up glucose and produce energy, and we feel well. When insulin stimulates fat cells in PCOS women, the binding levels of insulin appear normal, but further down the line, the uptake of glucose into cells becomes impaired. Insulin resistance causes hyperinsulinism and hyperandrogenism in ways that are not yet fully understood. One may trigger the other. An excessive intake of refined carbohydrates is, however, the true culprit.

It is felt by researchers that insulin somehow interacts with LH, and this interaction causes the ovaries to increase production of androgen hormones such as testosterone. High insulin stimulates testosterone while low insulin decreases testosterone. Zinc balances testosterone levels along with vitamin E. Insulin-like growth factors (IGFs) in the ovary promote insulin-like metabolic effects. It is felt that insulin and LH may halt the maturation of the dominant follicle at 5–8mm. This, of course, makes the woman become anovulatory – there is no ovulation and egg release cannot occur, so no pregnancy can happen. Fertility is thus compromised in women with PCOS.

Another mechanism may occur in women with endometriosis who eat an excess of refined carbohydrates, and have poorly functioning liver and pancreas cells. We know that many of the drugs given to women with endometriosis can lead to liver enzyme problems so these levels should always be checked; the GP should always run blood hormone level and fasting glucose tolerance tests.

Once again, we come into the realm of tests that all GPs should be offering to women with reproductive disorders. At present, most women have to fight for adequate treatment when it should be *de rigeur*. The moral of the story is that, if you are trying to achieve a pregnancy, too many sugary and starchy foods are bad news for the ovary, and an excess may even prevent ovulation.

Orthodox treatments use the oral contraceptive Dianette tricyclically, but new research suggests that antidiabetic drugs, such as metformin, also help to reduce androgen levels. These work by reducing both insulin resistance and circulating insulin levels; they also lower androgen levels, which reduces the hirsutism and male pattern baldness. They regulate the menstrual cycle back to normal and support fertility. However, they do come with side effects, such as nausea, diarrhoea, appetite suppression and reduced uptake of vitamin B12.[9, 10]

Obesity is thought to be related to insulin resistance and hyperinsulinism. Some 50 to 60 per cent of women with PCOS are overweight and weight loss in these women can be extremely difficult whatever they do. Conversely, 40 to 50 per cent of women with PCOS have a normal body build.[11]

In classical PCOS, the woman is overweight with severe androgenism (hirsutism, male pattern baldness and acne). Insulin suppresses sex hormone binding globulin (SHBG) in the liver and gut, which leads to increased testosterone. Concentrations of SHBG are low and periods are wildly erratic, being months or years apart. These women may develop acanthosis nigrans. Other women with PCOS are of normal weight, often have regular menstrual cycles and very little androgenism. This may be a result of the beginnings of insulin resistance and not true PCOS, and will respond well to nutritional treatment.

Increased levels of leptin, the protein hormone produced in fat cells that reduces appetite, can trigger an increase in LH and FSH, a Japanese study has shown. The theory is that if leptin can be decreased, it will affect the receptors on mRNA which help to decrease body weight and improve reproduction. GALP (galanin), a peptide, can target the leptin and cause levels to decrease.[12]

PCOS may well be a genetic 'strength' that has developed over the ages in times of famine. A slow metabolic rate is very economical in its use of energy. In hunter–gatherer communities when food was scarce, extra abdominal fat was protective of fertility and survival. It may have developed as a step towards sustaining human survival. Researchers always refer to genetic PCOS as 'the thrifty gene'.[13] The higher androgen levels would have provided more strength to gather food, and subfertile periods would have prevented the birth of extra mouths to feed in times of famine.

The milder form of PCOS may be common, but the more severe form associated with obesity may be a reaction to triggers in the environment and heightened unnatural stressors. Extra abdominal fat seems to be related to higher levels of LH, oestrone and androstenedione, and also higher fasting glucose-stimulated insulin. Hirsutism appears to be worse when these hormones are higher. Research suggests that women who opt for a vegetarian diet rich in soluble fibre show lower levels of blood androgen hormones than those on normal Western diets. This is probably because soluble fibre is much better at binding to oestrogen and helping it be escorted from the body.

In endometriosis, it is essential to have any excess oestrogen removed efficiently from the body, so the choice of rich soluble-fibre foods is important. These include green leafy and red vegetables, fresh fruits and oats, with a selection of legumes, nuts and seeds. This is really only going back to a more Stone Age-type diet, one that is full of natural foods as opposed to preprepared and processed foods that contain hidden additives, colourings and preservatives which may, in combination, interfere with normal hormone levels. In addition, exercise has been shown to reduce levels of LH and FSH and bring them back to normal.

The cysts in PCOS produce testosterone that is converted by the body into oestrone. Elevated levels of LH are seen when testosterone is high. If FSH is low, this gives rise to elevated oestrogen and stops the cells in the follicle from producing testosterone from the oestrogen. When that happens, ovulation does not occur. The balance is very fine and depends very much on foods in the diet, such as good oils and proteins, on which the steroid hormones are based. High FSH in turn gives rise to low oestrogen, a condition that is more usual in menopause or after IVF treatment, when the ovaries have been repeatedly overstimulated.[14]

Another theory suggests that PCOS might be triggered by adrenal androgens being produced in excess at times of stress. The adrenal glands produce adrenaline to give us extra energy at times of stress. Androgens (such as testosterone) are converted to oestrone in fatty tissue, which causes the blood levels of oestrone to rise. Raised oestrone causes excess LH and a deficiency of FSH. As high LH triggers the ovary to produce androgens within the follicle, a cycle begins which may continue for too long. This in turn alters the delicate relationship of the steroid hormone balance.

Increased adrenal activity mobilizes the fatty acids that depress glucose uptake by peripheral tissues, thereby reducing insulin sensitivity. Stress can also decrease chromium stores, which may lead to hyperinsulinaemia; the body compensates by releasing extra insulin to get blood levels back into balance.[15, 16] It is therefore essential to keep stress to a minimum. Assess what things are causing stress in your life and write them down on the left side of a sheet of paper. Then, on the right side, list the stressors that you can rid yourself of and take steps to remove some stress from your life.

The hypothalamus and pituitary glands in the brain control the ovarian hormones. If the hypothalamus secretes the wrong level of GnRH, the pituitary may increase LH production, which can trigger an increase in testosterone production in the ovary.

To date, there is not enough information on how all these hormones 'talk' to one another normally. Much is known of the effects of IVF drugs on hormone levels, but too few studies have been carried out on what is normal in women. The problem is that most women are or have been on the oral contraceptive pill (80 per cent of all American women) or steroid hormones as treatment for gynaecological conditions, or on hormone replacement therapy (HRT). Only a university department or institution with unbiased funding could take this type of research on board and, as most researchers are paid by pharmaceutical companies, funding for such pure research will be difficult to find, unless a wealthy benefactor who is without bias comes along.

It is a sad state of affairs that so little is understood of the normal hormonal balance of a normal reproduction system that has never been initiated into the use of drugs like oral contraceptives, steroids, GnRH analogues or HRT.

Emily F of London

I hope my story will encourage others to look beyond conventional medicine and discover that there are alternatives that work.

I have suffered from painful periods since I was 17 and must have seen at least 15 doctors, who all prescribed various, increasingly strong painkillers over eight years. I was told that it was quite normal to have painful periods – it was part of being a woman. By age 25, I was living in London and had joined another group practice of doctors, and was working my way through the insensitive ones. My periods were becoming more and more painful, and painkillers less and less effective.

I then met my friend Debs, who told me about the condition she suffered from – endometriosis – I had never heard of it, and none of the countless doctors I had seen over the years had ever mentioned that having painful periods could be a symptom of a medical condition. I made an appointment to see one of the doctors and suggested that I might have endometriosis. She agreed that it was a possibility and referred me to a consultant. Within a month I had had a laparoscopy and had been diagnosed as suffering from moderate endo and polycystic ovaries.

My consultant talked the options through with me and suggested that the best course of treatment would be Zoladex. While at the time I was happy with the way he dealt with me, and his suggested approach, I wish he had mentioned that there were non-medical avenues I could have explored. My experience with Zoladex was not one that I would wish to repeat – I had dreadful mood swings and was regularly depressed and inconsolable; I gained two stone in weight and suffered from hourly hot flushes. At the end of it, my periods were just as painful as they had been before the treatment.

The subsequent treatment prescribed was Dianette (an oral contraceptive) on a continuous basis – two or three packets, then a break. The periods were still very painful, but at least I could control when I had them, and the Dianette helped with the acne, which I had because of the polycystic ovaries. By the age of 30 I was still taking Dianette and various combinations of painkillers, but the pain was getting worse – to the point where I was seriously considering laser surgery (something I considered a last resort). I had also started to develop other health problems such as eczema, IBS and fatigue.

I then received details of the National Endo Society's 1999 AGM, where the speakers were to give talks on various complementary therapies; I decided to attend. The speakers were extremely informative and I came away determined to find a complementary approach that would help me. Soon after the AGM, my mother read an article in the Daily Telegraph, *which focused on a nutritional approach to relieving the symptoms of endometriosis. The interview was with Dian Mills and gave details of her book* Endometriosis: A Guide to Healing Through Nutrition. *My mother ordered the book and gave it to me for Christmas. I read the book from cover to cover – delighted that many of the other problems I was suffering from seemed to be related to the endometriosis and that I wasn't becoming a hypochondriac, as my doctor was making me feel.*

I made an appointment to see Dian in February 2000. Before the appointment I had to fill in a lengthy questionnaire about all aspects of my health, and I was embarrassed at how sickly I appeared. The first appointment was amazing – for once I could talk at length about how I felt without feeling that I was wasting someone's time. And Dian understood what I was talking about! Her suggested approach was to tackle my health goals one by one, dealing with my digestive problems initially (I was suffering from very sudden, violent and unpredictable attacks of diarrhoea), then focusing on the period pain and finally on my concerns about whether or not I was fertile. She suggested that I cut out dairy and wheat from my diet and prescribed what seemed like a long list of vitamins, minerals and supplements.

At first it was a struggle to find alternatives to dairy and wheat, but it soon becomes second-nature. It very soon emerged (via making mistakes when ordering from menus) that I was intolerant of dairy products. Knowing this made such a difference to my life – I had become scared of eating out or leaving the house too soon after a meal, just in case I had an attack of diarrhoea.

The first period I had after seeing Dian (I was still taking Dianette continously) was 50 per cent less painful than the last. By August of that year I had a pain-free period. It was incredible – after 14 years of pain. My energy levels had returned; my skin was better than I can ever remember it being and I had lost some weight.

Being concerned about fertility, my partner and I decided that we would start trying for a baby in September. I was expecting to be infertile, given my combination of endo and polycystic ovaries, and we decided that we couldn't afford to wait much longer as it could take a minimum of two years. To my shock and delight, I conceived in October and I am expecting a baby in four weeks' time!

So many people I have spoken to, especially those in the medical profession, have dismissed the benefit of a nutritional approach to dealing with endometriosis, but I would urge anyone who feels that conventional medicine has failed them to pursue it. In fact, I would encourage anyone who has just been diagnosed to try a nutritional approach before embarking on any medical treatment. It can be difficult to change your diet after years of eating whatever you wanted, but the benefits far outweigh the sacrifices you might think you are making.

Menstruation should occur at least three times each year with PCOS; otherwise there may be cellular changes in the endometrium due to the unrelenting levels of elevated oestrogen which could lead to cancer. Normal menstruation is once each month. Excessive bleeding at menstruation is usually due to an imbalance of iron levels, and iron EAP2 is the best-absorbed form which, if taken for two months, may help to stop heavy menstrual bleeding.

OVARIAN CANCER

Ovarian cancer is rare, thankfully. However, it is extremely serious as there are no symptoms until it is very advanced. By having ultrasound scans and internal examinations with a Pap smear, or with a CA125 antigen blood test, checks can be kept on anyone with a family history of ovarian cancer.

PREMATURE OVARIAN FAILURE (POF)

Approximately 4 per cent of the female population has premature ovarian failure, an endocrine disorder. For some unknown reason, these women suffer a loss of ova from the ovary. Suggested causes are endless. As the ova are produced while the baby girl is still within her mother's womb, so the problem may begin very early on. Clearly, the diet and environment of the mother during pregnancy is crucial to her daughter's health throughout her life. The ova may be dysfunctional, or there may be a chromosomal defect, Turner's syndrome, fragile X, metabolic dysfunction or viral infection damage. Autoimmune disorders may also affect ovarian function, or the ovaries may be removed at an early age.

Loss of ovarian function in this way may give rise to premature menopause if the hormone balance of the ovary is affected. We have seen how the follicle and corpus luteum produce the steroid hormones as a natural part of the menstrual cycle. With POF, this cycle is lost, so that the hormones do not function as they should. Periods often stop and hot flushes or night sweats may be commonplace. Sleep may become fractious, giving rise to mood swings, a low sex drive and bladder-control problems. Energy may be low and, of course, fertility is affected.

Two tests on the blood for FSH levels should be done one month apart. Normal FSH levels are 10–15 mU/ml and under; women with POF often have FSH levels above 40mU/ml, which is in the postmenopausal range. Health concerns are as in menopause – with the risks of osteoporosis, heart disease, thyroid problems, adrenal problems or diabetes.

Infertility for a young girl as a diagnosis can be utterly soul-destroying. However, 6–8 per cent of women with POF do become pregnant. Sound nutrition may aid the function of the ovary, endometrium and endocrine glands, and otherwise do no harm. Medical treatments include HRT and the oral contraceptive pill. Women's support groups can provide helpful advice (see p. 400).

KEYS TO COMBATING INSULIN RESISTANCE

1 Return to eating three regular meals each day. This is vital in order to allow the liver to rest and renew its hormone-releasing cells.
2 Reducing the levels of saturated fats, refined sugars, starches and alcohol is also crucial in combating insulin resistance.
3 Limit fresh fruit to two pieces each day to control fructose intake as the fruit sugar also travels through the liver to be processed.
4 Changing from fatty meat and dairy foods to oily fish and nuts and seeds can help to suppress the liver's release of saturated fatty acids.
5 Use only complex forms of carbohydrates such as oats, corn and rye, brown rice and legumes.
6 Forget high-sugar fizzy drinks and use filtered water or diluted fruit juices.
7 Try to cook many of your meals from fresh and keep convenience foods to a

minimum to reduce intake of hidden sugars and saturated and trans fats.

8 Avoid all bovine dairy products (from cows), and use dairy alternatives from goat's and ewe's milk products to maintain calcium levels. Some soya milk has added calcium.

9 Eat more oily fish, nuts and seeds, and legumes to obtain protein foods.

10 Exercise is a very important tool to prevent the dangerous overload of fat build up in the blood. Even a moderate amount of exercise can help to prevent this build up. Getting off the bus or parking the car further away from work in order to have a brisk, 20-minute walk each day may be just the thing. This will reduce the fatty build up in the blood.

COMPLEMENTARY TREATMENTS FOR PCOS

> The important thing is not to stop questioning.
>
> *Albert Einstein*

The herb *Vitex agnus castus* has been used since Egyptian times to normalize pituitary release of FSH and LH, and regulate menstrual cycles. It needs to be taken for four to six months to have an effect. The tincture form is the most potent, but tablets are also beneficial. These should only be taken under the guidance of a herbalist or nutritionist. Women with a pituitary adenoma or who are attempting pregnancy should not take agnus castus. You may take it in the three or four months before you wish to get pregnant, and then stop when you decide to try for conception.[17]

Vitamin E and zinc are known to balance testosterone, and pectin and guar gum are also thought to be helpful. Aromatherapy oils – geranium, bergamot, clary sage – may be used in the bath, and in base oil to massage the abdomen.

SUPPLEMENT REQUIREMENTS

These may be taken for three to four months to try and improve and correct menstrual function:

- Multivitamins/minerals
- Chromium polynicotinate
- Zinc citrate or methionine
- Digestive enzymes
- Bioacidophilus
- Evening primrose and fish oils

SUMMARY

1 Syndrome X or insulin resistance is related to refined carbohydrate consumption, and affects pancreatic production of the hormones insulin and glucose tolerance factor. All hormones work in relation to one another, and these hormones have a knock-on effect, leading to an imbalance of the steroid hormones of the ovary.

2 Hyperinsulinism triggers the follicle of the ovary to produce testosterone in excess. This stops the follicle from working properly. Women may become anovulatory.

3 Return to eating three regular meals each day, as this enables the liver to rest and renew its hormone-releasing cells.

4 Reducing the levels of saturated fats, refined sugars and alcohol is also crucial in combating insulin resistance.

5 Limit fresh fruit to two pieces each day to control fructose intake, as the fruit sugar also travels through the liver to be processed.

6 Change from fatty meat to oily fish, nuts and seeds to help suppress the liver's release of saturated fatty acids. Avoid bovine dairy foods. Research done in Florida suggests that the protein isomer in milk and that in the pancreas may have the same shape, and could lead to the immune system targeting the pancreas tissue if milk intolerance occurs. This may be harmful in the long term to insulin-producing cells.

7 Use only complex forms of carbohydrates, such as oats and rye, brown rice and legumes.

8 Forget high-sugar fizzy drinks and use filtered water or diluted fruit juices. Avoid all aspartame-containing foods.

9 Try to cook many of your meals from fresh ingredients and keep convenience foods to a bare minimum to reduce intake of hidden sugars, and saturated and trans fats.

10 Follow the supplement and diet programme for three to four months, combined with a 10-minute exercise regime before breakfast. Insulin levels are low on waking and this enables easier metabolism of fat cells during exercise. Ten minutes of aerobics or yoga before breakfast is equivalent to 30 minutes of exercise later in the day.

4 Coping with the pain of endometriosis

Nothing is too wonderful to be true, if it be consistent with the laws of nature.

Michael Faraday, Physicist

Pain is defined in the *Concise Oxford Dictionary* as 'suffering, distress, of body or mind'. The *Oxford American Dictionary* defines it as 'an unpleasant feeling caused by injury or disease of the body'. Endometriosis pain is dire, described by many as 'exquisite' because it takes over your life and colours your whole being, often leaving you stunned or unable to breathe. Pain is a signal that something is wrong within the body. Pain makes us adapt and do something to gain relief; it makes us react.

Chronic intractable pain, such as that from endometriosis, is exhausting. It saps our vitality and robs us of our pleasure in life. Doctors often diagnose and attempt to treat the cause of the pain, but they often fail to discuss the meaning of this pain so that we do not know what to expect in terms of our general well-being or our prospects for recovery. It is crucial that pain is taken seriously and not dismissed as being in the mind. Most women have great difficulty trying to explain to a sceptical doctor what is actually happening inside them. This adds to the anxiety, causing more tension and more pain.

Chronic pain is defined as 'pain which lasts for longer than one month and cannot be relieved by conventional treatment methods'. With endometriosis the pain may be intermittent, but it is real and causes much unhappiness and anxiety. Sometimes it becomes so overwhelming that death would actually seem a welcome relief. When ovarian cysts burst, the pain can be so unreal, so breathtaking, one almost wonders how the body can survive it. Being kept awake night after night by extreme pain wears out the nerves and leaves the sufferer feeling frail and battered. Struggling through day after day of pain wears down the soul.

Jo R of London

CASE STUDY

I can happily say that over the past few months since seeing the nutritionist many of my symptoms have subsided and I can now carry on a normal life. I was getting all the typical endometriosis symptoms, the bloating, abdominal pain, heavy periods and bad indigestion. After being careful with the foods I eat and cutting out wheat and reducing dairy foods, it has made an amazing difference. The fatigue has gone and period pains are a thing of the past. Really at first it sounded that cutting out some foods would be hard, but once you feel the effects, it is easy to keep to as you never want to feel so bad again. If to be well means I can't eat bread again, I can live without the bread. What I can't live with is the pain. I now take supplements on and off. Occasionally I lapse with the food if I'm eating out, but generally it is easy, and the way I feel now I do not want to give up and go back to those dark days.

WHAT CAUSES PAIN AND INFLAMMATION?

Pain is caused by inflammation. This is a protective mechanism in the body which is a local response around an area of damage to prevent or delay the spread of infection. It happens at a site of injury from stress, chemicals, heat, bacteria or trauma. The first reaction is for the blood vessels to dilate in order to increase the flow of blood to the site of injury. This gives the red appearance and burning sensations (with endometriosis this seems nearer to boiling point), which we feel after a cut to the skin. The mast cells (large cells in connective tissue) release histamines and prostaglandins which cause the inflammation. Histamine is a compound formed from an amino acid histidine and is found in all tissues of the body. It causes dilation of blood vessels and contraction (tightening) of muscles.

Small capillaries (blood vessels) in the area become permeable and fluids leak into the spaces between the cells, causing fluid retention (oedema) and localized swelling which puts pressure on the nerve endings, increasing the pain. At the site of the wound, zinc and vitamins C and A are always found as they are required for collagen production in order to build healthy new skin. The blood at the site of the inflammatory response clots (this uses vitamin K) to seal off the area and prevent us from bleeding to death. Clotting also stops the infection or damage from spreading into other areas of the body.

If bacteria are involved, chemotaxic chemicals (those which are on watch for danger) call for the 'immune army'. These include the blood cells called neutrophils, macrophages and lymphocytes which come to the injury site to fight the 'alien' danger. A pus-filled cavity may be formed, acting as a holding bay for dumping debris into, so that the white blood cells (macrophages) can come along and gobble it up.

With endometriosis much of the pain may be due to inflammation around the endometriotic implants. Once the immune army is called in and their chemical warfare begins, healthy tissue around the endometriosis may be bombarded with chemicals produced by immune cells – lymphokines, interleukins and interferons (*see* chapter 9 on the immune system). These white cells dump their chemical weapons onto the damaged tissues in an effort to remove the danger and to allow the body to heal the damage. The histamine release around the site also triggers more inflammation.

Other pain may be caused by adhesions between organs that pull and tug, leading to stabbing sensations. Yet more pain may be triggered as smooth muscle goes into spasm and cramp. With all three types of pain at the same time, the body becomes debilitated.

COPING WITH PAIN

Chronic pain is often frightening, debilitating and excruciating. When it subsides there is always a terror that it may return. Prolonged mild pain is totally fatiguing; it stops you from enjoying the normal things in life and leaves you feeling in despair. What do you do with pain? Do you go with it, fight against it or just learn to live with it? Fighting pain can be counter-productive as it causes us to tense up, when the best form of action is to try to relax. When we are relaxed the brain is able to produce endorphins, which are natural painkilling hormones.

We all have different ways of trying to cope with pain. When it goes on unabated for months on end, we take a battering. It is almost as if the psyche goes into hibernation in order to protect us. Getting through each day becomes a major achievement. Trying to find the energy to take a shower or prepare a meal can be exhausting and you may have to rest afterwards. It can be terrifying to be so ill and to discover there is no known cure. You either have to learn to live with it, which is not an option, or you have to take the bull by the horns and try everything which instinct tells you is right for you, at your own pace. Let this time become useful by reading and learning new things, making something good come out of the bad. That way positive things can happen. Not giving in to the illness, but turning it to your own advantage, stops it from ruling and ruining your life. Build on other skills you have developed over the years from hobbies or interests. With careful management on your part, you can take positive steps to regain your health. Apply the principles of relaxation, exercise and healthy eating.

Pain management treatment can be useful, but what works for one person may not work for another, so you need to persevere to find a strategy which works for you. Perhaps some of the following strategies may help you, as they have helped other women:

1 Gentle exercise
2 Acupuncture
3 Manipulation by an osteopath or chiropractor
4 Weight loss or improved nutrition
5 Hypnotherapy
6 Relaxation techniques
7 Counselling
8 Distracting hobbies or activities
9 Self-help support groups
10 TENS (transcutaneous electrical stimulation) machines from your GP. (These work best to reduce pain of medium intensity, such as period pain. They work for 10 per cent of patients and can help to reduce the need for medication.)
11 Medication
12 Surgery

The British Endometriosis Society (founded by Ailsa Irving in 1982) asked its members how they coped with pain. Ninety per cent of the women who responded used a wide variety of over-the-counter or prescribed painkillers. Many women used them constantly, although the majority took them only when the pain began to increase. Painkillers work more effectively if they are taken when the pain begins. Once extreme pain has taken hold, it becomes too intractable to shift. A few women took more than the recommended dose of painkiller, which can be very damaging to the liver and stomach. The women's most common complaint was that no painkiller ever took the pain away completely; it was merely dulled. A few women had been taking anti-depressants, some for several years. Non-steroidal anti-inflammatory drugs (NSAIDs) which may cause bleeding of the stomach lining; anti-spasmodics and analgesics were also mentioned. Some women drank alcohol with their painkillers, which is extremely dangerous.

DESCRIBING AND MEASURING PAIN

It is very important to find a general practitioner who will listen to your description of your level of pain and who will work with you to find the right type of painkiller. The chart shown in figure 4.1, drawn up by the American gynaecologist Arnold Kresch, may be used to show your GP the type of pain you suffer. Circle the words which closely describe your pain, to explain the type of symptoms which are present, and photocopy them for your doctor.

The diagram of three women (figure 4.2) which was also developed by Arnold Kresch, can be used to indicate where the pain is most severe. Write a 10 in the square where the pain is at its worst and radiate 9s around it. This way your GP can see exactly where the seat of the chronic pain lies, and this may help more effective pain-killing drugs to be prescribed.

Taking control into your own hands can help you cope. Endometriosis is so difficult to explain to sceptical individuals who have the philosophy 'Oh no, it's a woman's problem', and anxiety often can arise when you are unable to describe how the pain is creating problems for you. Certainly doctors need to be made aware of just how your pain affects your everyday life. When you are in the full throes of pain at 4 a.m. it is vital for the doctor to see you then. It is no good waiting until the next day when you are in recovery and crawling along to the surgery. The doctor needs to see the full effect of the pain in order to treat it correctly. If a doctor is unavailable, call an ambulance or get a taxi to the local casualty department.

It is crucial that you have a doctor you can trust, who is compassionate and who listens to your needs. He or she should be a part of your healing team. If you are coerced into unnecessary treatments, trust is lost and, once trust is lost, trauma and anxiety can delay healing. Indeed, anxiety and tension can worsen pain.

Appendix C (pp. 348–9) has a pain calendar for you to photocopy to chart your symptoms on a monthly basis. This will enable you to see if any patterns are repeated in each cycle.

What does your pain feel like?

Some of the words below describe your *present* pain. Circle ONLY those words that best describe it. Leave out any category that is not suitable. Use only a single word in each appropriate category – the one that best applies.

1	2	3	4	5
Flickering	Jumping	Pricking	Sharp	Pinching
Quivering	Flashing	Boring	Cutting	Pressing
Pulsing	Shooting	Drilling	Lacerating	Gnawing
Throbbing		Stabbing		Cramping
Beating		Lancinating		Crushing
Pounding				

6	7	8	9	10
Tugging	Hot	Tingling	Dull	Tender
Pulling	Burning	Itchy	Sore	Taut
Wrenching	Scalding	Smarting	Hurting	Rasping
	Searing	Stinging	Aching	Splitting
			Heavy	

11	12	13	14	15
Tiring	Sickening	Fearful	Punishing	Wretched
Exhausting	Suffocating	Frightful	Grueling	Blinding
		Terrifying	Cruel	
			Vicious	
			Killing	

16	17	18	19	20
Annoying	Spreading	Tight	Cool	Nagging
Troublesome	Radiating	Numb	Cold	Nauseating
Miserable	Penetrating	Drawing	Freezing	Agonizing
Intense	Piercing	Squeezing		Dreadful
Unbearable		Tearing		Torturing

Figure 4.1
Laparoscopic appearance of endometriosis, vol 1, 2nd ed, Resurge Press, Memphis,TN,1991, pp. 33. Reproduced with kind permission from Arnold J. Kresch, D C Martin, D B Redwine and H Reich.

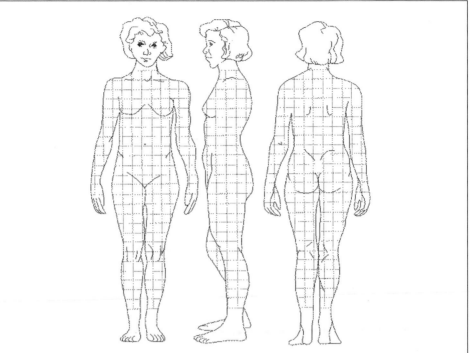

Figure 4.2
Laparoscopic appearance of endometriosis, vol 1, 2nd ed, Resurge Press, Memphis, TN, 1991, pp. 34. Reproduced with kind permission from Arnold J. Kresch, D C Martin, D B Redwine and H Reich.

COMPLEMENTARY THERAPIES

Over half the women in the survey had used complementary therapies to help control their pain. Nutritional supplements were used by the majority, with D,L-Phenylalanine (DLPA) being the most commonly used. Herbal medicines such as agnus castus, blue cohosh, raspberry leaves, slippery elm, violet leaves, peppermint and garlic oils were also mentioned. Homeopathic remedies had been used by some women and a qualified homeopathic practitioner can advise you on which remedy would be most appropriate for your symptoms. A variety of elixirs, such as camomile tea, raspberry leaf tea, arnica ointment, royal jelly, Bach Flower Rescue Remedy and Indian brandy, were suggested, and yet others used prayer and laying on of hands.

One-quarter of the women had used a combination of orthodox and complementary therapies. Winthrop, the pharmaceutical company, in their booklet *Managing Danazol Patients* by Richard P Dickey, PhD, MD (published by Winthrop in the USA), mention that irritability, nervousness, anxiety and emotional lability have been associated with a lack of vitamin B6. It also states that 'pyridoxine (B6) given orally 25–30mg per day may help to prevent headaches and visual changes in some cases'. So it is recognized by one drug company that a mixture of therapies may help. (Chapter 6 discusses the use of the drug Danazol as a treatment for endometriosis.)

A favourite way to treat pain was to curl up with a hot water bottle. Various techniques, like visualization, reading, having a warm bath, self-hypnosis tapes, watching videos and listening to music, or knitting could be employed to try to relieve the milder pain. Some women likened the pain to giving birth, but with no end product, and used the breathing exercises they had been taught for labour pains. The majority of women surveyed felt that trying to do some regular gentle exercise, such as swimming, walks or yoga, helped them most. One woman beat her cushions; another found solace in playing her flute.

VISUALIZATION

Dr Bernie Siegel of Yale University has written books about visualization techniques, which involves making mental pictures. You can imagine the endometriosis is gradually shrinking away. The author used to visualize fluffy white baby goats grazing on the endometriotic implants, making them shrink in size, or imagined a blue healing flame licking all around them.

Positive thinking is vital as it helps the body to heal itself. In illness there are often inadequate T-cells (white blood cells which attack the invading tissue, bacteria or virus). Stress is known to lower the production of T cells and B cells in the body, which weakens the immune system's response. Natural white blood cell production is known from research to be reduced by psychological factors. Sufferers of AIDS and cancers are seen to increase their white blood cell count overnight by visualization techniques.

However, it is the crisis which comes in the wee small hours which can be the most terrifying. The choice is between staying calm or panicking. Many women take extra painkillers or sleeping tablets. One woman reported, 'I take painkillers which make me sick and then I pass out' and another said, 'The pain is so overwhelming, I daren't even move and can't concentrate on anything.' Others moan the pain like a chant, or find that keeping warm is soothing. Yet others say their body just went into shock and shook uncontrollably; this is serious and a sign that the doctor should be called.

DEEP BREATHING

Steady deep breathing is very important, as hyperventilating (rapid and shallow breathing) can make pain worse. It interferes with the oxygen supply to cells which reduces their production of essential hormones, enzymes, energy and possibly endorphins. Hyperventilation means using the lungs to move more air in and out of the chest than it can deal with. Overbreathing is a reaction to pain and fright, but if it goes on too long, you can experience erratic heartbeats, dizziness, gut disturbances, pins and needles, muscle pain, clammy hands and a flushed face. Hyperventilation is caused by adrenaline pouring into the bloodstream, raising the heartrate, tensing the muscles and sharpening the senses so that we can escape from a potential danger. But if we are ill and in no danger, then hyperventilation begins to upset the acid/alkaline balance of the blood. Normal metabolism is altered, leading to exhaustion and depression. Hyperventilation was first described during the American Civil War, when soldiers were disabled by shortness of breath and irregular heartbeats. The trick to correct the breathing is 'Lips together, jaw relaxed, breathing low and slow'. It will take practice to get this right but perseverance could help your health improve.[1] Wearing warm, loose clothing and breathing deeply from the abdomen can make a difference to your pain.

SELF-HELP GROUPS AND POSITIVE THINKING

It helps to talk with someone who has endometriosis and understands your pain, which is why self-help groups can be so powerful in sharing different pain-reducing strategies. It is important to keep a hold on reality and allow yourself to be pampered a little. Allowing yourself to be ill and recognizing that you will get better helps to pull you through. It can be terrifying when the body goes out of control. We live in a world where we expect to be in control but, when nature takes over, it is very disconcerting. The body is always trying to heal itself and you can make a difference by the way you approach the treatment of pain. Settling into a comfortable position and staying still until the severe pain subsides is best. An occasional orthodox or herbal sleeping tablet to knock yourself out for the duration of the pain can also help.

Be positive about yourself, but allow yourself to grieve for the lost time. Your friends may be getting on with their lives and careers whilst you feel left behind. It is very important to know that the body can get well and that you just need to give it all the things it really needs in order to build itself up again. Persevere with your treatment strategies; when you have been ill for some time, the body needs time to heal, it will not happen overnight. It may take several months to totally heal, although some people feel much improved after a couple of weeks. We are all different.

At 4 a.m. when things look bleak and you feel very alone, remember that there are many women all over the world feeling the same at that very moment, and that you are not alone. Think of each other (mind meld) and pull each other through.

The treatment strategies chosen depends upon each person's physical make-up, medical condition, their personality and other factors, such as where the pain is seated. We hope that some of our suggestions will be of help to you. Remember that anxiety, anger and guilt can make pain worse; they are negative emotions, so try to be positive. It has been known for over a century that our emotional state influences our physical health. There is a new field of study looking into the mind-brain-immune connections, psychoneuroimmunology. It is known that the activities of the white blood cells of the immune system are influenced by the brain and nervous system, as there are receptors on each which receive messages from the others. What we think and feel are likely to influence the way our immune cells respond.[2] It is not understood how these areas influence each other and, as everyone is individual, it will differ from person to person. How we respond to the world and the pollution around us may affect our physical well-being. If we feel in control our bodies may cope better than if we feel out of control. Self-help is important because it makes us try to do something for ourselves and regain control over our health.

> The two foes of human happiness are pain and boredom.
>
> *Arthur Schopenhauer, Philosopher*

HOW TO COPE WITH CHRONIC PAIN

Some of the following ideas are suggested by the Chronic Pain Outreach Association in America:

1 Relax – listen to a relaxation tape or imagine a pleasant scene.
2 Do a distracting activity – reading, craftwork, etc.
3 Tell yourself that the pain is temporary and that it will pass.
4 Place a hot water bottle or bag of frozen peas on the pain site.
5 Make yourself laugh, watch a funny film.
6 Hold an involved conversation in your head.
7 Listen to your favourite music.
8 Try deep breathing or meditation.
9 Avoid stressful situations wherever possible.
10 Reduce tension by whatever means (even crying or shouting).
11 Notice the control that you do have (in whatever areas of your life).
12 Take a relaxing bath or shower.
13 Spend time in a very quiet room.
14 Use disassociation – become an 'observer' of your pain rather than feeling it as a 'participant'.
15 Use visual imagery to transform your pain into something different – a shape or colour, for example.
16 Focus your attention on a part of your body which has a different sensation.
17 Ask for the support of others.
18 Adjust your activity level gradually. Increase towards normal activity level over 3–4 days.

NUTRITION TO REDUCE PAIN AND INFLAMMATION

C
A
S S
E T
U
D
Y

Linda C of Surrey

After much trial and error I have changed my eating pattern to suit me, i.e. not combining foods and not eating foods that over a period of time have proved not to suit me (dairy, pastry, meats). I take vitamins and minerals every day and most of all I believe that a positive mental attitude to this condition has, along with the supplements, proved vital. I have had NO pain now for several years.

WHY CAN NUTRIENTS REDUCE PAIN?

Often diseases which are the result of vitamin deficiency are associated with unspecific pains. Changes in the central nervous system, and mucous membrane and skin inflammation are often highlighted in these conditions. While researching into endometriosis and nutrition, several research papers surfaced which showed that certain vitamins do possess analgesic (pain-relieving) and anti-inflammatory properties which correspond to those of orthodox medicines, but without the side effects. Pain is perceived as the body's alarm signal, showing that all is not well. For instance, severe vitamin C deficiency causes scurvy, manifested by bleeding gums, and considerable pain in the joints. If the need for vitamin C is corrected, then the symptoms diminish. Vitamin C combats inflammation and pain by inhibiting the secretion of prostaglandins which contribute to the symptoms.[3] Pain and inflammation which has its origin in a vitamin deficiency is best treated with that particular vitamin. Various other nutrients are known to play a role in relieving pain; these are the essential fatty acids from fats and natural cold-pressed oils, vitamins C, E and K and some of the B-complex vitamins, and D,L-Phenylalanine (DLPA), zinc, selenium and magnesium. If the body is subclinically deficient in certain combinations of vitamins and minerals, our responses to 'normal' pain could be heightened. By becoming optimally nourished we may be able to protect ourselves from the intensity of pain.

USE OF ANTI-INFLAMMATORY OILS OR FATTY ACIDS

Use of good quality natural oils may be a vital key to our disease. The choice of fats and oils used in cooking, for spreading and within pre-prepared foods, may have the most profound impact on our health and perception of pain. Most people know about saturated and polyunsaturated fats, but the key is the form in which they are found. Every cell membrane, all the steroid hormones and most brain cells depend upon oils (lipids) which our bodies process from the fatty foods we eat. In foods, oils can be found in two forms, cis oils and trans oils.

Cis fatty acids

In nature oil molecules are shaped rather like a horseshoe. This shape of molecule fits tightly with other phospholipids to form a strong cell membrane which protects the processes going on inside each cell. The membrane maintains the integrity of each cell and stops harmful chemicals from entering and damaging the powerhouses inside, which are working to produce proteins, prostaglandins, steroid hormones, enzymes and phospholipids. As these good quality cis oils make up almost one-third of brain tissue and every cell membrane, they are crucial to your state of health.

Your choice of these cis oils is therefore important. Look around your local healthfood shop for jars of extra virgin cold-pressed olive oils, organic butter and vegetable oils, such as sunflower, safflower and sesame, that are labelled 'unrefined', 'unhydrogenated' or 'cold-pressed'. Cold-pressed olive oil and butter are fine for light, shallow frying. For salad dressings use a mixture of extra virgin olive oil and some cold-pressed, unrefined walnut oil. Oils in tins are best, as light causes oil to go rancid. Fresh nuts and seeds are also an excellent source of cis oils. A handful of nuts and seeds or a tablespoon of cis oils each day will help to balance your intake of good quality oils. They aid thyroid function and your metabolism. Used in moderation they do not make you fat. However, if you have poor digestion (heartburn, constipation or diarrhoea) (*see* chapter 10) or a poor diet to start with so that you are unable to absorb enough of the nutrients needed to metabolize these essential fatty acids, then the digestion must be corrected and a digestive enzyme taken with each meal (*see* p. 194).

Trans fatty acids

Trans fatty acids are found when oils have been processed, hydrogenated or refined. They are often found in biscuits, cakes, pastries and margarines. Most vegetable oils on supermarket shelves have been processed, and so contain trans oils, which are implicated in breast cancer formation. Women with high levels of trans fatty acids in body cells have about a 40 per cent higher risk of getting breast cancer.[4, 5] When fats are processed, the molecule shape becomes more like a kink than a horseshoe. This fits loosely into the cell membrane, weakening it so that it is no longer effective at stopping harmful chemicals from entering the cell. This may damage the production of energy in the mitochondria and weaken defences against cancers. This may be why endometrial implants take hold.

Heat changes cis oils into trans oils, so deep frying is not advisable. You should avoid all oils which have been processed (hydrogenated), all oils which are rancid, and never use the same oil twice for frying. It is very important to read the label on oil jars and to buy only unhydrogenated, unrefined, cold-pressed oils. These are usually available only from your local healthfood store. It is in your best interest to avoid processed foods whenever possible, or to use convenience foods occasionally, but not every day. Being realistic, you will eat some trans fats, but try to keep them to a minimum.

Using and choosing good quality oils

There are three main fatty acids which the body uses:

- Linoleic acid – series 1 prostaglandins
- Arachidonic acid – series 2 prostaglandins
- Alpha-linolenic acid – series 3 prostaglandins.

Series 1 and 3 fatty acids have anti-inflammatory properties, and series 2 fatty acids can cause inflammation if not in balance with the other two. The body can make arachidonic acid from dairy products and the fat in meat, but it needs constant daily, fresh supplies of linoleic and alpha-linolenic acids from vegetable and fish oils as it cannot make series one and three vital fatty acids. If the daily diet is poor, the body supplies of these essential fatty acids will be extremely low.

Jane W J of Kent

I remember that the nutritional programme did make me feel much better. I still rely on the evening primrose oil. I really feel the difference in pain and PMT if I run out or forget to take it before a period. I take 1,000mg a day, upping it to 2,000mg a day in the immediate days before the period.

I conceived straightaway after the nutrition programme and, since then, my endometriosis has been in remission.

CASE STUDY

Essential fatty acids – the precursors to prostaglandins

Prostaglandins (PGs) are lipid (oil-based) hormones that have very important effects upon such body tissues as cell membranes in the reproductive system. The precursors to prostaglandins are the essential fatty acids (EFAs), arachidonic, linoleic acid and alpha-linolenic acid. Cis fatty acids should be the preferred source of oils in our diet.

The conversion of prostaglandins from EFAs depends upon enzymes, which are in turn nutrient dependent. If an excess of the wrong types of prostaglandins are produced by our tissues, this may lead to internal inflammation. Often the actions of one group of the PG system are in direct opposition to those of another.

There are three types of prostaglandins (*see* figures 4.3 and 4.4):

1 Series 1 prostaglandins are derived from vegetable oils and they have anti-inflammatory properties (linoleic acid).
2 Series 2 prostaglandins from dairy foods and fats within meat can cause inflammation to occur (arachidonic acid).
3 Series 3 prostaglandins are metabolized from fish and linseed oils and have anti-inflammatory properties (alpha-linolenic acid).

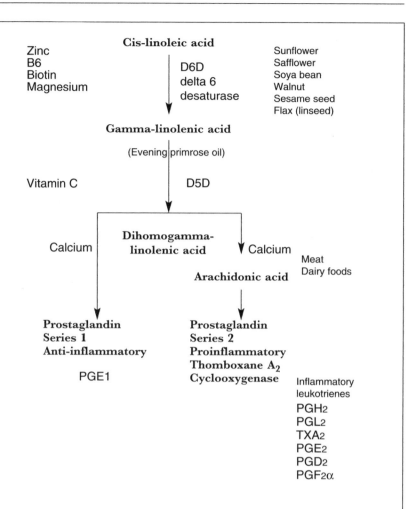

Figure 4.3
Metabolic pathway of the prostaglandin pathways for series 1 and series 2 prostaglandins.

Linoleic acid, which the body cannot make, comes from safflower, sunflower, hemp, soya bean, walnut, pumpkin seed, sesame seed and flax (linseed) oils. You need a fresh daily supply of this cold-pressed oil. Linoleic acid is the precursor of series 1 and series 2 prostaglandins. In your body, linoleic acid is changed, using nutrients, into gamma-linolenic acid (evening primrose oil). This is then changed again to dihomogamma-linolenic acid, which is the anti-inflammatory form, and also to arachidonic acid, which is proinflammatory. The vitamins and minerals which are required for their formation are listed.

The three different types of PGs need to be kept in balance (*see* figure 4.3), because they have a role in maintaining body homeostasis. (Homeo means same; stasis means standing still; homeostasis is the harmony within the body.) The body has an internal environment which has to be maintained within certain limits, for example, temperature control and the acid/alkaline balance, and it is constantly making adjustments to maintain this stable state. The body requires a rich mixture of gases, nutrients and water to control the temperature balance (here the thyroid gland in the neck is involved). It also needs fresh water to maintain health within cells. Health can deteriorate rapidly when this homeostatic balancing act is disturbed.

Thus, PGs possess both proinflammatory and anti-inflammatory properties. It has been suggested that more evidence 'appears to indicate that PGs from series 1 conceivably dominantly have an anti-inflammatory property, whereas the series 2 PGs may have mainly pro-inflammatory qualities depending on their local concentrations'.[6] Series 3 PGs are also anti-inflammatory. If you absorb enough linoleic and alpha-linolenic series 1 and 3 groups from good quality cis oils, you should be able to produce sufficient prostaglandin PGE1 which reduces the production of series 2 arachidonic acid (arachidonic triggers inflammation and pain in the body). Thus you can help to control internal inflammation just by eating the right sorts of oils. Evening primrose oil can be beneficial for some people; it tips the balance.

'Only the natural horseshoe shape cis form of linoleic and linolenic acids are able to contribute to the formation of PGs.'[7] Trans fatty acids which have been changed by chemical processing known as hydrogenation form a kink shape are not as effective in the formation of prostaglandins. Macrophages, often the predominant immune cells present during chronic inflammatory conditions, release PGs in response to inflammatory stimuli. In women with endometriosis the macrophage count is often higher than normal. If they release PGE2 more inflammation may occur (*see* chapter 9).

As an added bonus, PGE1 is able to stop blood cells becoming sticky; it can help to remove fluid from the body and can improve the functioning of nerves. It also has been shown to help immune cells in their work of clearing up cell debris in the abdominal cavity. These immune cells also need vitamin B6, iron and selenium.

Researchers think that an imbalance in the three different types of prostaglandins may be one of the causes of premenstrual syndrome and endometriosis pain. One piece of research shows that women with severe period pain, infertility and endometriosis had raised levels of prostaglandins series 2 (from arachidonic acid) in their peritoneal fluid, which could be the trigger for the inflammation.[8, 9] Therefore making the effort to ensure these oils are balanced in the diet is a good practical step to take.

Daily oil intake

How can you assess the daily intake of good quality oils in your diet and improve it where necessary? If your diet is very low in the oils from fresh nuts, seeds, good quality cold-pressed oils and oily fish, and very high in dairy foods and fatty meats, then the series 2 prostaglandins will outweigh those from series 1 and 3. The result may be internal inflammation and pain. A change in your eating pattern may be able to reduce this effect.

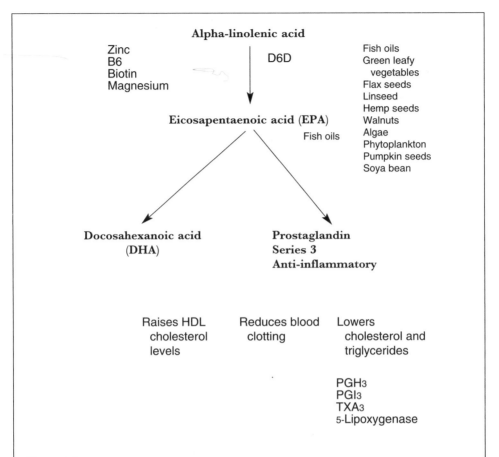

Figure 4.4
Metabolic pathway of the series 3 fatty acids down to prostaglandins.

Alpha-linolenic acid is found in flax seeds, hemp seeds, pumpkin seeds, dark-green leafy vegetables, soya bean, walnut and fish oils. The body cannot make this fatty acid so fresh supplies are required daily. Alpha-linolenic acid is the precursor of series 3 prostaglandins, which are anti-inflammatory. It is changed in the body to eicosapentaenoic acid (EPA). The enzymes require zinc, B6, magnesium and biotin to make series 3 prostaglandins. These are known to decrease blood pressure, reduce blood clotting, lower cholesterols and reduce internal inflammation. The vitamins and minerals involved in the process are listed.

Standard prostaglandin inhibitors (such as Ibroprufen) reduce all three types of prostaglandin, thus stopping the beneficial anti-inflammatory ones from working effectively.

Your body cannot take the steps to convert linoleic acid into gamma-linolenic acid (GLA) unless zinc, magnesium, vitamin B6, folic acid and biotin are absorbed from your diet. Vitamin C and calcium are then necessary for the final change into series 1 PGE1 and series 2 arachidonic acid. Evening primrose oil is very useful for some people as it bypasses the second stage of conversion, if the five nutrients are missing from the diet or being malabsorbed. Taken as a supplement, evening primrose oil can help to rebalance the three types of prostaglandins. The usual dose is four 500mg capsules per day. Too much stress, saturated animal fats, trans fatty acids and alcohol, can prevent the enzymes being able to change linoleic acid into a form the body can use to dampen down inflammation.

Practical steps you can take include:

1   Increase your intake of oily fish to twice a week.
2   Use one tablespoon of cis olive and walnut oils in, for example, salad dressing or soup once a day.
3   Reduce your intake of bovine dairy and red meat.

This helps to reduce the levels of arachidonic acid, which causes inflammation, while fish and nut/seed oils aid formation of the anti-inflammatory PGs. These good quality cis oils are essential in a well-balanced diet, and contrary to previous thought, they do not lead to an increase in weight. The fats which cause weight increase are the 'bad' saturated fats and trans fatty acids. The 'good' cis fatty acids aid body metabolism by supporting thyroid function. Researchers have observed that 'the more linoleic acid in the fat tissue, the less obese the person'.[10]

Barbara G of Essex

CASE STUDY

My endometriosis and period pains and periods in general are much better since being on a yeast-free diet and taking nutritional supplements, including GLA. I also eat oily fish (herring and mackerel), fresh 3–4 times each week. You can't beat fresh. Now I am recovered I will follow the same wholefood diet with a few extras such as a little bread. Efamol Marine has been extremely useful to me.

Fish oils

Fish oils are very important so long as they come from a reliable unpolluted source. Research on the effect of fish oils on endometriotic implants in rabbits with surgically induced endometriosis showed the sites of endometrial tissue shrank when the rabbits were fed fish oils: 'Proinflammatory prostaglandins in the peritoneal fluid were significantly lower in the fish oil group versus the controls. Total endometriotic implant diameter eight weeks after induction was significantly smaller in the experimental group versus the controls.'[11] The researchers concluded 'that dietary supplementation with fish oils can decrease the peritoneal proinflammatory prostaglandin production and retard implant growth in animal models'. Studies on the use of fish oils in women with severe period pains showed that the fish oils were effective at reducing pain. If you are vegetarian, you can use fresh edible food grade linseeds each day; grind and eat them with breakfast cereal.

The metabolism of essential fatty acids in the body to form anti-inflammatory prostaglandins is crucial. Essential cis fatty acids from both fish oils and unrefined, unhydrogenated cis vegetable oils are able to alleviate pain and inflammation in the peritoneal cavity and joints if taken for a sustained period at the right dose. People with arthritis or pelvic inflammatory disease can benefit from dietary supplementation with evening primrose oil, linseed oil (edible food grade), borage, starflower oil and fish oils. Always buy cold-pressed capsules from a reputable source. Some of the cheaper tablets can be ineffective and a waste of money.

Best quality oils to choose (all fresh cold-pressed)

Flax (linseed)	Pumpkin seeds	Soya beans
Fish	Walnuts	Seaweed
Sunflower seeds	Evening primrose oil	Sesame seeds
Almonds	Game birds	Hazelnuts
Cold-pressed oils in tins (e.g. extra virgin olive oil)		

Reasonable oils

Venison	Chicken	Mechanically
Eggs	Roasted fresh	cold-pressed oils
Organic butter in moderation	nuts and seeds	in glass bottles

Oils to use in very small amounts

Bottled hydrogenated vegetable oils	Dairy products	Pork
	Fried foods	Lamb
Beef	Hydrogenated margarine	
Butter		

Table 4.1
The quality of oils.
  Alcohol, sugars and refined starches all metabolize in the body to form fats which are stored in the body fat (adipose tissues). Fat cells produce oestrogen, which helps endometriosis to grow. Therefore, using only the good oils in moderation, and cutting out saturated and trans oils will help to control and normalize oestrogen production.

Jo R of Slough

Having suffered for years with extremely painful periods, mood swings, lethargy etc., I eventually sought complementary therapies. (After being diagnosed as having endo and being told that I needed a hysterectomy at 22 years of age.) Through cutting out all gluten foods, red meats and alcohol I found 110 per cent change for the better. Not only in my pain symptoms, but my monthly bleed would not be as heavy. My hair and nails became stronger and my overall health improved dramatically. Although I do feel the diet is difficult at times and slightly inconvenient, my whole attitude towards nutrition and health has changed. I think my mental health has improved too as I now feel stronger, more energetic and in control of my body. Thank you!

THE ROLE OF VITAMINS IN PAIN RELIEF

Vitamin C

Vitamin C, when combined with bioflavooids and digestive enzymes, has been shown in research to be more effective at reducing inflammation than non-steroidal anti-inflammatory drugs. An article about the research describes how 'Animal model trials looked at histamine-induced wheals in the peritoneal cavity. When given vitamin C, with bioflavooids and digestive enzymes they reduced the effect of the histamine. It was felt that this was due to the nutrients strengthening cells against agents which were causing the inflammation'.[12] Bioflavooids and vitamin C are known to have a beneficial effect upon immune cells. Vitamin C given to seriously ill cancer patients in a double blind controlled study showed that pain could be reduced significantly. Relief of pain using vitamin C has been shown in several other diseases. The way in which it works is not clear, but it may inhibit dopamine binding to membranes and inhibit prostaglandin levels. Low dietary levels of vitamin C in animal tests promoted the development of osteoarthritis. Relationships between vitamin E and vitamin C suggest that vitamin E may also be implicated in helping to reduce pain and inflammation. Together they thin blood, causing blood platelets to be less sticky. It has also been suggested that vitamin C 'has the property of a natural antihistamine and it reduces the severity of histamine attacks from internal inflammation, and may be able to detoxify excess histamine produced when the body is under stress'.[13]

Vitamin E

Vitamin E has an analgesic effect because it is able to inhibit pro-inflammatory prostaglandin production. In the 1970s research showed that '300 iu per day reduced muscle cramps and pains in the lower back'.[14] Studies also suggest that 'vitamin E has anti-inflammatory action as it protects lysosome membranes (internal cell particles which produce enzymes) from histamine and serotonin damage. It acts slowly to limit inflammation so needs to be taken regularly'.[15]

B-complex vitamins

Some vitamins are used alone, but often their synergy means that when they are combined they are more powerful. B-complex vitamins (B1, B6 and B12), when working together, have also been shown by research to exhibit an anti-inflammatory effect combined with an analgesic action: 'When vitamin B12 is taken with vitamin B1 and B6 they can together produce significant dose-dependent pain relief and inhibition of inflammation, comparable to the action of standard treatments in orthodox medicine, but without the side effects.'[16] Vitamin K seems to strengthen these effects; it has an anti-inflammatory and analgesic effect in animal models.

It is known from research that high doses of thiamin (vitamin B1) can suppress pain transmission, studies suggesting that there 'appears to be some relationship between thiamin and morphine'.[17] Vitamin B6 (pyridoxine) also has analgesic effects. If B6 is deficient, the amount of serotonin in the brain decreases and this can lead to depression. B6 helps to relieve the pain associated with premenstrual syndrome. It should always be taken with other B-complex vitamins as they work synergistically. The best absorbed form of vitamin B6 is pyridoxal-5-phosphate, which acts as a coenzyme in transforming tryptophan into serotonin. (Serotonin is a neurotransmitter which exists in high concentrations in the hypothalamus, a major gland in the reproductive system – people with insufficient levels show signs of depression.)

'Vitamin B12 was shown in three independent trials to have an analgesic effect when injected intramuscularly'[18] and when combined with vitamins B1 and B6, they produce an even stronger therapeutic anti-inflammatory and analgesic effect.

Tina R of Sussex

CASE STUDY

Before starting the nutritional programme I suffered with excruciating painful periods, back pain, heavy bleeding, bloating, extreme fatigue and mood swings. The pain could be described as worse than being in labour. Conventional drugs were unsuccessful. I have now been on the diet for three months. Almost immediately I felt an improvement in my health. As well as following a healthy diet I try to avoid wheat and dairy foods which I have discovered result in bloating and cause more pain. My last period was lighter and almost pain-free. I no longer suffer with bloating caused by allergies and intolerances. I have an increased level of energy and a feeling of well-being, and I now have a 'zest' for life and it feels great. My health is of paramount importance and I know I shall always have to take care. Nutritional support and advice has been invaluable.

MINERALS AGAINST PAIN

Magnesium

Magnesium is known to be necessary to the relaxation of muscles. It works to produce adenosine triphosphate (ATP), which produces energy in each cell. Without magnesium we would be plagued with cramps, spasms and convulsions. An adult needs 450–600mg of magnesium per day to maintain health. Magnesium plays a vital role in synthesizing myelin around the nerves, without which they become sensitive to pain. (Myelin is the protective fatty deposit which coats and protects nerves.) Magnesium also has an anaesthetizing effect on the central nervous system; therefore adequate magnesium 'is an important preventative against miscarriage and painful contractions of the uterus muscle'.[19] Magnesium malate is the best form to help with muscle relaxation and chronic fatigue; magnesium taurate is good for mental exhaustion and control of oestradiol; and magnesium EAP2 is beneficial for the heart. Different forms of magnesium are available in healthfood shops and by mail order.

Endometriotic implants, by their very nature, attach themselves to cell membranes on smooth muscle, thus affecting the way muscles relax and contract – endometriosis is a disease that has an effect on smooth muscle function. Little research has been done into this penetration into muscle fibres. However, research teams in Denmark and the Netherlands are preparing to look into this area. Muscle cramps cause some of the extreme pain of endometriosis.

Zinc

Zinc sulphate was given to 24 patients with rheumatoid arthritis in one trial in Washington University, USA. It is known from research that zinc has anti-inflammatory effects in the knee joint. An article reports: 'In a 12-week double blind trial using a placebo, patients taking zinc sulphate showed significant improvement for joint swelling and morning stiffness, and their personal impressions of their overall condition was high. Zinc is known to inhibit the immunologically induced histamine and leukotriene release from mast cells. Thus it can dampen down inflammation.'[20] The good cis oils require zinc for the body to metabolize them to form anti-inflammatory prostaglandins.

AMINO ACIDS

D,L-Phenylalanine (DLPA)

D,L-Phenylalanine (DLPA) has been well researched and its potential to reduce chronic pain is well documented. Its effects can last for months, even after treatment ceases. Some people experience a marked relief from pain in the first few days of taking it, but others find that it can take up to three weeks before chronic pain dies down. Phenylalanine is a naturally occurring amino acid. In nature this amino acid is found as the 'L' form, and the mirror-image 'D' form is man-made, and when both the natural and man-made forms are combined they can relieve pain. DLPA also acts as an anti-depressant and an appetite suppressant. It should not be taken as a occasional painkiller; it must be taken consistently over a period of time. DLPA works in 60 per cent of people. If it has had no effect after taking it for three weeks, then it is probably not going to work for you. But when it does work, the results can be excellent.

How does DLPA work? When we are injured, our brain begins to produce endorphins, hormones with properties that mimic those of the most powerful analgesic drugs. They are the body's own pain control system. For example, in people injured in road accidents, endorphins can prevent serious pain for several hours after the accident. DLPA works by reducing the levels of enzymes which normally break down endorphins, thus prolonging their effects in the body. The enzymes can also block the inflammatory effects of the proinflammatory prostaglandins.

Two DLPA tablets should be taken three times a day until the pain is reduced. The tablets can then gradually be reduced to a maintenance dose of one to two per day. The tablets should be taken 15 minutes before each meal if your blood pressure is normal (120/80mmHg or below), or 15 minutes after each meal if your blood pressure is high (140/90mmHg or above). Tablets are usually 375mg in strength combined with vitamins C and B6 to act in synergy. They are available on prescription from the NHS. Contraindications are pregnancy, breastfeeding, phenylketonuria, if you are taking monoamine oxidase (MAO) inhibitors as anti-depressants or if you suffer extreme hypertension (high blood pressure).

WHY DO NUTRIENTS HAVE THIS EFFECT UPON PAIN?

It is probable that nutrients activate certain enzymes and neurotransmitters involved with the perception of pain. Trying to achieve enzyme saturation point in all cells may be of benefit in promoting this anti-inflammatory and analgesic effect. (Saturation point occurs when the cells have the exact levels of vitamins, minerals and essential oils they need to work efficiently.) All enzymes use nutrients as co-factors in order to work effectively, so if the nutrient is in short supply, the pain control mechanism will not be able to work effectively.[21]

Vitamins can be seen as keys to metabolic pathways. The gate to each pathway within the body is shut unless that specific vitamin comes along with its key. All the enzyme and hormone reactions on the other side of the gate cannot take place unless that vitamin is present. If you eat well and your digestive system is able to absorb properly, you remain healthy. But if you 'snatch and grab' meals of dubious quality foodstuffs or you have a poor digestive system, then you may require supplementary nutrients to help you in the short term while your diet, digestion and absorption are improved.

USING NUTRIENTS TO CONTROL PAIN

Helena G of London

I would like to thank you for all your help. I have been keeping to my diet and taking the vitamins and minerals you prescribed for me. I must admit that I was sceptical at first about this kind of treatment, although I felt that it was worth a try since the treatment at hospital had not helped me at all. The diet did, however. It made me feel

CASE STUDY

more positive as I felt that I had some kind of control over my health. Then, following the treatment for just over a month, I began to see a vast improvement. I felt more energetic and suffered less pain. Gradually over the second month I felt better than I had in years. Not only had the pain decreased greatly and the stomach upsets ceased, but I had greater concentration and did not feel as weak. My relationship with my family and friends, and especially my husband, has improved as I am no longer as quick-tempered, irritable and depressed as I had been. Also since following your treatment, I have not had to take any time off work, and have found it easier to deal with the stress of my job. I was sure that I would lose my job. Thank you.

Research into other conditions shows poor nutrition plays an important role in the development of other diseases and the sensible choice of good quality food could pay you dividends.[22] We are all biochemically unique, therefore it is important for the individual to understand that what helps one person may not work in the same way for another. It has to be a trial and error approach. There are many treatments, orthodox and complementary, which others have found helpful. In chapter 11 (p. 255), we will look at which supplements can be taken safely and why they may be required. In chapters 11, 12 and 14, we will discuss the type of healthy eating programme you could follow and which foodstuffs you should eat regularly.

SUPPLEMENT PROGRAMME TO COMBAT PAIN

We have seen how important individual nutrients are in controlling degrees of pain within the body; how essential fatty acids can reduce inflammation and how vitamin C reduces histamine release. By maintaining a steady supply of good nutrients from food the body should be able to mute pain responses. Supplements may assist for a time to improve the body's fortitude. A selection of the following nutrients may help the body to cope with pain (*see* p. 255):

- Multivitamin/mineral
- D,L-Phenylalanine (DLPA)
- Essential fatty acids: omega-3 fish oils; omega-6 evening primrose oils (200mg per day)
- Magnesium malate
- Zinc citrate or amino acid chelate
- Selenium (non-yeast form)
- Vitamins A, C, E (antioxidants)
- Vitamins B1, B6, B12 (non-yeast form)
- Vitamin C with bioflavonoids and protein-digesting enzymes
- Proanthacyanadins
- Quercetin
- Resveratrol

SUMMARY

1 Regardless of what anyone tells you, the pain from endometriosis is REAL. Get your pain taken seriously. Try to reduce the pain symptoms through nutrition and use any method which helps to distract you whenever possible.

2 Photocopy and fill in the pain charts from Arnold Kresch and use them to teach your GP the extent of this very real pain. You can also chart your pain (*see* pp. 348–9) and see how it changes over time.

3 Take painkillers early on to reduce pain. Once it takes hold it is much harder to control.

4 Exercising at a level with which you can cope helps to increase endorphin levels in the brain. These are the body's natural painkillers. Do exercise such as gentle walks or pleasurable swims when you feel able, to build up endorphin levels.

5 Use relaxation and visualization techniques to aid your control of pain. Whatever works for you as an individual is the most important route to take. Feel comfortable about the techniques you try. If they feel wrong, stop using them.

6 Ask your GP or hospital for a TENS machine to try out.

7 Stay positive. You are going to beat this. At times when pain is overwhelming, this can feel nigh on impossible. Being positive helps to strengthen your immune cells to fight the endometriosis, which is essentially what is needed.

8 Let the time when you are incapacitated work for you. Use hobbies and skills you have acquired; you may be able to develop another career direction. Nurture your true friends. 'A faithful friend is the medicine of life' – *Apocrypha* 6:16.

9 Vitamins and minerals possess some analgesic and anti-inflammatory properties which may help combat pain. If you are very ill the effort of preparing and cooking food is almost impossible, but try to eat fresh nutritious food. As you begin to absorb the vitamins and minerals, the body can work more effectively to combat pain.

10 Vitamins C, E, K, A and B-complex, the minerals selenium, zinc and magnesium, amino acids and D,L-Phenylalanine, and evening primrose and fish oils all aid in the suppression of pain. Proanthacyanadins, found in blue and red berries, have strong anti-inflammatory and diuretic properties. Ensure that you are eating and digesting these nutrients and phytochemicals from foods in your diet. Remember that correcting the digestive tract is the first step. Consult a nutritionist for individualized advice.

5 Why is my fertility threatened?

All truth passes through three stages: First, it is ridiculed,
Second, it is opposed,
Third, it is accepted as being self-evident.

Arthur Schopenhauer, Philosopher

Everything you take for granted today was once revolutionary.

Professor John Crispo

How many infertile couples do you know? One? Maybe two? The rate of subfertility among couples of reproductive age in England and the USA is an amazing 15 to 20 per cent, about 1 in every five couples.[1] More than 2.4 million people in America alone have been robbed of the opportunity to conceive and have a family. It has been estimated that 30 per cent of subfertile couples may be infertile as a result of endometriosis.[2] One in 15 men and one in 10 women are thought to be struggling with their fertility – you are not alone.

Infertility is defined as lack of conception after at least 12 months of unprotected intercourse. This means that some couples may take up to two years to achieve a pregnancy, if 12 months is the mean. Infertility is a major health issue, often due to an illness, yet it receives very little attention from our society or from Parliament and Congress.

However, 65 per cent of these subfertile couples may be helped by drugs and surgery to achieve a pregnancy. By following the correct nutritional advice, the rate of success may be increased to 86 per cent, as shown by data from Foresight – the charity for preconceptual care.[3] Thus, help is available for the couple struggling with their fertility. By combining good nutrition and conventional medicine endometriosis patients enhance their ability to conceive. Everything that we put into our bodies has health consequences. Poor nutrition has detrimental effects on endocrine and reproductive functioning.

Endometriosis is a complex disease that appears to have several different mechanisms through which it may trigger subfertility. It is not clear if one or more of these mechanisms is the cause of the subfertility associated with endometriosis, but endometriotic implants have several different effects on the reproductive system.

In medical schools, few doctors are taught about nutrition, body biochemistry and metabolic pathways. If they were to spend time studying subjects other than physiology, anatomy and pharmacology, they would fail their board examinations.

What we need here is integrative medicine – medicine that merges the benefits of all approaches to healing patients. We must begin to heal the patient from within and offer the best from all Eastern and Western medical approaches. We need to make a paradigm shift to impartial evidence-based medicine.

ABDOMINAL ADHESIONS AND SUBFERTILITY

As the endometriotic implants grow and develop in the abdomen, where they do not belong, the body tries to surround them with fibrous connective tissue (scar tissue). The body does this in an attempt to isolate the implants and prevent them from doing harm by putting up a protective barrier. Adhesions can also be formed during surgery when abdominal tissue is traumatized. This fibrous tissue develops like moss growing on a stone and behaves like a Band-Aid on a wound. They solidify and thicken over time, and have the effect of making the implants stick to adjacent tissues.

Remember that blood is sticky and internal bleeding from the implant also forms adhesions, such that an implant may be stuck to several different tissues like a cat's cradle, as if we placed some very sticky glue-like gum in the abdomen and several organs became stuck to each other by the very sticky strands. For example, an endometriotic implant on the top of the uterus may cause the ovary and small intestine to become attached at the site of the implant. If the adhesions pinch off the Fallopian tube or if they cause a blockage of the opening of the Fallopian tube, they could obstruct the union of egg and sperm and prevent fertilization and conception, or cause an ectopic pregnancy, if the embryo can't travel to the womb. This type of obstruction can be easily diagnosed and surgically corrected.

However, this does not explain how patients with just a few implants and no adhesions can become infertile. Adhesions can also cause pain, as internal organs which normally slip and slide become firmly glued together. For example, if the bowel is stuck to a tender, painful ovary, flatulence could cause pain, and sexual activity may be uncomfortable due to constriction of movement. Operations, by their very nature, may trigger more adhesions to form even as others are removed – catch 22.

SECRETIONS FROM ENDOMETRIOTIC IMPLANTS

As we have already seen, the endometrium within the womb is a dynamic tissue that secretes a wide variety of nutrients and hormones required for normal conception. The endometriotic implants also secrete these same substances, but instead of depositing them into the lumen (centre) of the womb as normal, the implants release their chemical secretions into the abdominal cavity. Some of these substances, which are in effect strong hormones, could interfere with fertility. Recent studies suggest that endometriotic implants also produce cytokines.[4] These inflammatory immune cells are in the peritoneal fluid and, in patients with endometriosis, this fluid has been shown to be toxic to the preimplantation embryo. It also contains macrophages and growth factors.

PROSTAGLANDINS

One major group of hormones secreted by the normal endometrium is the prostaglandins. These are oil-based hormones found in nearly all the tissues of the body and are required for many bodily processes, including several stages of the menstrual cycle and pregnancy. Prostaglandins are required for ovulation, regression of the corpus luteum (ending the monthly menstrual cycle), sperm motility, immune interactions, contraction of the uterus at birth and menstrual cramps. Endometriotic implants and the endometrium of the uterus are the richest source of prostaglandin production in the body.

However, the problem with endometriotic implants is two-fold:

1   Prostaglandins are released into the abdomen instead of inside the womb.
2   Prostaglandin release by the implants seems to be out of phase with their release by the uterus. Prostaglandins are produced at the wrong time sending the wrong message.

For instance, there is a natural surge in prostaglandin F production at the end of the menstrual cycle, causing the effects of the corpus luteum of the ovary to die down and signalling the start of a new menstrual cycle. The endometriotic implants produce their prostaglandin surge several days after that of the womb lining. This may be one of the main causes of very early miscarriage. Approximately 31 per cent of biochemically detected pregnancies fail to atain viability; of these, 50 per cent are lost prior to the first missed period due to defective implantation. The majority (60 per cent) of lost pregnancies are due to chromosomal aberrations.[5] If a woman is a few days pregnant then the implant-produced prostaglandin F would wrongly tell the ovary to start a new menstrual cycle, causing the womb lining with the implanted egg to be sloughed off – an early miscarriage. Prostaglandins are messengers and like all messengers they sometimes get it wrong.[6]

Prostaglandins also play an important role in the contractions of the womb and Fallopian tubes. During the normal menstrual cycle the gentle contractions of the womb and Fallopian tubes aid the movement of egg and sperm to the outer third of the Fallopian tube where fertilization occurs. High concentrations of endometriotic implant prostaglandins at the wrong time could interfere with this and may prevent fertilization. An excess of PGF2 and PGE2 could cause contractions that are too strong and expel the egg too quickly. Series 2 prostaglandins are produced from the fats in dairy and meat products, and it is recommended that intake of these foods be kept to a minimum.

Series 2 prostaglandins are also responsible for the contractions of the uterus at the end of pregnancy, stimulating the powerful uterine muscle contractions required for the birthing process. Inappropriate concentrations of implant-produced prostaglandins could stimulate forceful uterine contractions (cramps) at the time of embryo implantation and lead to early expulsion of the embryo.[7] Indeed, in both humans and domestic animals, prostaglandin F is used clinically to induce abortion or to hasten the birthing process.

Series 1 and 3 prostaglandins, enhance the immune response and, as we will discuss in chapter 9, they may even modify normal immune interactions that could prevent conception. Prostaglandins also stimulate sperm motility, and high levels of proinflammatory series 2 prostaglandins could lead to early 'burn-out' of the sperm, preventing fertilization.[8]

Although prostaglandin secretion into the peritoneal cavity is required for the reproductive process, it is clear that too much of the wrong type of prostaglandin in the wrong place, or prostaglandin production at the wrong time, could easily interfere with fertility. Exactly how or even whether prostaglandins play a role in the infertility associated with endometriosis is not known, but they do seem to be involved.

PROTEIN PRODUCTION

The endometrium of the uterus and endometriotic implants have 'a prolific ability to produce hundreds of different types of proteins'.[9] Although the roles of all these proteins are not known, some of them are used by the body as nutrition for the developing embryo, and some function as hormones or trigger hormone release.

Various laboratory studies have shown that most of these proteins are produced by both implants and womb endometrium. However, two proteins have been discovered that are produced only by the endometriotic implants[10] – Endo I and Endo II. These two unique proteins may interfere with fertility. It is also possible that proteins that are common to both the uterus and implants, like prostaglandins, may be inappropriately produced by endometriotic implants, and have a bad effect on the reproductive system. These proteins may interfere with immune system surveillance so that implants are not removed by normal macrophages and natural killer cells. Isolated endometriosis stroma cells secrete more sICAM-1 than normal endometrium.[11]

ABNORMAL OVULATION

The monthly maturation of eggs and the process of ovulation may be altered in the patient with endometriosis: 'Women with endometriosis have been shown to have smaller, but many more, follicles maturing at the time of ovulation than controls'.[12] This suggests that the chemical secretions from endometriotic implants hamper the ability of the ovary to respond correctly to the message from the pituitary hormones, or that hormones secreted by the ovary do not give the correct message to the pituitary gland. Indeed, high prolactin levels are known to inhibit ovulation.

Under the influence of the pituitary luteinizing hormone, the follicular wall of the ovary close to the Fallopian tube thins and ruptures, releasing the ova. Endometriosis may prevent the completion of this ovulatory process. This inability to ovulate is called 'luteinized unruptured follicle syndrome' (LUF). In LUF syndrome, women have the normal sequence of endocrine events and a normal menstrual period, but their ovaries do not release any eggs at the time of ovulation.

This syndrome is difficult to diagnose since, from all external measurements (hormone concentrations and menstrual flow), nothing appears to be wrong. As the egg is but a single cell and the ovary wall repairs itself almost immediately after ovulation, the absence of ovulation usually goes unnoticed. However, some researchers have tried meticulously to check for ovulation with laparoscopic examination of the ovary at the presumed time of ovulation.[13] They found that the incidence of signs of ovulation was lower in endometriosis patients than in fertile control patients.

The precise means by which endometriotic implants adversely affect the development of the egg within the ovary is not yet known, but it is suggested that implant secretions, such as prostaglandins and excess natural oestrogens, or even oestrogens from outside the body (xeno-oestrogens), are damaging to conception. Non-steroidal anti-inflammatory drugs give rise to LUF, research has shown. In women with LUF syndrome, steroid hormone concentrations in the peritoneal fluid are much lower after the ovulatory cycle. It is felt that this may facilitate the development of endometriosis.[14]

IMPAIRED FERTILIZATION

In addition to an alteration in follicular development and ovulation, the actual quality of the eggs in women with endometriosis may be different. Various *in vitro* fertilization (IVF) programmes have observed that the presence of endometriosis in the abdomen, and especially in the ovary, adversely affects the appearance of the egg and decreases its ability to fertilize.

Normally the eggs have a yellowish appearance with a smooth oatmeal texture. The eggs of the endometriosis patient are sometimes dark brown in colour and have a granular texture. In 1985 Wardle noted that the fertilization rate of eggs from endometriosis patients was significantly lower than in patients who had unexplained infertility or blocked Fallopian tubes.[15] Again, this could be explained by the chemical secretions from the endometriotic implants which surround the ovary. Certainly it would seem that, from observation, women who have ovarian cysts should have them removed before undergoing ART (assisted reproductive technology). The quality of the ova is poor if 'chocolate' cysts are present and improves after they have been removed. More research is needed to look at this phenomenon. But it implies that women with endometriosis stand a better chance with ART techniques when their health has been improved.

Also, at the stage of conception, it is vital that the immune system does not react to the presence of the blastocyst. Normally, increased levels of progesterone from the corpus luteum quieten the immune system. Sperm appear in the Fallopian tubes 5–10 minutes after coitus, although some may take 48 hours. An organ on the head of the sperm releases enzymes which penetrate the ovum. If the woman's immune system is overactive at this time, both the sperm and blastocyst could be harmed.[16]

EARLY MISCARRIAGE

The most common time for a miscarriage to occur is during the first three months (trimester) of pregnancy. At this time, the embryo is developing into a fetus and is undergoing truly amazing and dramatic changes, including the formation of most of its internal organs. This is a critical period of development that requires an appropriate nutrient-rich environment, a healthy placenta and a very delicate balance between the various hormones of pregnancy. It has been suggested that women with endometriosis have a greater chance of miscarriage than women with other types of reproductive dysfunction: 'Miscarriage rates as high as 46 per cent have been reported in the scientific literature'.[17] This area is currently being examined by other researchers who have not seen as dramatic an increase in the miscarriage rate of endometriosis patients.[18] A high miscarriage rate among women with endometriosis would offer another explanation for endometriosis-associated subfertility.

Human reproduction is inefficient, with an estimated 50 per cent of conceptions failing, and 10–12 per cent of pregnancies ending within 12–14 weeks after the last menses. Many are associated with antiphospholipid antibodies, placental insufficiency, impaired fetal growth or fetal distress.[19]

However, the real enigma of a first trimester miscarriage is that if it occurs during the first six weeks of the pregnancy, there is a good chance that you may not even be aware that you are pregnant. You may think your period is late. It is very difficult to determine pregnancy rates in normal healthy women and in endometriosis patients. In fact, this lack of pregnancy information is one of the main reasons for the confusion in the scientific literature.

Regardless of whether or not there is a high miscarriage rate in endometriosis patients, it is imperative that you eat the right sort of nutrient-rich foods to try to ensure the maintenance of your pregnancy. Nutrition in both parents even before pregnancy has a profound effect on the state of the egg and sperm, as well as on the nature of the secretions within the peritoneal cavity. Your choice of foods, particularly fats and oils, may be a crucial factor as these affect the production of prostaglandins, cell membranes, steroid hormones, and neurotransmitters etc. (*see* chapter 4).

Thus, there are many reproductive problems associated with endometriosis, and scientific investigations have yet to determine exactly how endometriosis causes infertility. However, 40–60 per cent of women with endometriosis do appear to become pregnant. There are many positive ways that we can successfully attempt to correct the problem of infertility.

FERTILITY AND THE ALERT IMMUNE SYSTEM

'The leading question we should be asking here is whether or not the presence of antibodies can cause infertility and early miscarriage, by interfering with implantation.'[20] Reproductive tissues contain large numbers of immune cells and produce large amounts of cytokines, which are implicated in the fertilization process. Chapter 9 explains this in more detail.

To achieve pregnancy, sperm has to enter the body. The sperm can be judged as 'alien' by a woman's immune cells, because it is 'non-self'. If pregnancy is achieved, the woman's immune system has to adapt to the presence of 'alien' tissues growing inside her for nine months. However, there must be some mechanism which tells the female immune system that this alien tissue is not a danger to avoid damage to the embryo. Perhaps when the immune system is malfunctioning in endometriosis, this mechanism fails and causes an immune attack on the embryo and sperm, thus leading to infertility. Correcting or strengthening the immune system may help to achieve fertility. Healthy ovaries which produce the right amounts of progesterone are crucial in this process as progesterone dampens down a woman's immune system.

Scientists at University College London have discovered a protein (iscollin) inside sperm which is released as egg and sperm fuse, and starts a chain reaction that causes the embryo to form. Chemical interactions trigger calcium deposits inside the egg to vibrate and begin the cell-splitting process that leads to formation of the embryo. Defective sperm or eggs could not begin this chain reaction. This exciting area may lead to more research into egg quality in women with endometriosis.[21]

YOUR FERTILITY: NUTRITIONAL EFFECTS

Healthy parents usually have healthy babies. Once conception has happened, there is no changing what will be. We think of conception as the beginning of life, the time when sperm and egg collide and the magic of life begins. However, the egg and the sperm are not made in an instant; the parents' bodies have been working hard to prepare them for the previous three months. Women are born with all their eggs ready and waiting inside their ovaries (*see* p. 11). At birth, female babies have around one million eggs, but by puberty, only about 400,000 are still viable. Each month, five to ten eggs begin to ripen, but only two or three fully mature. Over the normal 28-day menstrual cycle, the mature eggs 'pop' out at ovulation and are sucked up by the Fallopian tubes to begin their journey to reach a healthy sperm. The ripening of the egg is supported by the mother-to-be eating a diet rich in essential nutrients.

Many ethnic groups have a period of time when a new bride is well fed before becoming pregnant; an early study on nutrition mentions how 'the Masai tribe had specific times for marriage to ensure that the bride had a few months on a nutritious diet'.[22] Even Queen Esther in the Bible had a special diet for a year before her wedding.[23] Leah became pregnant after eating mandrakes, which were believed to promote fertility.[24] In the book of Judges, an angel gave preconceptual advice to Samson's mother: 'Take care not to drink any wine or beer, or eat any forbidden food'.[25]

If the mother has a poor diet, consisting of highly refined foods, containing excessive sugar, fat and processed carbohydrates, the amount of nutrients available to the developing egg, or embryo, will be low. Poor nutrition at this time may lead to miscarriage.

Think of the womb lining as a nest. Birds build their nests to keep their young safe and warm; a place where they can be nurtured, fed and watered. A woman's womb plays a similar role. Each month the womb lining develops a lush, nutrient-rich, blood-engorged tissue; the womb is ready to receive the embryo and build a healthy placenta to supply all the nutrients the embryo needs to grow strong and healthy. If the mother's diet that month is poor, the womb lining will be poor, and a weak placenta is less likely to sustain an embryo. So the eggs and womb lining are both dependent upon a good diet.

Successful implantation depends upon a complex two-way 'conversation' between the blastocyst and the endometrium, which enables the embryo to implant at a site that is receptive. The nutrition producing hormonal balance, sperm and ova maturation, and a receptive endometrium, all at the same time, needs to be sound to achieve a pregnancy.

Wendy M of London

Years of undiagnosed endometriosis had led to the removal of a large ovarian cyst. Conventional treatments for the endometriosis and infertility had been to no avail. A visit to the nutritionist meant a substantial change to my diet and some vitamin supplements were taken. Within a few months period pains and bloating were less severe, PMS had virtually gone and I became pregnant. Yippee!

CASE STUDY

WHY IT TAKES 12 MONTHS TO MAKE A BABY

We have touched upon the nutritional needs of the mother, but what of the man, the father? He is not going to nurture the baby inside his body, but the health of his sperm is also dependent upon his diet for the three months before conception. That is how long it takes the testes to make healthy sperm. Too much alcohol, cigarettes and drugs, working with certain harmful chemicals, eating too many processed foods and too few vegetables and fruits may lead to sad-looking and possibly defective sperm. A low sperm count may be due to environmental factors, such as oestrogenic pesticides, but a poor diet will also lead to weakened or deformed sperm.

Research has shown that some chemicals can cause mutations to the sperm. Instead of the head of the sperm being oval, it can be too large or too small, or become pear-shaped, and these changes also cause chromosomal abnormality. Moreover, 'it takes 120 days for sperm production to recover after exposure to chemicals'.[26]

Putting a sorry-looking sperm into a starving egg and implanting the resulting embryo into a sick womb is a recipe for disaster. In the UK about 750,000 babies are born each year, but more than 40,000 are born early and are too small. One in 150 babies is lost through stillbirth, and one in four pregnancies ends in miscarriage, up to 60 per cent of which are due to defective sperm.[27] Every miscarriage is a bereavement, the loss of a loved one. It is a very unhappy and traumatizing experience for everyone involved. Time can heal the grief, but there is always a part of the sad experience which lingers on.

For a healthy pregnancy, a healthy diet and digestive system are essential. Your diet counts for both the potential mother and father. Let that be the message to remember. Healthy babies are what everyone wants most of all. All children deserve the best start in life and, by eating nutritious food for at least three months before you contemplate becoming pregnant, you are making a commitment to improve the health of your future child.

Mary F of Chicago

•
C
A
S
E

S
T
U
D
Y
•

I cannot for the life of me remember exactly what nutritional measures I made and what supplements I took (outside of evening primrose oil) when I was trying to conceive; it was three years ago. I wish I could be of more help because you certainly helped me! All I can tell you is that I believe that the nutritional measures you suggested played an integral role in my conceiving my second child.

I did have surgery for my endometriosis, but very little was found. After being on your suggested regime for three months, I conceived naturally and eventually bore a beautiful daughter. I only wish I had known more about nutrition and the role it plays in endometriosis when I was trying to conceive for the first time. I'd had a wonderful son, but not until I had taken an ART hormone therapy, which I would have liked to have avoided. You enabled my husband and me to complete the perfect family we always dreamed of having.

NUTRITION COUNSELLING

In 1971 Agnes Higgins described the Montreal Diet Dispensary Study: 'Twenty-three years ago, we were impressed by the research findings concerning the relation between maternal nutrition and birth weight, infant mortality and morbidity. Accordingly we decided to develop, for disadvantaged pregnant women, a nutrition counselling method that would compensate for individual differences in income, nutrition, weight, and special conditions of stress, with a view to improving the weight and condition of the newborn'.[28] Why then, so many years later, are we still debating the same point and not putting it into action?

Foresight (The Charity for Preconceptual Care of Great Britain), has looked at research by Dr Weston Price, Dr Francis Pottenger and Sir Robert McCarrison into the influence of sound nutrition on health.[29, 30, 31] Their conclusions are that the quality of the food you eat confers good health. Healthy food emanates from healthy soil and good farming principles. Dr Roger Williams also points out that we are all biochemically different and that individuals' requirements for recommended daily amounts of nutrients may differ due to their unique body biochemistry.[32] A recent study noted that 'in pregnancy it is known that nutrient requirements alter. Women on good diets are seen to have healthier babies than those on poor diets'.[33]

In the UK, Foresight has reported pregnancy outcomes for 367 couples who, from 1990 to 1992, followed their suggested nutrition programme. The average ages were 34 for women (22–45 years) and 36 for men (25–59 years). Fifty-nine per cent of the couples had a previous history of reproductive problems; 37 per cent had suffered from infertility for between one and 10 years; 38 per cent had had between one and five miscarriages; 3 per cent had given birth to a stillborn child. Of the children born, 40 were small for dates, 15 were of low birth weight, and seven were malformed. Forty-two per cent of the men had reduced sperm quality.

After both partners followed the Foresight nutrition programme, an astounding 86 per cent of the women had become pregnant by 1993, and 327 children had been born (137 males and 190 females), all of them healthy at birth. Birth occurred at a mean of 38.5 weeks of gestation and the average birth weight was 3,265gm (7lb 3oz). None of the infants was malformed and none had to go into special-care baby units.[34] This shows what can be achieved by dietary changes and by addressing genitourinary infections (such as chlamydia) which may be preventing conception. The programme involves no drugs and no expense save that of buying good food, and requires minimal guidance.

REPRODUCTIVE SYSTEM SUSCEPTIBILITY TO VITAMIN B-COMPLEX

The hypothalamic–pituitary–gonadal axis is highly sensitive to the intake of the B vitamins (*see* figure 2.1). This axis is the main highway along which the hormones (chemical messengers) travel. The vital hormone messages which pass from one end of the highway to the other must be correct. As a recent study explains: 'Low intake of B vitamins depresses gonadotrophin releasing hormone (GnRH) secretion from the hypothalamus and thereby affects the development of the eggs and sperm in the gonads (ovary and testicles).'[35] Moreover, as another source elaborates: 'Low intake of B vitamins may also slow down the ripening of the egg before conception and be affecting fertility. The hypothalamus in other mammals reacts to a severe deficiency of any of these B vitamins (particularly riboflavin [B2]) by inhibiting GnRH secretion and so causing infertility.'[36]

The liver has an important role in maintaining the body's oestrogen level within a normal range, and B vitamin deficiency may impair the liver's oestrogen-inactivating capacity. A healthy liver is vital for normal hormone balance.[37]

Many people eat a diet of overrefined foods. Convenience foods are low in essential nutrients, such as magnesium, zinc, selenium and iodine, which are removed during the food-processing techniques. Fresh, unrefined foods are always the most nutritious.

FEMALE ENDOCRINE HEALTH

The length and frequency of the menstrual cycle is an important biological marker when looking for toxic chemical effects on reproduction, but these effects are difficult to distinguish from the effects of poor nutrient intake. As a published report explains, 'The highest susceptibility to nutrient deficiency in the female ovary is during ovulatory maturation and embryonic development; the first 30 days after conception are crucial'. The research indicates that 'a 70-fold increase in sensitivity in the ovary (to nutrient deficiency) occurs between 11.30 a.m. and 7 p.m. on the day preceding ovulation. It is therefore calculated that the period of highest susceptibility could be as long as 60 hours prior to ovulation'.[38] This suggests that women should eat a healthy diet and reduce toxic overload at least one month before attempting to conceive, as should men. A recent study explains: 'Most of the defects in ova leading to miscarriage are already present in the embryo immediately after fertilization, and they have their origin in male and female ova and sperm before fertilization'.[39] This implies that the couple should both make sensible lifestyle changes for up to three months before trying to conceive to enhance their chances of achieving a successful pregnancy. The same study notes: 'The ova lie dormant from 15 to 45 years in a mother's ovaries until their turn comes to ripen, and when the dormant chromosomes are tightly packed and apparently very resistant to any external influence'.[40] Keeping chemical exposure to a minimum would seem to be advisable. If you or your partner work with or near strong chemicals, take the recommended precautions. The one-month period of ripening in the follicle before ovulation is the susceptible time-frame.

The future reproductive potential of the developing fetus can also be affected by your nutrition, and exposure to harmful chemicals before and during pregnancy. So avoid exposure to anything harmful; perfumes, bactericides, pesticides, petroleum, phthalates, household cleaning materials, paint strippers and some food additives – these could affect the health of your children and grandchildren. These chemicals may have a detrimental effect on the immune system. Use more eco-friendly products or non-biological versions of these products.

The Dietary and Nutritional Survey of British Adults in 1990 used a category of persons – eating affected by being unwell, which involved 9.5 per cent of women in the survey, aged from 16 to 64 years. Calorie intake in this category was some 18 per cent below average, with nutrient intake similarly reduced. The survey concluded: 'Ten per cent of women may not be eating well enough to sustain a pregnancy'.[41]

When recovering from amenorrhoea (cessation of periods due to poor nutrient intake), there are menstrual cycles that are too long and luteal phases that are too short. Research at the University of Sydney suggested 'a recovery period of at least six months from amenorrhoea before attempting a conception'.[42] This allows all the body systems to recover sufficiently from the lack of nutrients. It takes the individual cells some time to regain their full capacity and be able to work at what is known as 'enzyme saturation level', when all the enzymes are working at their optimum rate.

Research into restricted calorie intake has been done on monkeys at the University of Pittsburgh, and it was discovered that 'fasting for one day alone can change the hormone profile the following night'; moreover, 'missing a single meal could override the suppression of luteinizing hormone (LH)' ... 'The implication for slimmers is that even short-term deficiency can have a profound effect on endocrine function.'[43] Other studies offer similar conclusions, suggesting that 'restrained eating may be a marker for metabolic and emotional disturbances, and may also be associated with biological consequences, as the LH should take a message from the pituitary to the ovary. If suppressed, no message would be sent. Women with abnormal menstrual cycles experienced ovulatory disturbances including low progesterone and short luteal cycles'.[44, 45, 46] If you are restricting nutrient intake in order to lose weight, you may be damaging your chances of becoming pregnant.

BODY MASS INDEX

A body mass index (BMI) measure shows that women's weight:height ratio is a rough indicator of nutritional status. The body mass index chart has been designed as a result of feasibility testing. Low pre-pregnancy weight is a risk factor, with the risk increasing as the BMI falls below $24kg/m^2$. American data shows that 50 per cent of infertile women are below 20.7kg m^2. In a Hackney hospital study the mothers of the healthy weight babies had a BMI, on average, of $23.7kg/m^2$. A tool for determining BMI is based upon:

- Low BMI or underweight is $< 19.8kg/m^2$
- Normal BMI is $19.8–26.0kg/m^2$
- High BMI or overweight is $26.1–29.0kg/m^2$
- Obese is $> 29.0kg/m^2$

The BMI is a good general guide to fertility. Indeed, nearly 80 per cent of infertile women have been judged to be underweight.[47]

To work out your BMI:

$$BMI = \text{weight in kilogrammes} \div \text{height in metres squared}$$

So if you weigh 52.5kg and are 1.52m tall, your BMI will be $22.7kg/m^2$ which is just below the optimum range.

$$BMI = 52.5 \div (1.52 \times 1.52) = 22.7$$

In animal husbandry, it is well known that animals conceive on a rising body weight, not when weight is falling. All animals have a fertility threshold and in farming there still exists the practice called 'flushing': 'The practice of giving ewes which are in fairly poor condition an improved diet for a few weeks before mating so that they are in a rapidly rising condition when they meet the ram. Flushing is not fattening up; it means supplying all the essential nutrients to make the hypothalamus and pituitary gland (and ovaries) provide an excellent hormone profile'.[48] Dieting is a common cause of infertility. If the BMI is above 30, then fertility may be compromised. However, you need to lose weight first and then try to become pregnant when the BMI is around 23 to 28.

Claire C of London

In early 1996 I experienced dreadful pain on the left side of my stomach, which got worse midcycle and premenstrually, and I experienced some discomfort on intercourse. In March of that year, I was diagnosed as having pelvic inflammatory disease and was treated with antibiotics. The pain continued, but my husband and I were delighted to discover in September 1996 that I was pregnant. I suffered a miscarriage at 14 weeks in December that year, and after I had got over the immediate pain of that, Peter and I resolved to try to conceive again as quickly as possible.

In the spring of 1997, I was referred to a consultant gynaecologist because I was still suffering the same pain on the left side of my stomach, which a further course of antibiotics had not cleared up. I underwent a diagnostic laparoscopy and hysteroscopy in June 1997, which revealed extensive endometriosis and secondary adhesions, which were divided and ablated by laser. I underwent further laser treatment in August and October of 1997 because I was still in pain, and was told that I had extremely aggressive endometriosis, and was advised to conceive as soon as I could, because 'a pregnancy would be ideal to settle things down'.

Easier said than done, I thought! However, to our great delight, I conceived again in November 1997, but once again miscarried, this time at 10 weeks, in January 1998. After this second miscarriage, I resolved to try to do something about my endometriosis because conventional medicine was obviously not working for me. I read everything I could on the subject, visited every website I could find, went to a naturopath, had acupuncture and even visited a lady who claimed to be able to heal me and get me pregnant by hypnosis! By sheer chance, I came across Dian Mills' name one weekend in The Sunday Times, *and managed to get an appointment with her at the Institute for Optimum Nutrition in Putney – she seemed to me like the light at the end of a very long and dark tunnel.*

Dian spent an hour with me going over my history and my eating habits, and then devised a healthy eating plan for me and a regime of supplements, which I was to take for one month and then review. We agreed that my endometriosis did not seem to be affected by wheat or dairy products, as many people are, so luckily I was not advised to cut them out, but simply to increase other foods. I increased my intake of fresh vegetables, fish, live yoghurt, eggs, berries, nuts and seeds, and cut out citrus fruits, chocolate (as much as I could!) and caffeinated drinks; and reduced my alcohol consumption to less than five units a week. For breakfast I would eat (and still do) a chopped-up banana and pear, covered in live yoghurt and sprinkled with nutty and seedy muesli – yum! Lunch was salad with tuna or chicken, and dinner in the evenings was grilled fish or chicken with spinach, lots of garlic and herbs.

Dian prescribed vitamins C and E to work with the immune system and aid ovarian function; B6, magnesium and zinc to support the pituitary and ovaries; and evening primrose and fish oils (Efamarine) to aid hormone production and have an anti-inflammatory effect.

At the time I was working long, unsociable hours as a finance lawyer for a large US law firm, so had very little time to think about preparing food and making sure I had just the right ingredients. I'm certainly no Jamie Oliver in the kitchen, but there are so many interesting things you can do with food nowadays, and preparing a tasty nutritious meal does not have to take forever – just remember to always use the freshest ingredients, and get organized enough to plan what you're going to eat so that you're not snacking on things that are bad for you.

To our absolute joy, I became pregnant just over a month after my first consultation with Dian. The pregnancy was uncomplicated and stress-free (after I finally allowed myself to believe – when my consultant told me at 28 weeks that I was carrying a viable fetus! – that I was actually going to have a baby), and I continued my healthy eating habits all the way through my pregnancy. Our son Scott was born in June 1999, weighing a hearty 8lb 6oz, and at 15 months is still thriving.

In addition to Dian's 'bible' Endometriosis: A Key to Healing Through Nutrition, *I have invested in a book to help me get Scott into the habit of eating healthily –* Optimum Nutrition for Babies and Young Children *by Lucy Birnie. Both books are packed with tons of advice about how food can help you stay healthy, and interesting recipe suggestions which don't take forever to prepare or think about.*

Being diagnosed as having endometriosis is a sucker punch to any woman, but there is light at the end of the tunnel. I still have regular acupuncture, take my prescribed supplements and concentrate on eating healthily. Such was my success last time around, I have recently visited Dian to discuss a new regime to help me get pregnant again!

Good luck, and don't be at your wits' end – endometriosis is one thing where diet does make a difference, and it's enormously satisfying to know that you have had a hand in helping yourself get healthy.

NUTRIENT NEEDS OF OVA

It can be seen from research that most nutrients are essential to ovarian function. A low protein diet causes fewer ova to ripen or be released, as does a very high protein intake. Therefore moderation is the key. Research suggests a protein intake of 75gm (3oz) per day. The endocrine system needs the coenzymes riboflavin (vitamin B2), pyridoxine (vitamin B6) and biotin to metabolize proteins efficiently. Studies show that 'a low protein intake depresses GnRH secretion'.[49] Deficiency of thiamine (vitamin B1) inhibits ovulation. Optimum production of ovarian hormones requires the vitamins pyridoxine (B6), riboflavin (B2), folic acid, thiamine (B1), pantothenic acid (B5) and the minerals calcium and iron. B vitamins, magnesium and zinc are also important in the hypothalamus, the starting point for the process of reproduction.

Other researchers suggest the ovaries are rich in vitamin C, iodine and selenium, as well as B vitamins, magnesium, essential fatty acids and zinc. A good nutrient intake in the months before conception should therefore ensure that the reproductive system is in tiptop condition.

'LUF (luteinizing unruptured follicle), where the follicle does not "pop" out of an egg each month, has been reported in 79 per cent of women with endometriosis.'[50] One study on endometriosis and infertility states that riboflavin (B2) deficiency causes hormonal imbalances and is essential for liver clearance of the steroid hormones oestradiol (*see* chapter 9). Deficiency inhibits the LH secretion from the pituitary and GnRH from the hypothalamus. Riboflavin (B2) 'works closely with vitamin B5 and, if levels of vitamin B2 and B5 fall below 80 per cent, then the reproductive system fails'.[51]

Ann M of Lancashire

I must admit that I found the diet extremely hard to follow and after three weeks I reintroduced dairy foods; fruit and bread more slowly. But I became far more sensible about the foods I was eating. Even now, almost five years on, I don't eat as much creamy food or add sauces even though I don't feel I have a problem with candida overgrowth any more. I feel that the pain I was associating with my endo was due to disruption of my gut flora which came from long-term Danazol treatments. I was utterly miserable before the candida was diagnosed and treated. I have since had two successful pregnancies and we are expecting our third baby.

CASE STUDY

ZINC

A large percentage of couples who are referred to Foresight – the charity for preconceptual care – are found to be zinc-deficient. High levels of copper and low levels of zinc, often with low magnesium and/or manganese levels, are the most common findings, especially after using the pill or the coil.[52] Heavy metals, such as lead from petrol and cadmium from cigarettes, are antagonistic to zinc, as are high copper levels from excessive chocolate and tap-water consumption. If the potential parents work in an industry where they may come into contact with heavy metals, or toxic chemicals, they should use the physical protection provided by the employer. If excess wheat is eaten, phytic acid present in wheat binds to zinc and prevents it from being absorbed by the body, so wheat-based foods should be eaten in moderation.

FERTILE WOMEN'S DIETS

Researchers have also investigated what happens in fertile women with different eating patterns. Research at Hackney Hospital looked at the birth weights of new babies, and investigated what their mothers had eaten prior to and during pregnancy: 'Mothers of low birth weight babies had been eating meat, meat products, white bread, refined sugars and soft drinks in greater amounts. Mothers of the healthy weight babies had been eating nutrient-rich foods – three regular daily meals (breakfast being the most important), with wholegrain cereals, muesli, oats, nuts and seeds daily, eggs, egg dishes, wholemeal bread, dairy foods, and lots of fresh fruits and vegetables.'[53] A developing embryo or fetus requires abundant nutrients via the placenta in order to become a healthy bouncing baby. High-calorie, low-nutrient, refined foods were obviously detrimental to the developing baby in the womb: 'The hypothesis of the Hackney study, that the diet of the mothers of low birth weight babies had too few nutrients in their diets, was supported.'[54]

The most insidious type of infertility is caused by the body's inability to maintain a pregnancy. Conception may take place but the embryo may be unable to plant itself in the womb lining if this is inadequate owing to the mother having a poor nutrient intake. A developing fetus with a proportionately higher nutrient requirement may also fail to thrive if the womb lining is inadequate by day 15 of the preceding menstrual cycle. As we have seen, the placenta is formed by day 19, and has to filter nutrients from mother to child.

FETAL NEEDS

The fetus needs to extract nutrients from its mother in order to grow, but the mother herself has nutrient requirements, and has to limit the amount of nutrients available to the fetus in order to protect her own health. If the fetus absorbs too many nutrients from its mother, she could become ill. A balance has to be struck. Somehow in the process of evolution the fetal actions are opposed by maternal counter-measures: 'The general impression is of a mysterious symbiotic relationship, in which the mother and fetus conspire to realise the outcome that is so clearly desirable for both – the birth of a normal healthy baby.'[55] It can be deduced that 'if the mother is nutrient-deficient the fetus will struggle to survive'.[56]

CASE STUDY

Jackie H of Nottinghamshire

When I discovered that I had endometriosis I embarked upon a series of quests which I hoped would lead me to the desired goal – another pregnancy. A visit to a Foresight clinician advocated an anti-candida diet – no tea, coffee, sugar, chocolate, fruit for one month, and no yeasty foods etc. This alongside dietary supplements of vitamins and minerals, zinc and vitamin C. For the first two weeks I felt tired and suffered dreadful headaches and then started to feel better. However, the endometriosis symptoms did not abate and the much longed-for pregnancy did not happen.

My next visit was to a macrobiotic consultant. This time the diet was extremely strict and very narrow, unnaturally so. For a few months I lived off brown rice, oats, barley, organic vegetables, pulses, seaweeds, miso and very occasionally a small amount of fish. This regime stopped the pain and also my periods, but quite frankly was not a diet that I could stick to for any length of time. However, I did discover that organic vegetables tasted far nicer than ordinary vegetables and this is something that I have continued to include in my diet.

Vitamins, minerals and any other supplements were advised against. However, I did continue the Foresight vitamins and minerals as I considered the diet to be too restrictive – still no pregnancy.

In desperation I finally turned to you as my nutritionist to advise me in detail about foods and their effects on the body. I learned about the effects of gluten in susceptible people, the importance of cold-pressed oils and the link between animal fats and over-production of oestrogen in the body. For the first time somebody was actually taking time to explain the effects of food in detail. I modified my diet with the help of Dian and for the first time felt comfortable with how I was eating. She also prescribed vitamins and minerals, such as a multivitamin-mineral, zinc and vitamin B6, antioxidants, probiotics and a digestive enzyme, all tailored to my needs. I felt so much better and shortly afterwards became pregnant with my second child and surprise, surprise, two years later produced my third child! The gynaecologists had said that my endo was too bad for any pregnancy to take place. Throughout the various regimes I followed I learned something new about nutrition and these things I follow to this day, with the result that the endometriosis has completely cleared up and there has been absolutely no recurrence.

ROLE OF THE PLACENTA

The placenta forms at the time of contact between the blastocyst and the uterine membrane (endometrum). Even prior to implantation, there is an interaction among hormonal messages from the blastocyst, corpus luteum and endometrium. The blastocyst can synthesize protein hormones that are essential for its attachment.

A mother's pre-pregnancy nutrition is crucial to a healthy baby because it determines whether or not the mother will be able to grow a healthy placenta. Nutrients reach the developing infant in the uterus through the placenta, which develops in the first month of pregnancy. The placenta plays an active role in supporting the pregnancy: 'Far from being passive in its transport of molecules, the placenta is a highly metabolic organ producing some 60 enzymes of its own. It uses energy to fuel its work. The placenta's work consists of actively gathering up maternally produced hormones and nutrients of all description, and forcing them into the fetal bloodstream.'[57] The two bloodstreams are in close contact, separated by a space the width of three cells. This 'barrier' allows the transport of some substances, but is able to block others. The placenta itself also produces an array of hormones and other chemicals that maintain the pregnancy and prepare the mother's breasts for lactation.

Thus, the health of the placenta is a central consideration: 'If the mother's nutrition stores are inadequate during the time when the placenta is developing, then the placenta will develop poorly. As a consequence, no matter how well she eats later, her unborn baby will not receive optimum nourishment.'[58] This results in a low birth-weight baby, with a risk of adverse health consequences: 'After getting such a poor start in life, a girl or boy child may be ill-equipped, even as an adult, to store sufficient nutrients, and so may be unable to reach full developmental potential.'[59] The mother's body has to be prepared for a pregnancy by being well nourished. If you restrict your calorie intake, you run the risk of damaging the tissue which will develop into the placenta and the fetus.

NUTRIENT NEEDS

Vegetables make a major contribution to the intake of B vitamins and important minerals, including magnesium. As studies suggest: 'Vegetables were indeed the most important contributor of magnesium, with dairy produce in second place, and were more important than dairy produce as a source of B vitamins.'[60]

Eating patterns have changed so much over the past 40 years, from the consumption of regular meals with fresh vegetables every day to the non-stop 'grazing' on wheat-based snack foods. This snack food has much of its original nutrient content removed during manufacture, and often has to be fortified with synthetic nutrients. This type of diet can lead to low blood sugar (hypoglycaemia) and problems such as fatigue, irritability, dizziness and mood swings. New research shows that fruits and vegetables contain fewer nutrients than before as soils become depleted from overfarming (*see* chapter 11).

Many mothers do not have access to prenatal care and receive very little advice on diet and nutrition. Midwives legally cannot give dietary advice, and very few women see a dietitian. This can lead to poor health outcomes. Research in America shows that prenatal care is cost-effective: 'Saved dollars amount to $3.38 (£2.11) saved in direct medical care expenditure for every dollar spent on prenatal care.'[61]

There are three steps which will help to promote positive nutrition among women during pregnancy and lactation:

1 Increasing access to prenatal care.
2 Standard screening and intervention for poor nutrition, especially vital after the first miscarriage.
3 Delivering nutritional advice before pregnancy through school programmes in health and sex education classes.

It can be seen that it takes 12 months to make a baby, not just the nine months it is resident within the body. The quality of your diet during those three months prior to conception may well be crucial in maintaining and achieving pregnancy and producing a healthy child as the end result. The effort of eating well for 12 months is worth while for the lifetime of pleasure which children can bring.

That the maternal diet can influence pregnancy outcome even when energy intake is adequate is also well established. 'Burke and his colleagues looked at mothers who had eaten good/excellent diets: they gave birth to babies judged to be in good/superior health in 94 per cent of the time. Contrasted with mothers whose diets were classified as poor, and whose infants had good health only 8 per cent of the time.'[62] Diet is a vital consideration if a baby is wanted and needed so very much; diet is crucial to a baby's health as it grows and develops. Shouldn't we give our children a head start through correct nutrition? Every child has the right to reach his or her full potential.

Margaret and Arthur Wynn, a social scientist and scientist respectively, working from Hackney Hospital in London, have dedicated themselves to researching the link between the diet and infertility. They speculate that if a woman is infertile as a result of a poor diet and wishes to be fertile, two questions have to be asked:

1   What type of diet will replenish a couple's reproductive systems?
2   Can a woman and her partner be persuaded to consume a wholesome diet which can replenish them sufficiently?[63]

One study at the University of Mississippi suggested counselling by a qualified 'therapeutic dietitian' to promote fertility: 'Fertility was restored in 19 out of 26 women, who conceived spontaneously in due course. All the women had been underweight at the outset but were encouraged to gain half a pound per week. No drugs were prescribed.'[64] There is hope and although the process takes effort, it is not arduous.

Women in all social classes appear to eat very inadequate diets, to a point where the menstrual cycle is affected or suppressed. The main causes of anovulation are malnutrition, underweight and excessive exercise. Sometimes ovulation fails because of an underactive thyroid or pituitary tumours. Illness may be one reason for poor diet, but often it is the wish to be slim and attractive, in keeping with the socially accepted body image. This wish may be damaging to the fertility not just of this generation, but also of generations to follow.

The image of a healthy mother holding a healthy baby relies on the quality of life, hygiene, living conditions and sound nutrition surrounding them both. If eating well makes a difference, why not give it a try? There are no harmful side effects, just good health, as the evidence suggests: 'In the Hutterite culture (a Germanic organic farming community in the USA), fertility is used as an example of how high fertility can be when a population is healthy, stable and not using contraception ... producing 11 live births per married woman. Their infertility rate was only 2.4 per cent.'[65]

In one study, '55 per cent of all women in their childbearing years reported taking vitamin–mineral supplements rarely or occasionally'.[66] This research showed that 'women considered at the highest risk for nutritional inadequacy had lower rates of supplement use'. So the question must remain: should all women be given a supplement as part of a preconceptual care programme? Many doctors feel that this may prevent women from eating a healthy diet as they would rely on the nutrients in the supplement. But all the data suggest that women who already take supplements eat more healthily anyway, as they are giving more thought to their diet and nutrient intake. The design of appropriate individual supplement programmes should be considered, as many women self-prescribe and may not know the correct levels for supplementation. Healthy babies and healthy mothers would save thousands of pounds annually in health-care budgets, and would also lead to happier families in whom poor health was less of a problem.

SPERM QUALITY

Male infertility, particularly low sperm counts, is an increasing problem. A partner with a low sperm count may also require nutritional aid. Research on the subject states: 'The deteriorating quality of men's sperm has linked the problem with chemicals found in food, household products and the environment. Scientists are trying to find out why sperm counts may be falling. They have concluded that the chemical pesticides, which mimic female hormones, may also have contributed to rises in testicular cancer. The link is regarded as "plausible" by the Department of the Environment.'[67]

The suspect chemicals include pesticides; phthalates (a group of compounds that 'migrate' from plastic PVC wrappings and leak into such foods as cheese, meats, cakes, sandwiches and confectionery); phyto-oestrogens (plant oestrogens) occurring naturally in soya beans, which are widely incorporated into infant milk formula; alkylphenol polyethoxylates, used in detergents, paints and cosmetics; and ubiquitous industrial pollutants such as polychlorinated biphenyls (PCBs) which accumulate in fatty tissue. Even strong electrical equipment emits strong magnetic fields which may be detrimental to sperm health. Moreover, women working at VDU terminals also appear to have problems with fertility.[68]

'One man in 20 is subfertile' concluded an international study published by the Danish Environment Ministry and reported in the *British Medical Journal*.[69] The maximum sperm count a man can have is determined by the number of Sertoli cells, which provide nutrients to the developing sperm. As Sertoli cells are produced very early in life, a reduced sperm count implies that sperm damage is being done very early in fetal development, possibly via the mother's food intake and the environment. Moreover, 'spermatogenesis in the human takes 120 days to recover if there have been mutagens around. If the sperm are being damaged by chemicals the man must take precautions for the next three months whilst a new supply is being made.'[70]

Professor Niels Skakkebaek of the University of Copenhagen, Denmark, was the first scientist to observe toxic changes in human sperm. He says that exposure of the male fetus to high levels of oestrogenic chemicals in the first three months of pregnancy could be the vital trigger: 'It is quite clear from laboratory and clinical studies that pesticides of all categories may influence the immune system resulting in endocrine dysfunction.'[71, 72] However, much more research is needed to look at the effects of this pollution on hormone levels.

Once the sperm and ova have joined, the fertilized egg takes four to six days to travel along the Fallopian tube. By the ninth day, this blastocyst may comprise 1,000 to 10,000 cells and should then be able to attach to the uterus well. Faulty sperm will hamper this process.

SPERM NUTRIENT NEEDS

'Sperm counts of over 10 million/ml are classed as healthy, but nine million or below can bring problems.'[73] 'Some sperm enter the cervix within 30–60 seconds after ejaculation. Others are stored in cervical mucus and released continuously for two to four days. Of the millions of sperm entering the vagina, only 0.1–1 per cent reach the uterus. Of these, merely 1,000 to 5,000 sperm can actually be found in the Fallopian tubes. Excess sperm are removed through phagocytosis within 10–24 hours after entry.[74]

This is why a quiet immune system is essential. An overactive immune system damages sperm. Sperm have to be healthy to swim the long distances through the womb and Fallopian tubes. They encounter fluids on the way which may harm them so their outer skin needs to be strong. The head of the sperm is rich in zinc which helps to penetrate the ovum. This union of sperm and ovum triggers a cascade of calcium to flow all around the fertilized egg.

Subclinical deficiencies of various nutrients can affect sperm formation. Vitamin C protects sperm against free-radical damage, and the level of vitamin C in seminal fluid is much higher than in other body fluids. Vitamin E enhances the ability of sperm to fertilize an egg in test tubes. Zinc is critical in male reproduction (zinc and vitamin E increase testosterone levels, which is responsible for sperm production) and low zinc status may contribute to infertility.[75] Vitamin B12 also appears to improve both sperm count and motility, and deficiency is linked to sterility. Vitamin A deficiency causes abnormalities in sperm shape and, if the deficiency is prolonged, the spermatids and spermatozoa disintegrate. Selenium and iodine deficiencies are also associated with low sperm count. Magnesium deficiency is linked to mutagenic changes and infertility. Research suggests that 'manganese deficiency causes testicular degeneration'.[76] The amino acid L-arginine is essential for sperm production and motility, and L-caritnine levels appear to be high in the epididymis and sperm, which suggests that it, too, must play a role in male reproduction. These vitamins and minerals should therefore be supplemented in cases of male infertility, but not in excess: 'Excesses may also cause mutagenic changes so levels should be moderate.'[77]

It is wise to avoid excess fatty foods to ensure that the intake of harmful pesticide residues is kept low: 'Pesticides bind to fats and are to be found more commonly in fatty food. Once inside the body pesticides react like oestrogens, female hormones, and can upset the normal hormonal balance.'[78] The diet should be low in saturated animal fats, but some good quality cis oils such as flax seed (edible food grade linseed oil) and olive oils can be included. Eating organic food when possible can also help to avoid some pesticides.[79] In chapter 9 we will look at which supplements can be taken safely.

COPING WITH INFERTILITY

We all lose our fertility at some point in our lives. The poet Donald Justice says 'We must learn to close softly the doors to rooms we will not be coming back to.' Women with endometriosis may have to learn to close doors earlier.[80] However, the British Endometriosis Society's motto is 'Never give up.' Many women achieve pregnancy in the end.

Achieving pregnancy takes an average couple 18 months from the time they first start trying for a baby. This means that, for some couples, it may take two and a half to three years. There are many factors with endometriosis which can cause problems, but male infertility should always be investigated before female infertility, as it is less traumatic to treat. It responds well to zinc and vitamins C and E and evening primrose oils.

The trauma which some members of the medical profession can provoke by stating that endometriosis is a cause of infertility and that a woman 'can never get pregnant' can be too much to bear. The link between endometriosis and infertility is poorly understood. It is a hypothesis based on investigating the chemical secretions from endometriotic implants, which may well be correctable by diet. If one-fifth of the population have difficulty achieving pregnancy it may not be endometriosis alone that is causing the problem; it could be a combination of environmental factors. Ensure your lifestyle is giving your health the space, relaxation, exercise and nutrition you need to strengthen all your body systems. The negativity and mental anguish that couples have to endure from pessimistic, gloom-laden health professionals can be unbelievable. Yet, some women with endometriosis have had as many as five children. Just try to get your body healthy again. Miracles can and do happen.

Vicki D of London

In late September I went to see a nutritionist in a desperate state. Over three and a half years, I had undergone four IVF and ICSI procedures, countless inseminations with ovulation induction drugs and two major surgeries for endometriosis costing $100,000. My husband and I then moved from New York to London in July before undergoing a fifth IVF and ICSI procedure. Our NY doctor was by then also recommending donor eggs!

I felt very sick and run down and sought nutritional advice at the end of September. After three months on a healthy eating regime, I started to feel much better than I had in years. On January 15th my period was quite late and I took an at-home pregnancy test. Much to my joy and disbelief it was positive. My husband and I had prayed for a natural conception and we cannot express our joy and gratitude.

Nutrition does work! Our son was born in October, at 9lb 1oz, and is thriving. Two years later, Anne-Marie was born, at 7lb 12oz, after following the nutrition programme again.

•
C
A
S
E

S
T
U
D
Y
•

When a woman wants to hold her baby in her arms and her partner wants to look into the eyes of his child, but they are unable to have children, an enormous cavern, a yawning gap, permeates their lives. This can generate the tremendous stress of monthly trauma, of frustrated longing and desire. A cycle of distress which continues as each menstruation begins and hope ends can create chaos with relationships. This can be doubly so with endometriosis if painful or difficult intercourse (dyspareunia) is also involved, which can cause distress and despair in itself. It robs us of a joy and comfort in life, particularly if you are desperately trying to get pregnant.

Disbelieving GPs and rushed consultants may not take the time to help. In addition, many GPs are too embarrassed to talk about painful sexual intercourse. Ask for counselling and referral to a sexual therapy clinic or a clinical psychologist if you feel the need. Talking through the problems and getting the right sort of help is very important, although, when desire is there and the pain is real, referral to a psychiatrist is not the answer. You and your partner lose all spontaneity for sex, as deep pain sets you on edge and you expect the worst before it happens. When internal organs that are meant to slip and slide are glued together firmly with adhesions, and internal muscles are tense and inflamed, agony ensues. (Evening primrose and fish oils help to reduce the inflammation, and magnesium relaxes the muscles.)

However, there is a great variety of alternative ways of sexual intercourse other than penetration, and many other ways in which we can show our love for one another. Healing can make this all come right again.

> Understand that happiness is not based on possessions, power or prestige, but on relationships with people you **truly** love.
>
> *Life's Little Treasure Book on Joy*

KEEP TALKING

Communication is the most important thing. If love is strong and friendship profound, then keep talking to one another. Don't brush your deep distress under the carpet or try to ignore the problem. Talk things through, cuddle and cry together. Being together is the important thing, and recognizing that this is no one person's fault. You will overcome this problem, there is hope.

Two men's experience

'My partner was diagnosed as having a cyst on her ovary. As a result she had surgery, and the cyst and the ovary removed. I took the time to read up on endometriosis while my partner was in hospital. Needless to say it was a traumatic experience to see the effects major abdominal surgery and general anaesthetic had on someone I love and care for. What was worse than seeing her look ill were the mental images of her being virtually sliced in half. I so wanted to do something to stop the suffering, but I felt so totally helpless and useless. All I could do was be there for my partner, to offer her support and also gain as much information as I could on endometriosis.'

'Endometriosis does really test a relationship. It also shows how sexist the medical services are – seeing "women's complaints" as some form of neurosis or hysteria. What can a partner do?

'1 Become informed – find out what endometriosis is, so you can offer a more understanding ear.
2 Support your partner in any way you can. I was fortunate in having understanding

management and colleagues who allowed me to juggle my work shifts so that I was able to offer my partner the care she needed.

3 When your partner tells you about the various pains, etc., take her seriously. This is so important in a society which does not take women's health seriously.'

Women are more likely to talk this problem through with one another. Often it is the male partner who suffers in silence. At a psychosexual workshop for partners held in Brighton more than 40 couples found help by talking this through together. It was refreshing for so many people to be open about their sexual frustrations, and it removed the feelings of isolation which many had felt.

A husband's advice

'My wife was diagnosed as suffering from a disease called endometriosis. It sounded so, well, diseased! By becoming informed it provided us both with answers to questions which I am sure many other couples have agonized over. "Why can't you have normal periods? How can it hurt to make love?" Being naturally shy I have not found it particularly easy to make the first move in discussing what is, after all, a very personal subject dealing with period pains, painful intercourse and the like. However, what I have found is that it is absolutely vital for your relationship to put aside such traditional taboos and express your willingness to discuss such matters. It helps to show your partner just how much you care.'

Sharing stories and experiences in a group of people who are going through the same problems can help a great deal in coming to terms with how they affect one's life. A good book to read is *On Death and Dying* by Elizabeth Kübler-Ross. It explains how the pain we feel when someone dies can be comparable to the pain, depression and anger that infertile people go through. It is the mourning for a child who has never been born, but who lives in the soul, which hurts the most. Understanding this may help to put things in perspective for you; trying to appreciate life around you which may occur as a blur as the years pass while you try for a baby. Hold on to what you have around you, the love of family and friends.

One lady explained it this way: 'There were other things that we did to get over not having children. We started to make the choice our own rather than something that happened to us. We began to recognize that life was good when you are child-free. We took a few trips alone together and started to do the things we had put off just in case we had a baby. I finally returned to my artwork, something I stopped doing during my eleven years of infertility. I am now able to concentrate again and to paint for several months during the summer when the art school is on holidays. My husband started playing hockey and baseball, and we both started skiing and working out regularly. We began to focus our attention on each other and rejuvenated our relationship. Let's face it, when sex becomes a monitored chore during the infertile years, it takes a while to get your love life back on track. Now the focus is on each other rather than wondering if this will be the time that you get pregnant.'[81]

Part of feeling better has to do with giving up the anguish related to infertility and getting on with life. Setting new goals, perhaps making a career change or learning new things can open up a new world. Take the time and energy previously spent trying to have a baby and channel it into new adventures. Many couples struggle to survive the pain of infertility together, and because it has overwhelming negative influences, it tends to drive couples apart rather than bringing them closer together. Find time to return to the love that brought you together in the first place.

Believe it or not, there is life after infertility, and it can be an enriching experience. The biggest step is deciding when you have had enough and then taking your new life one day at a time. What is so difficult with infertility is living in limbo for years. Once the decision to stop treatment is made you will be amazed at how much better you will feel. Regaining control over your life is a wonderful thing. *Sweet Grapes: How to stop being infertile and start living again* by Jean and Michael Carter, published by Perspective Press, is another good book to read.

SUBFERTILITY

The endocrine system appears to monitor nutrient intake. If we fall below a certain level, the reproductive system stalls. A rising body weight from a diet full of fresh foods is very important – three regular meals each day, beginning with a nutritious breakfast. A selection of the following supplements may be supportive while diet is adjusted:

- Multivitamin/mineral
- B-complex (non-yeast based)
- Magnesium malate
- Iodine (kelp)
- Selenium (non-yeast based), with vitamins A, C and E as antioxidants
- Zinc citrate or gluconate
- Digestive enzymes
- Evening primrose and fish oils
- Bioacidophilus

NB Once you are pregnant, you should only take a multivitamin/mineral supplement containing 2,000 IU of vitamin A only, along with evening primrose and fish oils.

SUMMARY

1 The subfertility rate is high (15–20 per cent) in couples around the world, and endometriosis may be one contributory factor, causing infertility in some 30 per cent of all subfertile couples.

2   Endometriosis-induced infertility can be due to adhesions, early miscarriage (and vice versa), endometriotic implant secretions and anovulation (no ovulation), or impaired fertilization.

3   Nutrition will help improve your fertility. Nutrients are required for a healthy reproductive system. (Look up www.makingbabies. com for more information.)

4   The body matures the sperm and ova months before conception takes place. The health of your partner's sperm and your eggs and womb lining are dependent on your nutrient intake. Putting a sorry-looking sperm into a starving ova and implanting the resulting embryo into a sick womb is a recipe for disaster.

5   To sustain a pregnancy you need a healthy body weight:height ratio (body mass index). Fertility improves on a rising body weight, not when the weight is falling.

6   To improve your fertility, you need to eat nutrient-rich foods – three regular meals daily (breakfast being the most important), with wholegrain cereals, muesli, oats, nuts, seeds, egg dishes, wholemeal bread, dairy foods, and lots of fresh fruits and vegetables, especially green leafy ones.

7   A healthy placenta has to be made to house the fetus for nine months. The only way nutrients can reach the developing baby is through the placenta. To prepare the body to build a healthy placenta each month the diet must be nutrient-rich all the time that you are attempting pregnancy.

8   Fresh, unprocessed foods are always the most nutritious. Chapters 9 and 10 will explain the dietary changes necessary to improve the health of the reproductive system. Changes in your diet will help enhance fertility.

9   Never give up. Take time out for yourself and your partner. The pain and distress of subfertility is damaging to the immune, nervous, digestive and reproductive systems. It is very important to give yourselves time and space, and keep talking to one another.

10 Do things for yourself that you enjoy. Set new goals and create new 'moments' one day at a time.

THE RECIPE FOR MAKING BABIES

Take:
>1 healthy sperm
>1 healthy ovum
>1 healthy womb

Add:
>Relaxation
>Water
>Fresh air
>Nutrients
>Natural daylight

Mature for three months, then mix and gestate for nine months at 37°C in a non-toxic environment.

Dian Shepperson Mills

6 Many treatments, few cures?

Remember the 15th century proverb that summarizes the purpose of medicine: 'To cure sometimes, to relieve often, to comfort always'.

W M Burch, Endocrinology (3rd edn),
Williams & Wilkins, 1988

The true enigma of endometriosis is that we do not have a definitive cure for the disease. However, we do have access to many therapies that can ease the pain and symptoms of endometriosis and, in some cases, help the subfertile patient. Endometriotic implants may first have been described by Aristotle thousands of years ago. Ancient writings appear to describe the random appearance of the implants and their adhesions in the abdomen of women. Indeed, Egyptian papyrus texts speak of 'the wandering womb', an apt description if ever there was one!

Here we are, over 2,000 years later, and we still do not have a 'miracle drug' that will selectively destroy endometriotic implants. As already discussed, the problem facing modern scientists who wish to develop a cure for endometriosis is that endometriotic implants grow, look and behave like the normal endometrium of the uterus. Any drug that would destroy the implant would also destroy normal endometrium. Finding a cure sounds impossible, but recent research shows that there are subtle ways in which the implants differ in their behaviour from true endometrium, and it is possible that drugs that only target endometrial implants can be developed. The cure needs to target the 'rogue' tissue and leave the normal endometrial tissue intact. In the best case scenario with the body's immune system working normally, it should just remove the rogue cells.

Before we look at the role of nutrition or some of the non-traditional therapies as an aid for coping with endometriosis, let us look at what is available from your gynaecologist. In modern orthodox medicine, five main types of therapies are available:

1 Drug therapies
2 Surgical therapies
3 Pregnancy induction
4 Analgesics
5 Antihistamines

Any one or combination of these therapies can be used to treat endometriosis, dependent upon whether the treatment is meant to reduce pain or assist conception, or both. The choice of treatment is also influenced by the wishes of the woman and her age. In the majority of cases, endometriosis symptoms often diminish with the advent of menopause, so an older woman might not want an aggressive therapy like surgery, but may just want to decrease her pain symptoms with analgesics or through complementary therapy treatments. Likewise, a young woman in her teens would not want to subject herself to drastic surgery or use pregnancy as a possible 'cure', and she may prefer one of the drug therapies.

Ann W of Sussex

After being on different drugs on and off over the past 15 years, it is difficult to remember what did what. But I can remember you did suggest cutting out cow's milk and trying goat's milk. Following the diet and supplements did overall make me feel better in myself.

CASE STUDY

DRUG THERAPIES

The drug treatments usually mimic the beneficial effects of either pregnancy (high levels of progesterone) or menopause (removal of ovarian steroids). During pregnancy and the menopause, it has been noted that endometriosis becomes less active and may 'die back'. Drug treatments therefore try to mimic these natural chemical reactions in the body, by altering hormone levels so that they are the same as they would be during pregnancy or menopause.

PSEUDOPREGNANCY DRUGS

The word 'pseudopregnancy' means false pregnancy and, in this therapy, the hormones of pregnancy are administered in an attempt to mimic the beneficial effect of a natural pregnancy on endometriosis.

Birth control pills

Some success has resulted from women taking large concentrations of birth control pills containing synthetic oestrogen- and progesterone-like hormones. These combination pills are taken continuously over several months so no menstrual period occurs. The constant exposure of the endometriotic implant to progesterone and the lack of the cyclic pattern of the oestrogen hormones of the menstrual cycle cause the implants to thin out or 'die back'. Unfortunately, the implants do not disappear entirely; they lie dormant, like volcanoes, and they usually reappear after withdrawal of the treatment.

The drug treatments merely suppress but do not cure this problem. To elicit a cure, we have to find the real cause. However, these drugs can give respite from the symptoms of endometriosis and, for women seeking to have children, they may open up a window of opportunity in which they can try to conceive, whilst the endometriotic implants lie dormant.[1] As soon as the pill or GnRH tablets are stopped and whilst the endometriosis has subsided, the woman may find it easier to conceive over a six-month period.

For some women this type of hormone therapy reduces, and sometimes removes, the pain of endometriosis. Shrinking the patches of 'rogue' tissue may stop the implant producing harmful chemicals which alter surrounding tissue, and cause inflammation. This treatment is popular with young women, especially teenagers, since they feel it is more socially acceptable to take birth control pills than to take a hormone drug treatment for reproductive problems. However, the high doses of hormones, especially the presence of oestrogen, have side effects that makes this treatment undesirable for some women, who becomes bloated from water retention, suffer from migraines, have breast tenderness, or unwanted weight gain. Some effects are less obvious: 'The contraceptive pill changes blood biochemistry, so that higher levels of vitamin A and copper begin to circulate, but the levels of B-complex vitamins and zinc are lowered.'[2] Hormone preparations also disrupt the balance of our 'friendly' bifido gut bacteria, the very ones which protect the endocrine and immune systems.

A more direct way of mimicking pregnancy is to administer long-acting progesterone-like drugs such as Depo-Provera (medroxy-progesterone acetate). This treatment requires hormone injections only once every three months. However, the difficulty with long-acting progesterone is that it accumulates in fat tissue, and in some women, especially obese women, it may take a year after stopping treatment for menstruation to return. For this reason, women who want to become pregnant may not want to be exposed to long-acting progesterone.[3] On the benefit side, long-acting progesterone does not usually have the side effects attributed to birth control pills, although some weight gain and bloating may occur. As with the Pill, long-acting progesterone can reduce the symptoms of endometriosis by suppressing the cyclic activity of the endometriotic implant and impairing its growth. The implants and symptoms can recur after therapy ceases.

Short-acting progesterone has also been used successfully as a pseudopregnancy drug. In women who desire fertility, these drugs are preferred over the long-acting progesterone treatments because reproductive cycles start more promptly after cessation of treatment.[4]

The efficacy of taking birth control pills as a preventative measure against endometriosis has been questioned: 'Some 80 per cent of patients in the Brisbane research trial (looking at women with active endometriosis) had taken oral contraceptive pills. Fifty four per cent were pregnant and many had lactated, so prior pill use, pregnancy and lactation do not necessarily protect against the development of endometriosis.'[5]

Two new studies suggest that oral contraception is associated with an increased risk of endometriosis, but this finding is based on a selected population. However, other studies have shown that an increased sensitivity to oestrogen may lead to the development of endometriosis in some women.[6, 7, 8]

Progesterone cream

Mexican wild yams (and mistletoe) contain a substance known as diosgenin. When the yam undergoes a technical process in the laboratory, diosgenin becomes the product sold as 'natural progesterone'. It is very important, if you wish to try this type of treatment, to read about the form of the cream, which is available only on prescription in the UK. Small amounts of the cream are applied to various sites on the body during the second half of the menstrual cycle.

Progesterone is a steroid hormone, produced naturally in the body by steroid synthesizing cells, that is required for pregnancy. It makes the uterus relax and inhibits the ability of oestrogen to cause cramps. The progesterone from yams is not natural to the body. The structure of progesterone is the same for all animals. The term progestogen refers to any substance that has the same biological activity as progesterone. A progesterone-like substance derived from a plant is technically defined as a progestogen.

Progesterone has many effects on the body. It alters the electrical activity in the brain and in large doses acts as a sedative. When progesterone was first discovered at the University of St Louis, USA, its effects were tested on rabbits. The first doses given were high, as the researchers had no idea what normal levels were. Although there were no serious side effects, the rabbits actually fell asleep.

Progesterone also increases body temperature (it is thermogenic). Since progesterone increases naturally after ovulation, this thermogenic effect is sometimes used to determine if a woman is ovulating. Many women with endometriosis have reported a lower body temperature, of around 36°C, and normalized progesterone levels may assist them by helping to correct their temperature regulation.

The purveyors of 'natural progesterone' creams attribute cures for endometriosis, PMS, fibrocystic breast disease, uterine fibroids, ovarian cysts and osteoporosis to these products. Studies have been done on osteoporosis and do show benefits. More research is needed, however, to see exactly what is happening to the endometriotic implants when these creams are used. We would all like a cure to be forthcoming.

Wild yam, which contains diosgenins, that has not undergone processing has an oestrogenic action whereas wild yam diosgenin that has undergone processing has a progestogenic action and is known as a natural progesterone. For this reason, it is very important to have your hormone profile taken before using natural progesterone creams to make sure you are in need of it. You will not ovulate and are not likely to conceive with this programme, using the creams, from day 7 to day 28, the accompanying leaflets suggest.

PSEUDOMENOPAUSE DRUGS

'Pseudomenopause' means false menopause. Since the symptoms of endometriosis usually disappear once menopause begins, several drug treatments have been developed that mimic menopause. The hallmark of menopause is the absence of ovarian hormones and the absence of menstrual cycles. Natural menopause involves the gradual winding down over several years of hormone production from the ovaries. Pseudomenopause drugs rapidly shut down the ovary's ability to produce oestrogen and progesterone, but the effects are reversible. Without the cyclic exposure to these hormones, the endometriotic implants should shrink and die back. These treatments can be very effective in reducing pain symptoms and may help the subfertile couple. However, pseudomenopausal drugs have some serious side effects that many women find unacceptable to live with on a day-to-day basis. The side effects of each drug are explained in the following sections.

Danazol

The major hormone used as a pseudomenopausal drug is Danazol, which has a chemical structure similar to the male hormone testosterone. It can be taken as a pill once or twice daily. Danazol causes a hypo-oestrogen (low oestrogen) condition. How Danazol causes this is complex and not clearly understood, but the drug appears to have several effects which lead to a decrease in size of the endometriotic implants.

Danazol has the following actions:

1 It prevents the formation of some steroids by the adrenal gland and ovary, thus preventing the production of oestrogen.
2 It acts directly on the endometriotic implant to prevent its growth.
3 It inhibits the production of LH and FSH by the pituitary gland, which removes the major endocrine stimulus to oestrogen production by the ovary.[9]

Furthermore, Danazol treatment usually stops the menstrual cycle in the majority of women who take it. The lack of cyclic oestrogen and progesterone production inhibits the regrowth of the implants.[10] In short, the low oestrogen and the testosterone-like action of Danazol set up a hostile environment for the growth and development of the implants.

Jacky H of Nottinghamshire

My diet helped me with the effects of Danazol. I started taking Danazol in August and had the normal side effects. I put on a stone in weight, and suffered from severe muscle cramps and joint pains. Then I had a flare-up of thrush so decided to go onto a yeast-reducing diet. For three weeks, I cut out all yeast-based foods and took garlic tablets. The thrush went and so did the muscle cramps and joint pains. After three weeks, I reintroduced bread into my diet and back came the cramps as bad as before. I was on Danazol for nine months and now, so long as I avoid yeasts, I have no cramps or joint pains. I eat soda bread, which is easily obtainable.

CASE STUDY

Unfortunately, Danazol is not heaven-sent, and some women may experience aggravating side effects. As a result of Danazol's testosterone-like structure, it has side effects that reflect the action of male hormones. Some women complain of muscle cramps, acne, bloating, decreased breast size and, in rare cases, voice changes, hair growth on the face, an enlargement of the clitoris, headaches and nasal congestion. If voice changes, migraines and clitoral enlargement occur, the drug should be stopped immediately after consulting your doctor.

Another rare complication from Danazol treatment is liver problems, including an elevation of liver enzyme levels that can lead to the patient turning yellow (jaundice). Changes in the digestive enzymes in the liver may affect digestion in some sensitive people. When Danazol is taken for more than six months, liver enzyme function tests should be performed by the general practitioner.

Lesley B of London

As I refused to take Danazol when I was first diagnosed, I took the nutritional path to quell the pain and tiredness. After a few weeks it began to reduce symptoms, which fluctuated according to stress levels mainly caused by work situations. I have continued to use supplements, increasing the calcium and zinc, and trying such things as Gingko biloba *and* Echinacea. *As I still smoke and the balance of my lifestyle is still lopsided (always was, always will be!), I am prone to a low immune system whatever I swallow. But I believe that you definitely are what you eat. My message to endo sufferers would be to take whatever medical route you think is best for you, but in addition, try nutrition and look at your lifestyle. The supplements need to be of good quality and the amounts taken should be correct for your needs, enough to be of value. Thank you for all your support.*

C A S E   S T U D Y

Although most women do not suffer many side effects from Danazol, those who do can be devastated. Young women especially are concerned with the masculinization effects of Danazol since the changes to facial hair, voice and clitoral growth are not easily reversible. Also, the excessive weight gain causes many women to diet, thus reducing their nutrient intake even further. Up to 20 per cent of calcium can be lost from the bones, but this change is usually reversible. Pregnancy rates and pain relief after Danazol treatment appear to be reasonable, and because of this, some women risk the side effects.

GnRH analogues

Another group of pseudomenopausal drugs are GnRH analogues. GnRH stands for 'gonadotrophin-releasing hormone'. This is the hormone from the hypothalamus in the brain that controls the release of the pituitary hormones, FSH and LH (*see* chapter 2). The co-enzymes for its release are dependent upon zinc and vitamin B6. The GnRH analogues are synthetic compounds that look very similar to natural GnRH, but are chemically modified to make them more powerful and longer-acting than natural GnRH. GnRH analogues inhibit the ability of the pituitary to secrete FSH and LH, thus switching off ovarian function.[11]

Since LH and FSH are the hormones that stimulate the ovary to produce oestrogen, withdrawal of LH and FSH analogues leads to a hypo-oestrogen condition. As stated before, oestrogen stimulates growth of the implant and low oestrogen levels lead to a decrease in the size of the endometriotic implant. There are two types of GnRH analogues, the GnRH agonists and the GnRH antagonists.

The analogues most commonly used today are GnRH agonists, which stimulate the pituitary to produce LH and FSH. However, for the treatment of endometriosis, excessive amounts of GnRH agonist are administered, and the pituitary becomes overworked and exhausted by this sudden and rapid stimulation – and eventually fails to respond to any signals. This lack of response by the pituitary leads to decreased production of LH and FSH.

The GnRH antagonists, on the other hand, directly inhibit the pituitary gland from producing LH and FSH. It seems that the GnRH antagonists are better suited for the treatment of endometriosis. Unfortunately, GnRH antagonists have serious side effects, such as hives, which hamper their use as a therapy.

Although GnRH analogues do not have any male hormone-like effects, both Danazol and GnRH analogues induce the typical side effects associated with menopause. These side effects include headaches, hot flushes, sweating, vaginal dryness, painful intercourse, nervousness and moodiness. Research has shown that women may develop panic disorder and/or major depression while receiving GnRH agonists for treatment of endometriosis.[12] GnRH analogues may also trigger bone loss (osteoporosis), but this bone loss is usually reversible and bone density may return to normal after the treatment ends.

These drugs should only be taken for a six-month period because of the drastic loss of calcium (up to 20 per cent) from the bones. Sometimes 'add-back' hormone replacement therapy (HRT) is used alongside to try and halt the bone loss. Discussions at the World Congress on the use of GnRH analogues suggest that they should NEVER be used by teenagers, who have pituitary glands which are only just developing a menstrual cycle pattern.

SURGICAL THERAPIES

The surgical approach to endometriosis treatment involves either the selective removal of endometriotic implants or the complete removal of the reproductive organs. In both cases, we are talking about invasive procedures that are potentially painful, possibly expensive and somewhat traumatic. However, surgery may be very effective for some women.

LAPAROSCOPY

The selective removal of endometriotic implants is usually done through a laparoscope (figure 6.1). This is a fibreoptic device, containing a telescope and a fibreoptic light, that allows the surgeon to work directly on the reproductive organs through a small incision in the belly button (navel). In a laparoscopic procedure, the abdomen is filled with an inert gas, the pressure of which pushes the intestines out of view. This also enlarges the peritoneal cavity so that the surgeon can see the organs clearly and can move them around to find the patches of endometriosis.[13]

By making a second puncture in the abdomen, the surgeon can insert a grasping instrument that enables him to manipulate the organs. The laparoscope sometimes contains a laser or an electric probe that can be used to burn away the endometriotic implant. The laser is a high-energy light source powerful enough to burn tissue; it is so fine that it can cut sections from a single hair. The strength of an extremely fine laser can be more accurately controlled than that of an electric probe, and the physician has much better control of the depth of cellular destruction. The laser can also be used to remove endometriotic implants from areas which are not easily reached with an electric probe. This operation is less invasive than a laparotomy, but it still carries the slight risk of side effects. The use of anaesthetics always poses some risk and a careless operator could harm the bowel or one of the major blood vessels, although this is *very* rare.

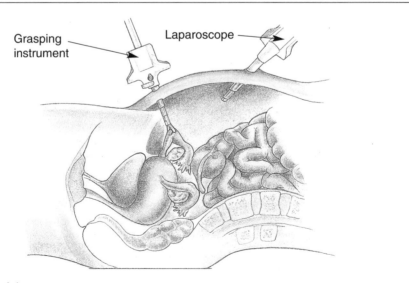

Figure 6.1
Cross-sectional diagram of a woman's abdomen showing the placement of the surgical instruments used during a laparoscopic examination.

It is a good idea to combine the laparoscopy with laser treatment, diathermy, cauterization or excision to avoid having to undergo a second operation at a later date, with all the additional trauma and double-dose of anaesthetic in the body that a repeat operation entails. If you are booked in for a laparoscopy, check with the surgeon and let him know that if endometriosis is found, it can be lasered away rather than having a second operation later. Many doctors video the procedure so that a record can be kept for future reference. This can be useful when several doctors are involved with your case.

In addition to burning away or removing the implants, the surgeon can cut apart any adhesions that are present. As discussed before, adhesions are connective tissue bundles that attach the organs to each other. If the adhesions cover the Fallopian tube or twist the Fallopian tube away from the ovary, their removal may restore fertility. Adhesions may also stretch pain receptors in nerves and their removal can reduce pain. Some surgeons also cut the sensory nerves to the uterus to relieve pain; however, this may affect bladder function and the ability to achieve orgasm. These various types of surgery may be very effective in some women.

In women with mild endometriosis, pregnancy rates after surgery of 60 per cent have been reported, with a significant reduction in pain symptoms. Most women can return to a normal life two to three days after the procedure, which is a more rapid result than having to wait for the weeks involved in drug treatments. Most pregnancies that result after drug or surgical treatment occur five to 18 months after treatment. If pregnancy does not occur during that period, then the chances of getting pregnant may be reduced unless other methods of treatment are tried. This failure to conceive is primarily due to the regrowth of the endometriotic implants after treatment. Because of this, some physicians like to couple surgery with various drug treatments to extend and enhance the effects of therapy. Remember that drug and surgical treatments only suppress symptoms; only rarely do they cure the disease. Unfortunately for the majority of women, endometriosis may recur up to 18 months after drugs and surgery.

HYSTERECTOMY AND OOPHORECTOMY

In desperation to alleviate the extreme pain, some women elect to have their ovaries (oophorectomy) and uterus (hysterectomy) removed. This can be very effective in removing pain symptoms, but is a drastic action that obviously cannot be undone. This type of surgery will overnight make a woman menopausal whatever her age, and she will have to contend with the rapid onset of the extreme symptoms of menopause. Natural menopause can take up to seven years, as the ovaries gradually cease their function. The hot flushes and mood changes associated with menopause can be aggravated after a complete hysterectomy (hysterectomy and bilateral salpingo-oophorectomy) since the procedure involves the abrupt removal of the ovaries and hence ovarian hormones. This procedure should not be entered into lightly, and trying the least harsh treatment method first (such as nutrients and diet) and working up can prevent this more drastic action.

Laparotomy, which may be used for hysterectomy or exploratory surgery, involves a four- to five-inch cut in the abdominal wall at the bikini line. Some hysterectomies can be done via the vagina or by laser laparoscopy. Myomectomy is the surgical removal of fibroids when the woman wishes to conserve her uterus. Endometrial ablation is where the womb lining, the endometrium, is burnt away. Both are alternatives to having the uterus removed.

The lack of ovarian steroids after a complete hysterectomy and oophorectomy can also lead to rapid bone loss (osteoporosis), especially in women with a family history of bone loss with ageing. The sudden loss of oestrogen slows calcium deposition in bone. Because of the menopausal and other side effects (such as sweating, vaginal dryness, painful intercourse), a woman who has had her uterus and ovaries removed should think about taking supplemental oestrogen therapy or HRT. It is often recommended that women with endometriosis should wait at least six to nine months after hysterectomy and oophorectomy before taking HRT to allow any endometrial implants on the peritoneal cavity walls, bowel or bladder to die back. Immediate use of HRT gives the body access to more oestrogen, which could trigger these endometriotic patches to become active again, causing the pain to recur.

In some cases, women who have never had endometriosis or period pain symptoms will suddenly develop endometriosis after being given HRT patches. More research is necessary to discover exactly what is triggering the disease to take hold, but it is clear that an imbalance of oestrogen levels are the key factor.

In the USA, 33 per cent of women have had a hysterectomy by 60 years of age; in Australia, 20 per cent of women have undergone the procedure by age 50 and, in Britain, 20 per cent have had a hysterectomy by age 55.[14, 15, 16] Many doctors feel that one-third of hysterectomies performed because of excessive bleeding are unnecessary. Hysterectomy as a panacea for endometriosis has come under considerable scrutiny in recent years. It is a complex procedure and should not be entered into lightly.

The uterus has multiple functions. It is a significant source of prostaglandins and several other hormones. Research suggests that it regulates ovarian hormone production via these prostaglandins, enzymes and the feedback loop to the pituitary gland. The uterus also produces prostacyclin, a hormone which prevents platelets in the blood from clumping together to form clots. Prostacyclin is therefore protective against heart disease.[17] Hysterectomized women who retain their ovaries develop a much higher risk of cardio-vascular disease than women who have never had a hysterectomy. They are also at greater risk of osteoporosis and depression.[18] Dr Donna Shoupe, professor of obstetrics and gynaecology at the Women and Children's Hospital in Los Angeles says that the commonly used statement that 'you don't need our ovaries so we'll just remove them' should be replaced with 'your ovaries protect you from many diseases, they are valuable and are not easily replaced'. There is no other organ in the body where clinicians would argue for removal of a functioning, healthy organ, with the rationale that the patient can take a pill every day for the rest of her life. Ovaries work differently after menopause and still produce some hormones, which protect women from osteoporosis, heart disease, depression and Alzheimer's disease, and promote wellbeing and energy. They should be conserved.[19]

The uterus is an important sex organ. Research by Masters and Johnson shows that, at orgasm, the uterus contracts and rises, undergoing a series of contractions which may be helpful in transporting sperm to the Fallopian tubes. At hysterectomy, some of the nerves connected to the uterus are severed. These nerves also supply the clitoris and upper thigh.

Dr Stanley West, an infertility specialist at St Vincent's Hospital in New York, states that 90 per cent of all hysterectomies are unnecessary and that the only appropriate reason for this procedure would be for treating cancer of the reproductive organs.[20] Laser laparoscopy and conservative surgery are clearly preferable to hysterectomy for the majority of cases of endometriosis.

Take your time to make the decision, find out as much as you can about it, and discuss it in depth with your partner, doctor and other women sufferers. Recent information shows that pelvic damage can ensue.

Cathryn F of Manchester

I was 24 when I found out I had moderate/severe endometriosis, diagnosed by laparoscopy. I'd had excruciatingly painful periods since I was 15 that frequently resulted in my blacking out, nausea and vomiting, and severe contraction-like pain. I had seen doctor after doctor, and been given all manner of explanations that mostly revolved around 'you just have painful periods, get used to it' or 'it's just your body settling down', and all sorts of treatment suggestions, including prescriptions to every kind of pill and analgesic. There was even the suggestion that I have a baby (at 16) and that I take up football.

None of these helped at all and it took great courage, hope and a lot of persuasion to keep going back to traditional medical services. I believed that my body's pain was an indicator of a problem with my physical health and, because of the organs it was affecting, that my fertility was also likely to be affected. I found it impossible to find anyone who would take my concerns about my physical health or particularly my fertility seriously. 'You must be ovulating or you wouldn't be experiencing this pain, so don't worry about it.'

My consultant prescribed Zoladex – injections in the stomach for six months – but I derived absolutely no benefit from this. In response to my questions about diet and nutrition, my consultant told me that endometriosis is a chronic, degenerative pelvic disease which had nothing to do with diet or nutrition, and as there was nothing I could do about it, I should stay away from the 'cranks' at the Endometriosis Society. He believed that surgery was the only option for me.

I had a more positive experience with alternative therapies. I tried acupuncture, which seemed to alleviate some of the more intense pain caused by the 'contractions', and I also tried traditional herbal remedies. I cannot say how I would have been without the herbs; they may have stabilized my hormonal system, but I noticed no obvious signs of improvement with them. I had tests done to determine my nutritional status and took the recommended

CASE STUDY

supplements. I also made a lot of changes to my lifestyle – changed my job from working as a child psychologist to working as a marine ranger and researcher with wild dolphins. All in all, however, the endometriosis was still greatly interfering with my life. Two days per cycle were completely written off; the blackouts and severe pain were still frequent and, due to the unpredictability of my cycle, I never had any idea when the pain would hit me.

I researched as much as I could on the Internet, and read any material I could find to try to learn from other women's experiences. A lot of the case studies I came across related amazing transformations overnight in response to one or other remedy. I didn't give up, but my hope for a miracle cure was more or less dead. All the nutritional information I found focused on minimizing dairy, sugar, caffeine and alcohol, and taking supplements. For two years, I improved my diet, reduced all the problem foods and took handfuls of supplements, but with little noticeable improvement in my health or pain levels.

I came across Dian's book and made an appointment. I cut out dairy completely and took more supplements – no change. Then Dian mentioned that some women found that cutting out wheat made a great difference. I had never heard about this in all the research I had done. I agreed to try it for one cycle, expecting absolutely no improvement.

I could not believe the difference when my period came round. I was hopping and skipping about – absolutely no pain, no blacking out, no nausea, no nothing! I reintroduced wheat the month after (still not really believing), and back came the pain. I have been wheat-free for nearly one year now and worried that the pain will slowly creep back, but it hasn't. I still get very tired and 'spaced out', but there is no pain. Eating wheat-free takes a little more thought and preparation, but there are some good recipe books around and some great alternatives to wheat flour.

I still don't feel that I understand the cause of my endometriosis. My periods are still irregular, and my fertility – if I believe the medical doctors – is severely compromised, but my life is now my own. It has given me new hope and reminded me again that I do not need to aim for or settle for anything less than optimum health. My hope now is that I can find the key to my fertility. Thanks, Dian.

PREGNANCY INDUCTION

Having a child is a life choice, not a treatment for endometriosis. The high levels of pregnancy hormones seem to suppress endometriosis in most cases. Unfortunately, this is a Catch-22 situation – endometriosis appears to impair fertility while pregnancy inhibits endometriosis. But pregnancy is not always desirable at a time when a woman's reproductive system appears to be very sick. Looking after a baby while in pain from endometriosis is not a life choice many women would want to make. The benefit of pregnancy in reducing endometriotic implants has been noted in many cases, but the duration of this benefit after the child is born is highly unpredictable. Some women go for years after a pregnancy with no symptoms of endometriosis, while others have endometriosis symptoms as soon as one month after the birth of their child. Discussion and information should be key factors in helping to make the right decision. There are many considerations: 'breastfeeding every seven hours for two years has also been suggested to keep endometriosis at bay'.[21]

For women with endometriosis who want to have children, getting pregnant would have the double benefit of conception with remission of endometriosis symptoms. The two major medical treatments for enhancing the chances of getting pregnant are:

1   Ovarian superstimulation coupled with interuterine insemination (IUI) or normal intercourse.
2   *In vitro* fertilization (IVF).

These techniques are called assisted reproductive technology (ART).

Another path to follow would be nutritional medicine – healthy eating and taking nutritional supplements for four to six months before attempting a pregnancy. This third path is *natural*, with no side effects other than improving wellbeing. It enhances the couple's reproductive health, which can only be of benefit to the forthcoming child.

ARTIFICIAL INSEMINATION OR INTERUTERINE INSEMINATION (IUI)

There are several drugs a gynaecologist can administer that stimulate the ovary to produce more and larger follicles and improve your chances of getting pregnant. The two major types of drugs used to stimulate the ovary are either drugs that 'fool' the pituitary gland into producing extra FSH and LH, or drugs that contain FSH and/or LH. Once the physician has stimulated the ovary to be more active, at the anticipated time of ovulation, the patient can then either have sexual intercourse or undergo IUI. FSH may either be recombinant human FSH or a genetically engineered form of FSH. Discuss their use with your consultant.

The benefit of artificial insemination is that a larger number of sperm can be placed close to the area of fertilization and thus increase the chances of getting pregnant. The drugs used to stimulate the ovary can be quite expensive. However, the increased chances of pregnancy offered by IUI may be desired by many couples. One possible drawback to ovarian stimulation is that the high levels of steroids, such as Clomid, Pergonal and Gonal-F, present during this procedure can also stimulate the endometriotic implants and increase the symptoms of endometriosis as well as enlarge ovarian cysts. This is again a Catch-22 situation. Being informed is vital in order to make the right personal decision. Read and research well.

Questionable evidence has been presented that suggests the high concentrations of reproductive hormones that are present during ovarian superstimulation may be harmful to ovarian well-being. Dr Kamal Ahuja of the IVF fertility centre at Cromwell Hospital in London has cited 60 studies in the *Journal of Human Reproduction*, representing hundreds of cases of ovarian cancer reported worldwide that may be linked to fertility drugs.

IN VITRO FERTILIZATION (IVF)

ART treatments involve risks, as research has shown: 'Both the mothers who conceived multiple gestations by means of IVF and their neonates are at an increased risk of having multiple morbidities. The IVF infants had longer hospitalizations, respiratory distress and had to be given oxygen therapy. It is concluded that IVF couples are at increased risk of giving birth to low birth weight infants.'[22] It may be that couples wish to run these risks and try to become pregnant by artificial means. In any event, all the ethical dilemmas should be explained by the staff at each unit to couples thinking of undertaking these procedures. Other research has looked into the risk to mothers who have been exposed to the fertility drugs involved in IVF procedures, as there have been concerns that these procedures may be associated with breast and ovarian cancers. The suggestion is that long-term follow-up examinations of these women should be undertaken to analyse the risk statistically.[23]

The authors of this book would recommend that couples try the least harsh method first, which would involve healthy lifestyle changes to diet, patterns of exercise and relaxation – all of which cost very little – before embarking on costly IVF procedures. By taking the simple option first, there is nothing to lose and everything to gain.

It is interesting that women are given ovulation-blocking drugs to prevent pregnancy. Then, later on in life, when the ovaries are inefficient, they are offered drugs to overstimulate the ovary.

In vitro fertilization (IVF) is a complicated and very expensive procedure. It can, however, be a means of getting pregnant. The reason that IVF is effective is related to the aggressive nature of the procedure. In IVF the ovary is superstimulated to produce an excess of eggs (rather than just one) and these eggs are removed from the ovary before ovulation by inserting a needle through the wall of the vagina and directly into the ovary, under ultrasound control.[24] The eggs are sucked from the ovary into a test tube, placed in a dish with the sperm and sometimes fertilization occurs. The resulting embryos are then transferred, by a long thin tube, through the cervix and into the uterus. These procedures can be physically, emotionally and financially stressful and have less than a 10 per cent success rate for women with endometriosis. (Remember, in the endometriosis patient, the peritoneal fluid contains the chemical secretions from the endometriotic implant which may damage the egg or sperm and prevent conception.)

Many scientists and physicians have debated whether or not IVF has any substantial benefit in getting the endometriosis patient pregnant.[25] Research has indicated that IVF has the same benefit as Danazol in increasing the pregnancy rate – 10 per cent. However, other research suggests that the older endometriosis patient (over 35 years of age) has a better chance of getting pregnant with IVF than any other treatment.[26] Patients with autoimmune antibodies benefit more from IVF plus immunosuppressive drug treatment.[27]

Despite the cost of treatment, success cannot be guaranteed: 'Treatments cost several thousands of pounds or dollars so that only couples with sufficient disposable income can afford this path. Live births following IVF treatments range from 23.3 per cent to 4.8 per cent at clinics in Britain, the national average being only 14.2 per cent.'[28] This means that the top rate is 23.3 live births for every 100 treatment cycles. Almost 20,000 women in the UK had test-tube baby treatment in the year ending March 1995. Costs range from £3,000 to £5,000 per cycle, but financial concerns are not the only consideration: 'Since the Human Fertilization and Embryology Act came into force in 1991, more than 500,000 human embryos have been created. Fewer than half are used in treatment and by March 1996 about 20,000 babies had been born.'[29] It is suggested that 'nutritional medicine should play a role in handicap prevention and medical treatment of infertility alongside IVF and GIFT'.[30]

There are concerns that use of these techniques is increasing too rapidly. Researchers at a Dutch university in 1995 found that the fetuses of five out of 12 women conceived through micro-assisted fertilization received the father's male infertility genes.[31]

Speroff and Walsh (1987) quote healthcare costs for infertility in the 1980s as $200 million (£125 million) per year; it must now be much more.[32] Combining orthodox fertility treatment with sound nutritional principles can only have beneficial consequences for both the health and the wallet. In England the highest average success rate for IVF is 23.3 per cent; in the USA, this is nearer 30 per cent. In combination with nutritional counselling, this rate could increase greatly. One only has to look at the Foresight success rate of 86 per cent when nutritional advice is given together with eradication of genitourinary infections. Costs are much lower for nutrition consultations (£30–£50 per hour) than IVF treatment, and for fresh foods and supplements for a few months. The cost per IVF is, on average, £1,750 per cycle.

With IVF, it is now recommended that no more than two embryos be placed in the uterus to avoid multiple pregnancies. The chances of having twins is around 15 per cent.

NUTRITIONAL IMPACT ON FERTILITY IN ASSISTED REPRODUCTIVE TECHNOLOGY

Vitamin C is vital to uterine health. In Japan, it was found that 'when giving women who fail to ovulate vitamin C at 400mg per day combined with Clomid [ovarian stimulation], all the women ovulated. It potentiated the effect of the Clomid [ovarian stimulation]'.[33] It is also seen from research that 'vitamin E prevents miscarriage by allowing the embryo to attach firmly to the uterine wall and a normal placenta to develop around it'.[34]

Clomid has side effects such as weight gain, breast tenderness, abdominal bloating and discomfort. Perganol likewise notes oedema as a side effect.[35] Zoladex and Danazol list weight gain as a side effect.[36] These side effects can have far-reaching consequences: 'Women placed on these medications are often found to be uncomfortable with the amount of weight gained and put themselves on a reducing diet, thus cutting down the essential nutrients available to them.'[37] At a time when women are seeking to become pregnant, they are reducing their nutrient intake. This would appear to be the very worst time to try to diet. IVF treatment is expensive; in addition to the treatment the couple should concentrate on eating well to maximize the chances of a pregnancy. Remember that fertility increases with a rising body weight and decreases with a falling body weight.

ANALGESICS

Painkilling drugs can be taken to reduce the pain of endometriosis, and coping with pain is dealt with in detail in chapter 4. The most common pain suppressants are anti-prostaglandin drugs (such as aspirin, Motrin and Distalgesic). These antiprostaglandin drugs inhibit the production of prostaglandin E and prostaglandin F, which are produced in large amounts by the endometriotic implant. Unfortunately, the disease itself is not affected by analgesics, so endometriosis will continue to develop unchecked, but with a reduction (dulling) of pain symptoms. Because of this, analgesics are usually used in conjunction with the other therapies. Analgesics may also contain caffeine: 'Caffeine is a weak stimulant that is often included in small doses in analgesic preparations. It is claimed that the addition of caffeine may enhance the analgesic effect, but the alerting effect, mild habit-forming effect and possible provocation of headache may not always be desirable.'[38]

ANTIHISTAMINES

Antihistamines (which inhibit histamine production) can be short acting and in high doses have the disadvantage of causing drowsiness. As histamine release can be quite strong around endometriotic implants, antihistamines can sometimes be beneficial in pain reduction. Some antihistamines must never be taken with grapefruit juice. A substance in the juice called furanocoumarin attaches to an enzyme in the small intestine, which normally breaks down drugs. Prescription drug doses take account of that process, but because the furanocoumarin in the juice blocks this enzyme, it greatly increases the potency of the drug.

Drugs taken for allergies, high blood pressure and heart disease can therefore be too strong.[39] (If you take antihistamines, ask your pharmacist for advice about the brand you use.) Vitamin C is also a powerful antihistamine and this may be why it appears to reduce endometriosis pain in many women, especially when combined with bioflavonoids.

ETHICAL DECISIONS ABOUT TREATMENTS

With so many different and sometimes drastic treatments available, it can be bewildering as to which way to turn and which direction to choose: 'Decisions can only be made on a basis of information and if a woman is not properly informed about the diagnosis or treatment of her condition, her chances of making a meaningful choice are diminished.'[40] Doctors often use highly technical language which makes it difficult sometimes to follow their gist. The doctor and consultant are in their roles to heal, and they may find it very difficult, even uncomfortable, to be faced with a patient who has a disease for which there is no cure: 'Doctors have been trained to be positive and helpful to patients and they do not like to send them away empty-handed.'[41] Knowing that with the placebo effect 30 per cent of people may get well even when given sugar tablets, many GPs are reluctant to be totally honest about drug side effects.

There is at present no definitive medical cure for endometriosis, but if you become informed and work with a nutritionist, you might be able to relieve the pain and subfertility. Women often comment that their quality of life improves after nutritional counselling.

The shock of being diagnosed with a chronic condition brings its own anxiety and fear. Modern Western medicine conforms to our cultural myth that the body can be controlled; we always want to believe that someone can 'make it better'. In a clinical situation, lack of knowledge, lack of information, or lack of instruction, can provoke even more anguish.

Informed consent is extremely important, and there are ethical choices for both doctor and patient to make before choosing the treatment most appropriate to you as a unique individual. Building up a relationship of trust and confidence with your doctor is vital.[42] Providing information can itself lessen the pain, anxiety and tension. No doctor can do anything to a patient without his or her consent, and coercion should never be used. Each woman has a right to know how the drugs and surgery will affect her body, so information should be forthcoming from the health professional in each case. If a consultant expects you to comply to treatment without you being fully informed, you may need politely to question further about the efficacy (effectiveness) of the treatment.

The law ensures that your doctor should not have a hidden agenda when prescribing your treatment: 'Doctors, dentists and pharmacists who accept inducements to prescribe or supply medicines and other health products will also face fines of up to £5,000 or, in the most flagrant cases, a maximum of two years in jail. The move is in response to the increasingly lavish scale of gifts and other rewards being offered by some pharmaceutical companies and wholesalers, in an attempt to win orders. Offers which alarmed ministers include competitions with prizes of holidays or video cameras, and in one case bottles of wine simply for ordering a particular medicine. A government minister agrees that the public does not expect health-care professionals to be influenced in their decisions by incentives to prescribe or supply particular medicines.'[43] In America the American Medical Association has also clamped down on such practices.

Never assume that you are being given all information available, always dig a little deeper. Some charities are controlled by drug company interests and will only give one side of the story in order to boost sales. There are always two sides to a coin.

Health professionals should always work towards the good of the patient. Pellegrino, a medical ethics expert, gives his sense of the patient's good as 'the good most proper to being human', and that this 'involves the right to make choices, to plan for one's future and aim at goals, so that each individual is given the respect of patient dignity and human freedom'.[44] Whatever decision is made, it should come from the information given by the medical staff involved in a patient's case. Never be afraid to ask for more information if it is not clear.

The final decisions can only be guided with competent discussion between you and your consultant. 'They focus their (and our) attention on cures and imminent cures, on successful medical interventions, research funding and medical care and are more directed toward life-threatening conditions than toward nursing for chronic illness and disabilities'[45] is a criticism that has been levelled at the medical profession. Try to achieve a balanced exchange of information: 'The medical intervention should be modifying the disease using the craftsmanship of the physician or surgeon. Plus there is the sense of good as the patient's own concept for his or her own good, which takes into consideration what the patient feels is worth while and in their best interests.'[46] Most people know little or nothing about how to live with long-term or life-threatening illness; how to communicate with doctors and nurses about these matters; or how to live with uncertainty and pain when doctors cannot make them go away. Patient support groups have arisen to fill this gap for people suffering from every type of illness and disability. Some forward-thinking doctors even run doctor/patient forums to share information about how diseases impinge on life.

We need to consider the ways in which we create new life. The practice of IVF means that thousands of embryos are created, some of which are implanted, others are used for research, others destroyed. With HFEA approval, embryologists decide which ones are to be screened out. At the extreme, IVF can be a bad science with unscrupulous multi-million pound pharmaceutical companies using children like commodities.[47] Yet, with nutritional guidance, eating well and using supplements for three months, women who have tried IVF without success have become pregnant. Try this simple, healthy route first before resorting to other treatments.

We need to aim for preventive medicine, to prevent the endometriosis and infertility from taking hold in the first place, but also to encourage all health professionals to listen and respect what the patient feels is right for her as an individual.

> Human destiny is bound to remain a gamble, because, at some unpredictable time and in some unforeseeable manner, nature will strike back.
>
> *Rene Dubos,* Mirage of Health, *1959*

Studies show that, in America, 'at present hysterectomy is the most performed major operation for American women between the ages of 15 and 45; the average age of elective surgery is 35 years. In 1985 one million women were given hysterectomy and over 35 million American women have had hysterectomies. Over half these women had their ovaries removed as well, even if the organs were not diseased. A half of all women in the USA have undergone hysterectomy by the age of 65 years.'[48] In the UK the situation is not dissimilar: '... 53 per cent of general practitioners believe that hysterectomy should be used only as a last resort in menorrhagia; 14 per cent of all UK women will have a hysterectomy before the age of 65 to solve this problem.'[49] The level of hysterectomy varies widely from country to country and from area to area: 'In California, barely half of all women will carry their uterus to the grave, whereas a gynaecologist in Saudia Arabia may do no more than one hysterectomy per year. Perceived abnormal bleeding accounts for 70 per cent of all hysterectomies in premenopausal British women. About one woman in seven will decline a hysterectomy if she can be shown to have blood loss in the normal range.'[50] We all have to ensure that only essential hysterectomies are performed and that other treatment options are always offered. Informed choice is your key here. Ensure that you are always given sufficient information to make the right choice for your unique circumstances. Choose only that option that feels right to you. Always take the time to read your consent form completely and be sure that you agree fully with all the terms before any surgical procedure is undertaken. You can write on the consent form which treatments you agree to and which ones you refuse to undergo.

All treatment decisions should be made on the basis of knowledge as to how they may affect your future health. The outcome is important as it impinges on the rest of your life. Try to become informed and make an informed decision. Join one of the endometriosis support groups around the world, as they will support you and keep you informed.

COMMUNICATING WITH YOUR DOCTOR

Making yourself understood during the few precious minutes you have with your doctor is vital. You will need to understand his or her point of view in order to communicate effectively. Express yourself articulately. You may need to take along a list with helpful reminders on points you wish to raise. You could also jot down any advice you are given. You will then be in a position to discuss your treatment options and explain any anxieties you may have. Occasionally the doctor may record on cassette the advice which he gives, so that the implications can be fully understood when listened to again in the comfort of your home.

Many people are overawed by doctors' authority, since they are experts in their field and have so much knowledge. One often feels obliged to accept their suggestions without question. This only becomes a problem when we feel unhappy about a particular treatment. However, you have rights as an individual and as a patient, and there are many ways in which you can help yourself become more assertive in expressing your needs and desires.

Concrete steps you can take include making sure that you have the right doctor and becoming educated yourself about endometriosis. Local endometriosis groups usually know which doctors in their locale are the most sympathetic to the symptoms you experience. By understanding the symptoms and treatments available for endometriosis, you will be able to converse intelligently with your doctor. Analyse what your aims in treatment are – having a baby or eliminating endo-related pain. Explain these goals to your doctor and persist in finding a way to achieve them. Indicate any self-help methods you are using. In this way you should be taken more seriously.

Obtaining feedback from partners, close friends or those in a similar predicament can also be useful. It helps to put all the ideas and options into perspective. Other women with the condition may have been along the same route as you and can offer sympathy, as well as make practical suggestions. Talking through the options will help you to clarify your own position. As a unique individual, your decision depends upon what you consider right for you. Always listen to other people's ideas and experiences, but you must then analyse every fact before deciding which path is the best one for you to take. We all have a sixth sense and know in our hearts what is right or wrong for us. Follow your instinct as to what is appropriate for you.

Finally, if after this much effort on your part, you are not receiving the kind of health care you require, you may consider asking for a second opinion. It is no sin to disagree with your doctor and should you be unhappy with any of the advice you are given, you are entitled to ask for an appointment with another doctor. The following checklist may help you:

- Is the doctor giving you respect as a person in your own right?
- Does the doctor believe that all the symptoms you describe are related to endometriosis, or does he/she suggest that you are exaggerating the pain, or that other conditions may be complicating the diagnosis? Are you being taken seriously?
- Do you feel reassured that your doctor is listening with compassion to all the symptoms you are describing. Does he/she believe what you are trying to explain?
- What happens when your problem becomes urgent? Does the doctor see you quickly or do you have to make an appointment days ahead?
- When your GP responds to you, is he/she expressing things in ways you can understand, or is he/she spouting jargon?
- Can you put your trust in this doctor?
- Does this doctor have your complete faith when it comes to operations? Has the doctor been open and informative about the surgical techniques and drug treatments beforehand (especially important if this is a new technique or part of a drug trial as medical ethics are then involved)?
- Do you feel confident that this doctor is open and honest with you about all the treatments which may be available? Any doctor should be comfortable with being a part of your healing team. If not, change doctors.

When you are chronically ill, it can be difficult to appear self-assured, and doctors often misconstrue the distress of the condition as a woman being weak and emotional. Taking a friend along to the consultation for moral support can be helpful under these circumstances. Feeling drained is often a part of this disease pattern; the body is ill and trying to tell us that it needs nurturing back to health. Don't feel guilty about being ill. Just listen to your body. Perhaps it is asking for a rest.

MEDICALLY TRAINED DOCTORS AND NUTRITIONAL ADVICE

Be aware that your doctor may not have received much training in nutrition: 'On average medically trained doctors only spend between 7 to 14 days during their 7-year training actually studying aspects of nutrition.'[51] However, most nutritionists have spent three to four years studying their subject, some many more. Nutrition is crucial to health and is the mainstay of preventive medicine. When the World Health Organization states that over one-third of all cancers develop as a result of poor diet, we wonder what other illnesses we could avoid if we all ate healthier diets.

A recent report indicated that only 20–25 per cent of medical schools run nutrition courses. Nutrition was perceived as a 'soft' topic and was not considered as a science amongst physicians. It was found that 'nutrition knowledge was low amongst physicians in practice and that this decreased with the number of years in practice. Lack of time was cited as a barrier to doctors discussing disease prevention with patients and many doctors had little confidence in their ability to change health behaviour in their patients.'[52] Dr Alan Levin, a doctor of environmental medicine in the USA, states that, 'Even today in the medical schools, preventive medicine and nutrition are very, very minor courses. Everybody laughs at them ... The important things are pharmacology, internal medicine, surgery, and how to deal with a disease once it happens. They are not concerned with altering people's diets or environments so that they don't develop a disease.'[53] Doctors do not study body biochemistry or metabolism, so they do not understand the way nutrients work as part of enzymatic and hormonal systems.

The World Health Organization stated in 1973 that all doctors should work alongside a nutritionist and yet, over a quarter of a century later, there is still no sign of this. Nutrition is complementary to orthodox medicine and the one can help the other. The main problem is that nutrients are natural, and drug companies cannot patent natural products like vitamins and minerals so they cannot make money from their sales. Only formulated chemical drugs invented by pharmaceutical companies and unique to their laboratories can be formally patented, enabling big profits to be made. Food is often seen by governments as a commodity, not as a health-giving substance. It is sold for profit, not for health, so food standards often fall short of what our bodies desire. Meldrum states that, 'nutritional therapies ... improve both health promotion/prevention and treatment/care services at no extra cost in the short term and with the prospect of a reduction of costs in the medium to long term'.[54]

Trained nutritionists work with their clients to assess biochemical individuality by looking at nutritional status, using blood and tissue tests. They work on a one-to-one basis to correct any imbalances and resolve symptoms. They examine the root of the problem to elicit a cure, rather than just suppress symptoms, and will, for example, look at strengthening the immune and reproductive systems. They support the client through changes in eating patterns, encouraging the choice of foods which are nutrient-rich rather than high in empty calories, thus improving nutrient intake; and they may suggest nutritional supplements for three to four months to help correct imbalances.

Consultations with a nutritionist normally last for one hour and people are seen on average four times. To be effective, nutrition requires perseverance and skills in food choice, and this comes with encouragement. With face-to-face, one-to-one guidance and counselling, clients feel the support and see the results of nutritional medicine. It is a delight when women return exuberant after a couple of months to say what a massive impact changes in eating patterns and supplements have had on improving their quality of life. They have more energy and normal pain-free peiods once we discover what is triggering the pain. If doctors and nutritionists could work together towards improving health, great leaps in healthcare and particularly fertility treatment could be made.

Nutrition consultations should be part and parcel of all healthcare programmes. This is particularly important after stillbirth and miscarriages. Seek out a well-qualified nutritionist in your area and talk with him or her. Most practitioners offer a free 15-minute consultation first to consider the options open to you.

If you try, you might. If you don't, you won't.

W Pickles

SUMMARY

1 There is no known medical cure for endometriosis at present.

2 Traditional medicine can suppress endometriosis symptoms with a variety of strategies including: drug therapies which stimulate pseudopregnancy or menopause to suppress endometriotic implants; surgical therapies which remove the implants; pregnancy induction; analgesics or antihistamines to dull pain.

3 Become informed. Whatever decision is made should be based on the information that you have been given honestly by the medical staff involved in your case. Also read books, scan the internet (*see* www.makingbabies.com, www.nutrition.us.com and www. endometriosis.co.uk) and talk to other women.

4 A good line of communication must be established between the endometriosis patient and her physician for trust to develop.

5 Medical treatments can be beneficial if the patient has faith in her doctor's care and knowledge. If you think your doctor needs more knowledge, there are a vast number of information leaflets provided by endometriosis associations around the world. Their aim is to help educate health professionals in the immensity of the impact on life from this disease.

6 If you have seen more than four physicians, then nutrition is a possible answer. See a nutritionist for a full assessment of the underlying nutritional imbalances.

7 Work with your body to help it to heal. It needs clean, fresh water, natural daylight, rest and relaxation and, above all, fresh, unadulterated food free from chemicals, pesticides and additives.

One who eats whole food will be strong and healthy.

Okinawan proverb

7 The holistic approach to endometriosis

Edison's electric lamp is a completely idiotic idea.

Sir William Preece, FRS
Post Office Chief Engineer, UK, 1876

Truth is not known until it happens. Some holistic therapies work whether they appear to have a scientific reason behind them or not. There are things in heaven and on earth which our science does not yet understand.

Your health is dependent upon fresh air, clean water, a variety of nutritious foods, your living conditions, cleanliness and good hygiene. We have a modicum of control over these things. We cannot change the genes that we have inherited. But it is suggested by some research that 'whilst nutrition (or specific nutrients) cannot negate one's ultimate genetic fate, it can modify the time frame during which the characteristics of this fate appear. Some nutrients turn on or turn off the expression of specific genes, and genes can affect the use of specific nutrients'.[1]

Your body is not just a set of disparate organs. Modern medicine has broken the body into compartments for treatment, but that is not how the body works. Each system is linked to the other by receptor cells which send chemical messengers to each other. It is like networking, or living in symbiosis – you scratch my back and I'll scratch yours. If one system begins to fail, the others will rally round and take the burden to allow healing to take place. The body works as a whole and we have to treat it as such.

How do you really feel? When we ask someone the question 'How are you?', the majority of people politely say, 'I'm okay, thank you', even when what is going on in their mind may be totally different. They could have a backache, headache, sore throat, or indeed any of a myriad of minor problems that often lurk behind our usual facade.

It is amazing that we tend to ignore what our bodies are trying to tell us. The headaches, bad period pains, constant infections and sore throats, stomach aches and that awful tired feeling (as though you are up to your knees in a tin of treacle) all happen for a reason. Why do we consistently ignore these warning signs? This is our body's way of letting us know something is going awry. In fact, sometimes the body positively shouts at us. But we ignore it as life rushes past at an alarming rate, and we have to keep up, so we push ourselves to the limit.

Life has far more stressors and strains than ever before. Worrying about where the next meal is coming from is not so much of a problem any more. We do not have to chase our prey or go out gathering and foraging; it is all neatly packaged in the supermarket. We go along and pick out the ready-made meals, place them in our home freezer and take them out when we need them. In the evenings when we return from work we are often too exhausted to cook anyway.

If we are ill and have to take time off work, it is the pits. We feel so guilty knowing our desk will be covered with mountains of outstanding work, so we rush back to the normal routine before we are properly cured. People often return to work too soon, before the immune system has restored itself to a strong position, ready for the next onslaught of bacteria and viruses to hit our systems. In the olden days there were convalescent homes where we were allowed to be ill, and where the staff nursed us back to health over several weeks. Good food was served and, as we began to heal, we worked in the gardens growing fresh vegetables for our meals. That brief respite from daily life with clean air and good food allowed the immune system to renew itself. That really was a holistic approach.

A holistic approach to illness can cover different angles. There is not much point in trying too many therapies at once. You need to choose one or two therapies with which you feel comfortable. We all have a sixth sense which many of us try to ignore. In order to be 'in tune' with our own bodies' needs we have to sense what is best for us. This is a part of being true to yourself – knowing what feels right and what feels wrong.

> In order to know the future, it is necessary first to know the present in all its details, as well as to know the past. Today is what it is because yesterday was what it was. And if today is like yesterday, tomorrow will be like today. If you want to be different, you must make today different.
>
> *G I Gurdjieff (1915), Mira*

Seena M of Devon

I decided to follow the 'complementary' path of treatment for my endometriosis and infertility which included acupuncture, homeopathy and nutrition. In addition I had the support and prayers of my husband, friends and family. I now have two extremely healthy, bright children – Verity, aged 3, and Henry, 8 months. I fed Verity till she was 18 months and intend to do the same with Henry. I have had no more pain despite my periods returning about 8–10 weeks after both births and, considering they were both by Caesarean section, I feel incredibly fit and healthy. Which therapy helped the most? I'm sure they were all just part of the whole but the results are wonderful and five years ago it was difficult to contemplate such a happy end to my story. Thank you.

CASE STUDY

It helps to know that you are not alone with the pain of endometriosis, that while you are curled up with a pillow in bed, other women are in pain at that same moment.

Some women find joining a support group helps to share the steps forward, or at least talking with the local group leader for support.

Endometriosis is like a game of snakes and ladders. One day you feel so ill and the next you feel 'normal'. It is so good to feel normal again, you can overdo it and relapse the following day. There is a trick in knowing when to rest. Giving in to pain can be distressing and many women tend to push themselves too hard. The immune system renews itself when the body is at rest, so quality time for yourself is valuable to the healing process.

Knowing how to help yourself heal is also important. A combination of orthodox and complementary medicine may be suitable for you. Sometimes a medicine will work for you and at other times it won't. One treatment style may be useful on its own, but occasionally two will enhance each other. Because we are each unique human beings, what works for one person will not always help another. But modern medicine tends to treat us all the same, even when it is so obvious that we are completely different, inside and out. You need to find the right path for you by a process of trial and error.

As Charles Duell (Director of US Patent Office, 1899) believed: 'Everything that can be invented has been invented!' But there is much we still have to learn about the workings of the human body. Even the workings of some of the drugs offered to you for endometriosis are not fully understood. There are many paths left unexplored, and one of them is the role of nutrients in the endocrine and immune systems. As drug companies can make no money from selling these nutrients, they see no point in doing the research.

The term 'biochemical individuality', coined by Dr Roger Williams, implies that each of us has a subtly different body biochemistry. Organs are slightly different shapes; enzymes work at different levels; drugs work in slightly different ways.[2] But finding the combination of therapies that is right for you is where your sixth sense comes into play – listen to what your body tells you feels right.

RELAXATION

Every day you need to take 'time out' for 20 minutes and allow yourself space to just be. Relaxation time is very important when the rest of life is so stressed. Your body requires a period of rest each day to recharge the immune system. Research has shown the body heals much faster while we are asleep. At first it can be nigh on impossible to relax if you are used to doing everything for everybody. Choose something to help you relax. Lie in the bath with favourite music and candles; go for a walk; spend time on a hobby you really enjoy; or spend time with a valued friend – just sharing life can be very valuable. Let the world rush by you for a change, while you step into your own area of peace for your special moments. We stretch ourselves to the limit and those few minutes of relaxation, which you deserve, may help your body to begin to recover. Do not feel guilty, everyone is entitled to some time for themselves. Your body deserves a rest for healing purposes. Be kind to yourself, as you are unique in the universe.

Liz N of Yorkshire

I have continued to eat a healthy diet based on the principles you outlined. I have also bought the books Optimum Nutrition *and the* Fatburner Diet *by P Holford. This has helped my overall general wellbeing and I try to do regular exercise to keep fit, and get fresh air and natural light to help my psychological state. Overall this strategy (including the vitamin supplementation) has helped me to keep my endo under control. Certainly the other symptoms, such as PMS, mood swings, irritability and anxiety, have all decreased. I use homeopathy and reflexology, both of which improve my feeling of wellbeing to a limited extent but they did not affect the underlying endo.*

EXERCISE

If possible, take a short walk after your evening meal as this will aid your digestive processes as well as help you relax. You could take up an exercise (this does not have to be as hard as aerobics and jogging). A gentle walk or swim will help your muscles increase their mitochondria (cell organelles which produce energy, *see* chapter 2). The more mitochondria you have in your muscles, the more energy you can make.

Exercise not only tones the muscles and keeps the heart and lungs fit, it also stimulates your digestive tract to help you digest food effectively and excrete harmful substances more rapidly. You are also making the lymphatic system work by triggering movement of the lymph, so that the white blood cells of the immune army move around the body.

Exercise also raises the levels of endorphins (brain chemicals which act as natural painkillers) in the bloodstream, which also help to elevate your mood. Feeling positive can help to stimulate the immune system. Exercise also aids the proper excretion of oestrogen and cholesterol from the body. Research has shown that oestrogen and cholesterol when bound to fibre are excreted in greater amounts when exercise is undertaken (*see* pp. 196, 212 and 282), which prevents them from recirculating and causing health problems.

If you are in great pain from endometriosis you may not feel like aerobics or jogging, but gentle walks, swimming for pleasure or yoga may help to move stiff muscles. A short, brisk walk of 20 minutes, three times a week, also helps to put calcium into bones to prevent osteoporosis. If you exercise in daylight and eat sufficient zinc- and vitamin B6-rich foods, then your pituitary gland functions effectively to produce the hormone signals necessary for ovarian function.

Never stress the body with too much exercise, be moderate. Over-exercising is stressful and uses up the body intake of B vitamins, zinc and magnesium, the very nutrients the pituitary and ovary most require. (This is why athletes and ballerinas who train constantly and are underweight often have amenorrhoea [lack of periods]. Their BMI is too low and they may become deficient in nutrients vital to the ovaries.)

NATURAL DAYLIGHT

Research has revealed the importance of natural daylight for health: 'The retina of the eye and its zinc and vitamin B2 level are crucial in the formation of hormones. When the eye registers the presence of light, a signal is sent to the hypothalamus in the brain. The hypothalamus then begins to produce hormones that trigger the pituitary gland which, in turn, instigates production of the sex hormones by the ovaries. The pituitary produces gonadotrophic hormones which stimulate the ovaries or testes to produce the female and male sex hormones.'[3] We all require 20 minutes of natural daylight each day on the retina of the eye to begin this process. If you work in an office with fluorescent lights, it is important that you escape at lunchtime and take a walk, especially in the winter months when we travel to and from work in the dark: 'Fluorescent lights impair the function of the pituitary gland ... in natural daylight the ovaries can produce their oestrogen and progesterone.'[4]

Research appears to confirm the connection between natural light and the good health of the reproductive system: 'There is a positive correlation between follicular fluid melatonin and oestradiol. This suggests that melatonin may be involved in the regulation of hormone production in the ovaries.'[5]

Female animals have breeding patterns that are seasonal, as bright light triggers oestrus in some animals. Whether humans have a seasonal breeding cycle remains unanswered. Anecdotal evidence reports that Eskimo/Inuit women cease menstrual cycles in winter. In Finland, the light summery months of June to September have the highest rate of conception. The rate drops during the dark winter months of November to February.[6]

The connection between natural light and female reproductive health in particular was highlighted in a study of women undergoing IVF treatment: 'Follicular fluid samples were obtained from the largest pre-ovulatory follicle of 120 women undergoing *in vitro* fertilization, and were examined for melatonin levels. The concentration of melatonin and progesterone during the autumn and winter (dark) months were significantly higher than those of the spring and summer (light) months. By contrast, oestradiol concentrations were significantly lower during the dark months than during the light months. There was a positive correlation between follicular fluid melatonin and progesterone concentration, and a negative relationship between melatonin and oestradiol. This suggests that melatonin may be involved in the regulation of hormone production in the ovaries.'[7] We can conclude that natural light and zinc intake are very important to our fertility.

HEALTH'S INTANGIBLES

Some researchers feel that there is a mind–body connection to health, and that the pineal gland in the brain may be the link. But whatever the link, the body has an amazing ability to heal itself if we allow it time and space and fill it with healthy air, food and water. Research scientists know that there is a 30 per cent recovery rate from the 'placebo' effect. (A placebo effect is a positive therapeutic effect claimed by a patient after receiving a dummy tablet believed by him to be an active drug.) This may be because they are taking part in a clinical trial and feel they are actually doing something positive to help themselves, or they feel someone is taking care to help them try to get better. One correlation between mind and matter is the disappearance of a serious medical problem when a patient falls in love. Whatever one chooses to call this mental shift, it may be a master key that unlocks healing. Belief, be it healing shrines, drugs or whatever, is a major factor in recovery.[8]

Whatever this mystery factor, it would appear that the combination of trying to help yourself to get better and having someone care that you do get better has a profound effect on health outcomes.

> Behold the turtle: he only makes progress when he sticks his neck out.
> *James B Conant*

RELAXATION TECHNIQUES

Sleep can be elusive when you are in pain. Try going to bed and listening to some favourite music to lull you to sleep, or buy a relaxation, self-hypnosis or sleep tape to talk you through the relaxation techniques. Consider magnesium supplements – 'Magnesium might be of benefit both in calming you down and in helping you sleep at night, as it is a natural tranquilliser with no side effects and no possibility of addiction.'[9] One company (*see* p. 396) produces a pain tape which helps to calm pain down, and they also produce sleep/relaxation/health tapes. There are many ways in which you can try to help yourself and they are not difficult or expensive. Visualization therapy (*see* p. 59) has helped many people with cancer and it may work for you. Prayer can be a powerful tool for some people, as can healing circles.

When you are extremely debilitated and life looks bleak, when friends are getting on with their lives but you are stopped in your tracks by intractable pain, then positive thinking is needed to lift you up. One helpful relaxation tape suggests very simply: 'Stop hating the part of the body that is letting you down. Rather look upon it as a sick little child and love it better.'[10] This has the immediate effect of softening your feelings towards yourself. Hating bits of your body for ruining your life is no help to recovery. What you need to do is accept yourself as being ill, and try to love yourself better. Pamper yourself, put yourself first for a change, get the environment right, reduce the stressors, and let go of the pain and terror and cast it away. By doing all the positive things you can to move forward, even if at first it is only inch by inch, the first steps on the road to health can be taken.

COMPLEMENTARY THERAPIES

A variety of complementary therapies have become popular and may help you to control the symptoms of your endometriosis. (If you wish to further your knowledge in this area, please see the reading list provided at the end of this book.) This section will look briefly at therapies which have helped some women.

NB Always ensure that you are using a qualified practitioner who is insured to treat you. They should have a certificate displayed in their offices and belong to their governing or regulatory body.

Lorraine W of Avon

I was diagnosed with endo after a laparoscopy 18 months ago. After nine months of various hormone treatments and no improvement, I went to see a herbalist. My symptoms were irregular cycles (36–72 days), heavy and painful periods (8–10 days), PMT for two weeks before the period began, weight gain but inability to lose weight, listlessness, distressing hair loss, and spots, irritability and sudden bursts of tears for no apparent reason.

After initial herbal medicine and vitamins and minerals, my condition started to improve. I began an anticandida diet – no fruit for one month only, no refined sugars, no yeasts – and I excluded dairy products as I felt I had an intolerance to them.

It's been five months since I began the diet and I have noticed a big improvement in my condition. My last period was almost pain-free with no PMT. The cycle was 35 days only and the bleed lasted only 6 days. My hair is growing thicker, my skin is improving, and my energy level has increased so much that I can now do a six-mile bike ride each night and keep fit with Callanetics twice a week. I am still taking some vitamins. I have no dairy products, no yeast products, and am trying to keep refined sugars and caffeine to as low a level as possible. My diet is mainly raw and steamed vegetables with stir-fries. I try to follow the Hay system – not mixing starch and proteins – and my digestion has greatly improved and so has my temperature. I always felt cold before.

• C A S E

S T U D Y •

Vis medicatrix naturae – Honour the healing power of Nature.

Hippocrates, 460 BC

ACUPUNCTURE

Many women with endometriosis have been helped by acupuncture. In this ancient Chinese therapy needles are stuck into certain known pressure points or invisible energy channels called 'meridians', which are believed to run between the organs of the body. The needle manipulation is said to unblock channels of energy in the body (called 'Qi'). The body is viewed as a balance between opposing forces, 'yin' and 'yang'. Yin is passive and tranquil, representing darkness, coldness, moisture and swelling. Yang is aggressive and stimulating, representing light, heat, dryness and contraction. Any imbalance is thought to be a cause of illness, for example, too much yin can cause dull aches, pains, chilliness, fluid retention, discharges and tiredness. Always consult a qualified practitioner. Letters after the name include MBAcA, FBAcA, MIROM, MRTCM, MTAS, BAAR, LicAc, BAC, DrAc (*see* p. 392).

AROMATHERAPY

Aromatherapy involves treating illness with essential oils extracted from plants, which are believed to have medicinal qualities. Essential oils are produced by tiny glands in the plants, and these oils are distilled and dissolved in alcohol. In Britain the diluted oils are used mainly for massage treatments or are added to baths, cold compresses or used as inhalations. They are absorbed through the skin into the bloodstream and work internally. You should never swallow the oils. A trial using aromatherapy with sufferers of endometriosis was undertaken, using specific oils. Over half the women in the study experienced a reduction in pain and depression, and had an improved sense of wellbeing. The oils of geranium, bergamot and clary sage are thought to support the reproductive system (*see* p. 51).

BACH REMEDIES

Bach remedies are a series of 38 preparations from wild flowers and plant extracts, first made by Dr E Bach in 1915, and they are available from most good healthfood stores and pharmacies. The remedies are used to treat the whole person, not just the illness from which they are suffering. Bach believed that the dew on the plants was impregnated with their medicinal qualities. He collected this dew, distilled it and dissolved it in alcohol to give to patients. The remedy is chosen according to the patient's psychological and emotional states. The remedies are sold in a concentrated form which needs diluting in spring water. Put four drops of the concentrate into a small amount of water or drop them directly onto the tongue. Bach's Rescue Remedy is popular with women with endometriosis as it seems to speed up recovery from stress, pain and exhaustion. There is no register of practitioners using Bach remedies, though some courses are offered.

BIOCHEMICAL TISSUE SALTS

Biochemical tissue salts are natural mineral salts in tablet form which are essential for health. A lack of these salts or imbalance can cause disease. These salts provide a small, easily absorbed dose to help the body heal itself by restoring the correct balances. There are 12 tissue salts prepared in a homeopathic way. Combination N is for menstrual pain; combination B is for nervous exhaustion, edginess, general debility, and aids convalescence. The tablets are lactose-based, and so are unsuitable for anyone with a milk allergy. They are prescribed by naturopaths, herbalists and homeopaths.

CHIROPRACTIC AND OSTEOPATHY

Using the hands to manipulate the body, chiropractors and osteopaths can correct disorders of the joints, muscles and spine. Spinal problems can cause referred pain in other areas of the body, e.g. the hip or leg. In some cases these problems can be the cause of period pains or constipation. Displacement of lumbars 4 and 5 (vertebrae in the small of the back) can be related to problems in the reproductive area as these hold the ligaments that support the uterus and Fallopian tubes. A twisted pelvis can lead to infertility, as the Fallopian tubes may be twisted away from the ovary, so correcting the tilt may be beneficial. Often, women find they have worsening backache after surgical operations. When the body is unconscious on an operating table being manipulated, sometimes the joints need correcting afterwards. The chiropractor makes greater use of X-rays and conventional methods like ultrasound than do osteopaths. Most chiropractors use the letters DC after their name, but from 1991, chiropractors trained at the Anglo-European College of Chiropractic at Bournemouth, UK, can use BSc Chiropractic. The letters MRO mean 'Member of the Register of Osteopaths', which is regulated by the General Council and Register of Osteopaths in Berkshire, England (*see* p. 399).

HEALING

Some people have the gift of healing by the laying on of hands. This usually is done by someone with a deep faith in their God, and who prays for healing power to flow from God through themselves into the individual seeking healing. Many healers can heal whether or not the person seeking healing is a believer. To find a genuine healer, work through a recognized church or try the addresses on p. 394. Many healings can hardly be called miracles, as they are understandable, given the connection between the body and soul. Spontaneous remissions of disease can and do occur. To understand why, we might have to wait until until our understanding of physics improves. Our bodies comprise chemical, magnetic and electrical impulses which may or may not be involved in the healing process. True healing could never be a part of a money-making racket, so avoid all dubious institutions and seek those which feel full of reverence and peace. Search for sincerity, not charlatans.

HERBAL MEDICINE

Herbal medicine treats the patient as an individual, with individual needs, and not just as another medical case history. Treatment is tailored to the specific requirements of the individual at that moment in time. Knowledge of the power of plants with healing properties has been passed from generation to generation. Indeed, it is the precursor of modern medicine – the use of digitalis (from foxgloves) for heart disease, willow (precursor of aspirin) for headaches, and blue cohosh (known as papoose root in the USA) for infertility. International scientific research not only confirms our knowledge of the healing powers of herbs but also enlarges it.

Trained herbalists have the letters MNIMH or FNIMH after their name, and can be found through the addresses on pp. 395–6.

HOMEOPATHY

Homeopathy first began in 1810 when Samuel Hahnemann discovered that fighting like with like seemed to help people heal. This was well understood by Hippocrates in the fifth century BC. He conjectured that illness symptoms were the body's way of fighting the illness. Hahnemann termed this new medicine 'allopathic', meaning against illness.

The homeopathic approach is based on the whole person, including their mental, spiritual, emotional and physical wellbeing. Therapists can be found through the Royal Homeopathic Hospital (*see* p. 396). There are five NHS homeopathic hospitals – in London, Bristol, Tunbridge Wells, Liverpool and Glasgow, and one private homeopathic clinic in Manchester. Each is staffed by medically qualified homeopathic staff.

HYDROTHERAPY

Easing yourself into a comfortable hot bath can have a very soothing effect on aches and pains. Hydrotherapy (water treatment) is much more specific in its use of water's properties to cure ailments. At the root of this belief is the feeling that water is the essence of life. We are, after all, 70 per cent water! In water's various forms (gas, liquid, solid, steam) it can be used to induce relaxation, to stimulate blood flow, to remove impurities, drugs or alcohol, to ease pain and stiffness, and to treat diseases. A list of accredited therapists can be obtained from the addresses on p. 396.

HYPNOTHERAPY

Somewhere between sleep and wakefulness is the state of consciousness that hypnotherapists use to try to improve a person's health and relieve pain. Hypnotherapists induce a trance-like state and use it to bring about physical or mental changes in the patient, but treatment by an unqualified hypnotherapist can do more harm than good. For a list of well-trained therapists contact the addresses on p. 396.

MASSAGE

Massage is one of the oldest therapies known to man, used since 3000 BC. Hippocrates wrote in 5 BC: 'The way to health is to have a scented bath and an oiled massage each day.' The use of massage helps to relax, stimulate and invigorate the mind and body. It also helps to improve the blood, lymphatic, muscular and nervous systems, helping to rid the body of waste products. Treatment by an unqualified masseur can do more harm than good, so contact the addresses on p. 398 to find a qualified practitioner.

NATUROPATHY

Naturopathy helps the body to heal itself, for example, by fasting after an upset stomach, sweating out a fever, or submerging a sprained ankle into icy water. Naturopathy uses chiropractic, diets, exercise, massage, osteopathy, hydrotherapy, relaxation and breathing. It also encourages people to think positively about good health, and to live life as naturally as possible amid the pressures of everyday life. Naturopathy tries to identify the underlying cause of the illness and sets out to treat this, using diet and other therapies rather than just suppressing symptoms. Each case is treated as unique and naturopaths seek to complement and support conventional doctors. A list of qualified practitioners can be obtained from the General Council and Register of Naturopaths (*see* pp. 398–9), and have the letters MRN and ND or DO after their name.

REFLEXOLOGY

Reflexology involves massaging the reflex areas in the feet. These correspond to the 'energy channels' known to acupuncturists. Gentle massage can unblock these channels, allowing energy to flow again and heal damage to the body. It originated in China and is said to help people with pain, digestion problems, period pains and osteoporosis. Therapists use the letters MBRA after their name (*see* p. 399).

SYSTEMIC KINESIOLOGY

Kinesis means motion, and kinesiology is the study of locomotion in relation to the structure and working of the muscles, for example, if leg muscles work properly then the knee will jerk when it is hit. This connection was recognized by a chiropractor in 1964. Systemic kinesiology works by correcting the motions of muscles and ligaments in the body.

Kinesiologists do not diagnose illness but look for imbalances or deficiencies in nutrition or energy, to locate physical problems. They give a light, fingertip massage to pressure points to stimulate the blood and lymphatic systems. This form of muscle testing gives a clear picture of a person's state of health. Practitioners can be found through the Academy of Systemic Kinesiology (*see* p. 400).

WALKING

Exercise is a vital factor to sustain good health. We know that it aids the process of excretion of oestrogen by the body. Once oestrogen is bound to fibre in the bowel, exercise can stimulate peristalsis and excretion. It also builds up 'feel-good' endorphins. Building up to five brisk 45-minute walks each week can benefit the reproductive, immune, nervous and digestive systems. Enthusiastic walkers stay fit and healthy.

YOGA

The postures and exercises which make up Indian hatha yoga are the best-known form in Britain. The philosophy stresses the influence of mind over body, and that mental and spiritual development are necessary to reinforce the benefits that physical exercises can bring. The movements are done slowly and never strained, creating an awareness of the body to allow a better relaxation of muscles. Conditions such as arthritis, backache and period pains may be helped. Breathing plays an important part in the exercises. Skilled yoga teachers can be found through the Yoga Biomedical Trust and the American Yoga Association (*see* p. 400).

CONCLUSION

There is a life out there to be led and if you suffer from endometriosis remember that this is only a phase in time when the body has succumbed to illness. The body needs a period of convalescence to heal; it needs looking after. Endometriosis is a jigsaw and you need to fit all the pieces together gradually, allowing each area time to heal. Everyone wants to be well very quickly, but when the body has taken a while to become ill, we have to be patient and work with it to achieve recovery.

Angela A of London

For my endometriosis, I have taken Chinese herbs and vitamin and mineral supplements for about a year to help balance my hormones. Finding the correct balance to resolve my problem with hair loss is a challenge. Improving my diet, like stopping chocolates and coffee, cakes and biscuits, and increasing good healthy foods, has been the key. However, if I follow a stricter regime I feel even better. Gone is the horrible debilitating pain that put me in bed for a couple of days each period month. The terrible sharp drowning pain that went on and on is gone. All I have now is mild discomfort if I don't take some supplements such as the GLA.

CASE STUDY

Try the various techniques we have discussed – relaxation, gentle exercise – and work with good friends and caring family members to help pull you through. Recovery doesn't happen overnight. Most people, when they are ill, expect to go to the doctor and take a tablet to put everything right. Endometriosis is not like that. It is far more complicated because it is systemic; it affects the whole person, not only the reproductive system. Begin to help yourself, and these positive actions may start to pull you out of the vicious circle that the pain of endometriosis can drag you into.

Your body does not want to be ill and it is constantly trying to heal itself. Endometriosis is nothing that we have done to make ourselves ill; it appears to be a combination of factors – environmental pollution, hereditary factors, poor diet, poor digestion, lack of exercise and relaxation in this mad world we inhabit. The body is out of balance and it needs rebalancing. You have the power to do that, and the time taken will be well worth it because it gives you your life back again. Go ahead, try it.

> If you do not take the time to be well, you WILL take the time to be sick!
>
> *Lindsey Duncan, Nutritionist*

SUMMARY

There are a number of holistic therapies that appear to help with endometriosis, pain and infertility. We have looked at several, and they all are worthy of investigation if you feel that they may be of value. You must ensure that each practitioner holds recognized qualifications and seek advice from the organizations listed at the end of this book. Books on each speciality are available from local libraries.

1 Your health is dependent upon fresh air, clean water, cleanliness, nutritious food, good living conditions and hygiene. Assess your needs and do what you can.

2 Listen to what your sixth sense tells you. By becoming in tune with your body's needs, it helps you to judge what feels right and what feels wrong. You have the power to help your body heal – it is always striving to be well. Illness is not natural to it. Be gentle with yourself.

3 Every day allow yourself 20 minutes of 'me time'. When you can, just be.

4 Choose a treatment which feels right for your needs and try it for at least three months to give it a chance to work.

5 Ensure that you have 20 minutes each day in natural daylight to aid the function of your pituitary gland so that it can send the right messages to your ovaries.

6 Try going to bed and listening to some favourite music or a relaxation tape to lull you to sleep. Magnesium helps you sleep at night, as it is a natural tranquilliser.

7 Feeling positive can help to stimulate the immune system. Try to take the positive step of recognizing that part of you is ill and sickly and needs looking after.

8 Exercise increases the excretion of oestrogen from the body. Research has shown that oestrogen bound to fibre is excreted in greater amounts when exercise is undertaken.

9 Be kind to yourself, look upon your ill body as you would a sick little child and love it better.

10 Love and be loved – Always *amo tu*.

8 The nervous system and low moods

> Therapeutic success rarely comes from depressed pessimistic patients.
>
> *R Anderson*

The combined symptoms of endometriosis day in and day out can lead to both mental and physical exhaustion. Women often talk about being too drained to even talk to someone on the phone, and just wanting to curl up in a heap and sleep until they feel well again. The crucial aid to recovery is to regain some quality of life that the full-blown disease decimates. Being so tired all the time, suffering constant acute and horrendous pain, being unable to work effectively, and the loss of physical touch if intercourse is painful can be extremely depressing. Many doctors immediately think, 'Ah, clinical depression', and slam women onto anti-depressants, and tell them that the problem and pain is all in the mind.

Clinical depression usually involves feeling suicidal, but many women with endometriosis do not have that depth of depression. Often the depression is not clinical – it is grief at the loss of normal functioning in daily life, what is termed 'despair depression'. The light at the end of the tunnel is still there, but you simply do not have the energy or wherewithal to reach it. Despair depression is labelled 'dysthymia', a Greek word for despair. It may be reactive – from the loss of a true love to reading the bad news in the daily headlines – or it may be due to a skewed body biochemistry.

Labelling the medical file 'in need of psychiatric help' still carries a stigma in the eyes of some employers and, with dysthymia, it is more like reactive gloom. Winston Churchill suffered from it and termed it 'the black dog days'. Indeed, 8.5 per cent of the populations of the UK and the Nordic countries, when questioned, claimed they often felt down in the dumps. The people in Spain, Italy and Greece appear to suffer from less dysthymia, possibly due to their traditionally close family ties and having loving people who rally round each other at times of crisis. In Spanish hospitals, doctors have to push through ranks of family members before they can reach the patient.[1]

There are nutritional ways to support the nervous system through trauma and avoid taking strong drugs and medications. Friends and family support can bolster up the psyche.

We understand very little of the brain's working mechanisms and so much has yet to be discovered. However, all illness has a basic theme: the brain's chemical balance becomes imbalanced and things are not working as they should. But this does not automatically mean it is a psychiatric problem. The problem can be a biochemical one that is affecting the brain's biochemistry and, in many cases, it just requires the right nutrients to correct the disrupted biochemistry and thus enhance mood, improve neurotransmitter function, increase energy and help the body muscles to relax. Besides, anti-depressants often have side effects that can make the endometriosis worse, as they often have adverse effects on the gastrointestinal tract, disrupting the gut flora, and may cause harm to the gut membrane and liver enzyme function, thus upsetting the absorption of crucial nutrients upon which the reproductive system depends.

Different cultures view depression differently. The Western medicalized pharmaceutical-driven culture sees profits to be made with the use of drugs, so that is the automatic first choice when someone feels low. In 1985 in the USA alone, 1,542,000 pounds of tranquillisers and 836,000 pounds of barbiturates were swallowed to treat illness.[2] Many Americans see a 'shrink' on a regular basis so this is not surprising. In Britain, we have more of a 'stiff upper lip' attitude and drugs are used for different reasons.

No biochemical tests are undertaken to see whether or not these sufferers have high copper, mercury or lead levels that could be affecting their brain biochemistry. Indeed, psychiatric treatment is based on subjective clues rather than objective laboratory tests to discover if the body's and brain's natural biochemistry has been disrupted. This is sad because much harm may be done when the wrong treatment is given, and ideas are implanted which are incorrect and lead to self-fulfilling prophesies – 'well, if the doctor says I am mentally ill, I must be'.

In India, there are many different varieties of stress disorder that are recognized, all stemming from four basic emotions – depression, elation, anxiety and fear. With endometriosis there are two which stand out as important – *baden mein dard* which means 'pain in the body', and *dil mein udas,* which means 'sorrow in the heart'. The pressure of life events, illness and traumas, whether physical or emotional, all take their toll, and if you are feeling below par and your coping skills are at rock bottom, you will not deal well as crises arise. The endometriosis pain within the body causes immense sorrow in the heart indeed.[3] In Latin, the term *acedia* was used in the fourth century to describe a person who was exhausted, listless, sad and dejected, and feeling torpor or apathy. In the 12th and 13th centuries, the term 'melancholy' was used to describe someone who was under stress with low energy and fatigue.

Neuroendocrine theories were developed by the likes of Newton and Boyle in the 18th century to describe a concept of fatigue that was often associated with depression; it denoted lassitude and weariness as a result of mental or physical exertion. By the 19th century, illness and idleness under the Protestant work ethic was viewed as a crime. In the mentality of some people, it is still viewed this way, which can be very hard with the endometriosis patient who, due to the high oestrogen effect, tends to look healthy despite the pain and illness.

This despair at one's lot in life and enduring of chronic pain that many doctors are unable to recognize as being as intense as it is, can permeate everyday life as you struggle to do normal things like go to work, keep a home and have a social life despite all the pain and exhaustion. But unless this has been experienced, it is difficult to grasp the forlornness that endometriosis wreaks on normal everyday life. Many health professionals have experienced no greater pain than a severe toothache, so they have no parameters with which to understand or comprehend the extreme pain that endometriosis sufferers endure. They have no means by which to measure the searing abdominal pain. Simple pleasures like shopping are gone because there is too much pain to allow you to linger and look at things; a walk in the country out over the hills may be impossible because a large cyst on the ovary can give so much pain on moving further than a few feet; holding the man you love in your arms and wanting desperately to make love, but knowing that it will cause intense internal pain making you unable to walk for the next two days, is soul-destroying. Couples suffer from endometriosis, not just the woman.

People often use stimulants in food to help them get through each day – coffee and strong tea, coke, chocolate and alcohol – and a few choose recreational drugs. These substances work by altering the neurotransmitter balance in the brain, thus affecting the nervous system and, in some cases, stimulating the adrenal glands to secrete adrenaline. When you drink coffee, research has shown that the brain may become more alert, memory may be improved for a time, and you will feel much brighter and able to concentrate more clearly. But coffee has a downside too. Later on, you will have to rush to the loo as caffeine is a diuretic and you will lose zinc, magnesium and calcium in the urine. People often feel more ill at ease and shaky after coffee, becoming more irritated by the smallest things and then needing another coffee to keep them going – it is addictive. So in the short term, it helps but, in the long term, it is detrimental to the nervous system.[4]

The classic behaviour of the depressed animal is to become submissive, its body immobile, and avoid the company of others. This is called the 'hurt animal syndrome', curling up in a corner – the Greta Garbo response of 'I want to be alone.' There may be an adaptive value to such behaviour during fear and illness, as immobility means that the victim is less conspicuous to predators. Heart rate is reduced and, in humans, there is a tendency to faint as an adaptive response. This response known as 'vagal death', where the heart rate is lowered rapidly at times of extreme shock – such as when a person freezes or a loved one dies – can lead to repeated fainting episodes.[5]

THE BRAIN

> Use it or lose it.
>
> *Anon*

The brain is a very sensitive organ. It is two-thirds fat and weighs around 3lb (1.3kg). This is where we store all our memories, in the limbus system at the core. How does it do that? Wouldn't we all love to know? Everyone has experienced a smell that suddenly triggers off a memory of another time and place associated with that aroma – a happy time, the evocative smells of a Shaker settlement, the lavender perfume of Grandma sitting in a rocking chair, a particular aftershave that reminds you of someone you love. Close your eyes and you can soon be with that person in your memories. After people leave you, the smell of their clothes lingers and this is often used to help ease the pain of bereavement by Cruse counsellors. Many supermarkets use synthetic smells to help us feel at home and relaxed so that we will spend more money – the aromas of freshly baked bread and percolating coffee lull us into buying more than we intended. We are told that these are the two smells that will help us sell a house when prospective buyers come to call! We remember childhood, music and friendships associated with specific aromas.

The brain communicates using neurotransmitters made from proteins. So, proteins and fats in the diet are crucial to the health of the nervous system – we heard this before with the hormones of the endocrine system and the enzymes of the digestive system. Neuro-transmitters move at great speed through the brain – we talk about brainwaves – passing from cell to cell and giving up their messages. Brain neurons are studded with receptor cells, molecules that dangle into synapses to snare passing neurotransmitters, like a fishhook snaring a trout.[6]

Some of them have links to other body systems, like cholecystokinin, a gastrointestinal hormone that resides in the gut. This hormone tells us when to eat and when to stop eating. It knows when we are hungry and when we are full, and it comes from the hypothalamus. We met the hypothalamus before in the endocrine system – it is the gland which sends GnRH to the pituitary and helps the ovary to function. As always, we see how everything in the body is so interlinked and intertwined that it is obvious that one system must have some effect upon another. In this case, the digestive system sends a message to the nervous system saying 'Stop eating now.'

The nerve cells in the brain and throughout the body are called neurons and these are protected by a fatty layer, the myelin sheath. They are connected together by branches known as axons, and some are short while others may be 1m long. The nervous system is almost like a roadmap and the neurotransmitters are like motorcycle couriers who carry the messages. If you touch this page now, that message will have travelled from your finger to the brain at 124 mph. We think carefully before we take some actions, but others we do involuntarily – like tapping your foot or scratching your hand when it itches.

The neurotransmitters are like hormones in that they are specific, like one particular key for one particular lock. Different neurotransmitters do different things in the brain and body. Most of the neurons are in the brain, but some travel down the spine, and nerves run throughout our body. Hence, if you cut your finger on paper, a little nerve makes you go 'Ouch! That hurts!' That is also why endometriosis hurts so much. The nerves in the abdominal cavity are sending the message to the brain that something is not right – the internal bleeding and inflammation, the adhesions pulling and tugging, or the ovary that is spewing out hot sticky liquid all over the delicate intestinal membranes. We can tell that something is wrong because of the searing pain. It is a signal from the body that we need to heed and try to correct by removing the cause of the pain. Modern medicine gives us painkillers and drugs to suppress pain, but often it will only be dulled, and may return with vengeance once the treatment is stopped.

BRAIN FUEL

How we feel and think, the way we can relax or feel tense, whether we are tired or alert depends upon the chemistry of the brain. If you feel abnormally tired and befuddled, then the brain is not working effectively. The fuel for the brain is glucose, a simple sugar that is used to fire up the system; approximately 20 per cent of the body's glucose is used by the brain for energy. When we feel stressed, the hormones from the adrenal glands, adrenaline and cortisol, are secreted in greater amounts, which causes more sugar from our body's stores to be released into the bloodstream. This is part of the 'fight or flight' mechanism designed to give us a boost of energy to get away fast from oncoming danger. However, in modern life, it happens much too often and we have nowhere to run when sitting exasperated in an office chair or traffic jam. Once excess sugar is in the bloodstream, it has to be used up or it may trigger syndrome X or hyperinsulinism. Once the sugar is used up, the body feels a lull and the brain is the first organ to suffer. You begin to feel a 'brain fag' and become irritated at the slightest thing.

The key to keeping the whole system on an even keel is to avoid eating simple sugars in cakes, biscuits and chocolate bars, and by eating more complex carbohydrates by snacking on nuts and seeds or fruits. These release sugar more evenly over the course of the day into the bloodstream so that there are no sudden highs and lows. Stress increases insulin, adrenaline, cortisol and oestrogen, and reduces progesterone, resulting in an imbalance in the main steroid hormones. This all sounds a very familiar story with the hormone balance profiles seen in endometriosis patients, doesn't it?

We need to know how to combat this illness in the brain, when the glucose, proteins and fats are not working as evenly as they should, and how to help our thinking become crystal-clear again and help the brain work effectively at reducing pain and our sense of despair. The neurotransmitters are crucial in this process. Some may make us feel happy and calm, others can make us feel agitated and aggressive, while endorphin levels help to balance our perception of pain. Dancing and exercise are a good way to release more 'feel-good' endorphins.

There is indeed an inner joy that some forms of music can release within us and this may be what aids the release of endorphins. Certain pieces of music can remind us of particular situations and people, like the soundtrack from the movie *The Mission*, Pachebel's *Canon* and Bon Jovi's *Always*. The Addiction Research Center in Stanford, California, reports that when people listen to music, they begin to feel euphoric. When they blocked the brain's endorphin receptors with the drug naloxone, listening to the music was much less pleasureable. Endorphins are associated with pain-relief, orgasm, and feelings of pleasure and happiness. They are the brain's natural opiates and are peptides.[7] Memory exists in the womb, research has shown. Babies who have been introduced to a piece of music while in the womb react by calming down and opening their eyes when that piece of music is played again after they are born. Certain songs bring back shared emotions. The memory for music stays with us even in cases of stroke and Alzheimer's disease, and lyrics can be recalled. This was demonstrated on the BBC2 TV programme 'Ever Wondered?', broadcast on 30 October 2001.

ELECTRICITY IN THE BRAIN

The messages carried by neurotransmitters have to jump across a gap from one cell to the next in the brain. These gaps are called synapses, and the electrical charge across the gap causes the neurotransmitter to be fired. This opens the next cell, where the message is accepted and passed on if necessary. The electrolyte chemicals of the brain – calcium, magnesium, sodium and potassium – are all found in our food. If you have ever had extreme diarrhoea and were in danger of severe dehydration (the loss of those minerals), you may have been given an electrolyte drink to restore the balance. Anti-depressant drugs increase the levels of particular neurotransmitters in the synaptic gap, for example, noradrenaline and serotonin.

Neurotransmitters fall into two groups: excitatory ones, which make us function and keep us alert, though in excess they can lead to agitation; or inhibitory ones, which make us feel calm, but which in excess may cause us to feel unhappy, depressed and despairing. Normally, the body has both the excitatory and inhibitory neurotransmitters in balance, and this helps us to feel well.

If, however, you take too many stimulants or are overstressed, too many of one type of neurotransmitter may be released at one time. This leads the body to reduce the number of receptor sites available for other neurotransmitters to try to halt the problem. In doing so, you feel as though more of the stimulant might help, and so a vicious circle of drug and stimulant use builds up. When a person tries to avoid the things they crave for a while, they may feel extremely low and develop headaches as there are insufficient receptor sites open for neurotransmitters to function at the normal balance. For instance, caffeine withdrawal can produce up to five days of bad headaches and cravings.

Once again the body in its wisdom likes balance, so when the system goes out of balance, we are in trouble. Amino acids from protein foods make up the neurotransmitters, of which there are more than 40, far more than the number of letters in the alphabet. If you think of the 26 letters in the alphabet creating all the words in a dictionary, you can then see how many combinations there can be. With 40 neurotransmitters, there are endless combinations of protein chains you can make. Protein and fat deficiencies, or the choice of poor-quality ones in the diet, can have serious deleterious effects on the workings of the nervous system.

EXCITATORY NEUROTRANSMITTERS

Adrenaline The release of adrenaline from the adrenal gland gives us a rush of energy and vitality, as well as the stamina we need to get through a busy day or that boost of energy when we need to go that extra mile. In the USA, this is called epinephrine.

Dopamine This catecholamine neurotransmitter is linked to alertness, concentration and happiness. Both adrenaline and noradrenaline are made from dopamine, which is dependent upon the amino acid L-tyrosine. There are receptors for dopamine in the eye, pituitary gland, hypothalamus and nigra cell area in the lower midbrain. Therefore, it may have an impact on the endocrine glands of the reproductive system.

Noradrenaline This is another catecholamine neurotransmitter that is dependent upon the amino acid L-tyrosine. When an individual becomes aroused or afraid, it becomes active. It also works in connection to the heart. In the USA, this is called norepinephrine.[8]

Serotonin The most talked about neurotransmitter, serotonin works by lifting the mood. Many of the pharmaceutical anti-depressants work by raising serotonin levels in the body. The amino acid tryptophan is a precursor of serotonin and is found in foods such as turkey. Serotonin is found in blood serum and induces a powerful contraction of smooth muscle, for example, in the intestines and blood vessels.[9] It is known to aid sleep and is involved in the regulation of body temperature. The structure in the brain with the highest concentration of serotonin is the pineal gland, where it is converted into melatonin, a hormone that is responsible for the day–night cycle and ultimately sleep.

Glutamate This amino acid neurotransmitter is responsible for exciting neurons to fire off messages. It works with specific receptors and appears to be responsible for cognition, memory, movement and sensation. It is also vital for the integrity of the mucous membranes in the intestines, where it prevents toxins from breaching the gut wall and eventually reaching the brain. Glutamate acts as fuel for the macrophages and lymphocytes of the immune system, and for protein synthesis. As with any substance, an excess can cause problems; glutamate excess has been implicated in many brain diseases.[10] (Glutamine is a part of gliadin, the protein part of gluten, so people who are gluten-sensitive should be wary of taking L-glutamine alone.)

INHIBITORY NEUROTRANSMITTERS

Acetylcholine This is not made from amino acids, but it does control mental alertness, memory and concentration. Vitamins C and B5, or pantothenic acid, and choline (another B vitamin) are its precursors. It also works in the contraction of muscles and coordination of movement, preventing clumsiness. Levels can fall with high stress hormones and ageing. Between the ages of 50–90 years, the part of the brain important for memory loses 20 per cent of its volume. Acetylcholine is one of the molecules through which neurons communicate clearly.

Gamma-aminobutyric acid (GABA) This helps us to relax as it calms the nervous system and controls the release of dopamine in the brain.

These inhibitory neurotransmitters promote a calm relaxed mood and tend to remove anxiety and depression. The amino acids that support their formation are L-tryptophan, L-glycine, L-taurine, L-tyrosine and L-histidine. Certain amino acids are believed to be the 'workhorse' fast transmitters in the brain. Some of them always seem to be excitatory – for example, glutamic acid and aspartic acid – while others seem always to be inhibitory – such as GABA and glycine. Glutamic acid, aspartic acid and glycine are amino acids that constitute part of the proteins we eat.[11]

The nutrients zinc, vitamins B6, B12, B1 and B3, and folic acid all work in the brain to produce enzymes that help the conversion of amino acids to neurotransmitters. There are also the electrolytes calcium, magnesium, potassium and sodium, which aid the firing of the neurotransmitters across the synaptic gap between each cell. Once more, we see that a variety of nutrients are required for the healthy functioning of the nervous system. Research completed in London at the Institute of Psychiatry and King's College Hospital showed 'that a third of all patients with either severe depression or schizophrenia were deficient in folic acid'.[12] Interestingly, the oral contraceptive pill also depletes the body of folic acid.

'ANTINUTRIENTS'

Lead is a neurotoxin, and its presence can interfere with the function of the brain and nervous system in many ways. It accumulates in the hypothalamus and hippocampus, so the avoidance of lead in petrol fumes and paints has long been acknowledged as important. High copper levels are related to mental agitation. Tapwater, chocolate and aubergines contain copper, but it is only when the levels are excessive that problems arise. Mercury has long been recognized as a neurotoxin. Hair mineral analysis can show whether levels are high in the body. These heavy metals can be chelated out of the body using other nutrients, such as vitamin C, zinc, selenium, pectin and alginates.

AMINO ACIDS IN NATURE

We all need to eat some protein foods every day to take in sufficient amino acids to aid the body's cells in the production of proteins for new growth as well as enzymes, neurotransmitters and hormones. A wise choice of good quality protein foods along with the essential cis fatty acids (which are cold-pressed) will ensure that the body has the right building materials to maintain good health.

To improve our sense of wellbeing, certain amino acids are essential:

L-Tyrosine For a boost of energy, to lift mood and improve thyroid function. This amino acid can have amazing effects when used carefully for short periods of time. It is a precursor of the neurotransmitters dopamine, adrenaline and noradrenaline, and of the thyroxine (for thyroid function) and catecholamine hormones. It aids pain relief in the brain. It can be used as an anti-depressant in its own right but, when overused, it may trigger headaches and mild elevations of blood pressure. Keeping a pot of tyrosine in the supplement cupboard for the bad day when you wake up feeling low and drained of energy is helpful in creating a feeling of calm. It can boost energy and wellbeing within a couple of hours. Stress exhaustion requires tyrosine, as it helps in the production of adrenaline. It can stimulate sex drive and decrease appetite.

Its long-term use is not recommended. It should not be used by those with cancerous tumours, high blood pressure, phenylketonuria or mental illness.[13] It has long been used by the US military for intense action in the field at stressful times. During its use, the brain builds up more dopamine receptors to catch this amino acid, which can reduce some depression states.

- 500mg once a day
- Food sources: rolled oats, cottage cheese, eggs, yoghurt, pork, chicken, turkey, duck, game and avocado.

L-Tryptophan To calm nerves, lift mood and promote sleep.

The use of pure tryptophan was banned at the end of the 1980s when a Japanese company produced this amino acid in the form of sleeping tablets where one component went wrong and made several people fall ill. It should be used with care. Tryptophan is a precursor of the neurotransmitter serotonin and the body can convert it to vitamin B3. It has been used in the past as an anti-depressant, and research suggests that it may act as a painkiller. It reduces the appetite for carbohydrate foods.

- 500mg per day
- Food sources: oat flakes, cottage cheese, almonds, eggs, pork, chicken, turkey, duck, wild game and avocado.

L-Taurine For relaxation, thus lessening anxiety and irritability.

This is manufactured from another amino acid in the liver – methionine. Women need taurine more than men, as the hormone oestrogen inhibits its synthesis in the liver. It interacts with bile salts, to maintain their solubility, and with cholesterol, to prevent gallstones. Greater concentrations of taurine are found in the pineal and pituitary glands after exposure to natural full-spectrum light. People deprived of natural light may become depressed and research suggests this could be due to low taurine levels.[14] Taurine is found in breastmilk, but not in cow's milk. It increases some of the effects of insulin and, because insulin can affect hypoglycaemia, taurine should be used with caution.[15] Taurine helps the cell membranes of the brain become more electrically stable and aids the release of neurotransmitters. Some problems of fertility may be related to taurine deficiency.[16] Taurine, manganese and zinc work closely together. It stimulates prolactin and insulin release.[17]

- 500mg per day
- Food sources: animal and fish proteins, particularly organ meats.

D,L-Phenylalanine (DLPA) An anti-depressant, painkiller and appetite suppressant.

As the precursor to tyrosine, this requires the presence of vitamin C for its metabolism. Phenylalanine stimulates the production of cholecystokinin (CCK), a gastrointestinal hormone that makes the stomach feel full after a meal, which sends a signal to the hypothalamus via the vagal nerve.[18]

Dr Seymour Ehrenpreis, at the University of Chicago Medical School, published a report on its use as a painkiller in 1978. Pain relief took from one to four weeks to reach optimum level when the D and L forms of this amino acid were combined. Patients with chronic pain have reduced levels of endorphins and DLPA appears to restore these levels to normal. As it does not interfere with the transmission of normal pain messages, the defence mechanism of the body is not compromised.

It has an anti-depressant effect that may be achieved within a few days once the supplement programme begins.[19] It strengthens the nerve cell metabolic pathways that produce the excitatory neurotransmitters noradrenaline and adrenaline. If the body can produce enough to meet your needs, it will more likely be able to withstand the mental and emotional stress that causes depression. If, on the other hand, your cells are depleted by poor digestion, they will not be able to 'charge up' the brain when mega-stress occurs.[20] Having sufficient DLPA also strengthens the effect of the pain relief.[21]

- 100mg before a meal, if blood pressure is normal
- 100mg after a meal, if blood pressure is high
- Food sources: soybeans, cottage cheese, fish, meat, poultry, almonds, brazil nuts, pecans, pumpkinseeds, sesame seeds, lima beans, chickpeas and lentils

GABA (gamma-aminobutyric acid) Works alongside glutamic acid and glutamine in all brain functions.

GABA can work as a fuel to both stimulate and sedate the effects of the nervous system, and suppress appetite and reduce blood sugar levels. Vitamin B6 and manganese are important in its formation.[22]

Other substances that may improve our sense of wellbeing are omega-3 and omega-6 oils, B vitamins, magnesium and acetyl-L-carnitine.

Siberian ginseng This is an adaptogen. Unlike Korean ginseng, the Siberian form is not oestrogenic and it therefore safe to use with endometriosis. It helps the adrenals adapt to stress and supports them.

Gingko biloba A compound in the leaves of the *Gingko biloba* tree reduces blood clumping in arteries, increases glucose uptake by cells, acts as an antioxidant, improves blood flow in arteries, veins and capillaries, and inhibits monoamine oxidase (MAO) in the blood, thus aiding neurotransmitter function. It helps to reduce dizziness and improves memory, the research suggests.

St John's wort This perennial plant has been used in the treatment of immunocompromised patients. The active compounds in the plant are hypericum and xanthrones, which act as MAO inhibitors, agents used to treat depression. Reports in the *British Medical Journal* concluded that St John's wort extract was effective in the treatment of mild-to-moderate depression when taken in doses of around 300mg/day. It should not be taken in conditions of extreme sunlight as it may cause a rash, nor should it be used by women taking oral contraceptives as it disrupts their action.

Valerian This has always been used as a tranquilliser, especially during the Blitz in World War II. It has also been shown to reduce spasms in the body. It is attractive to animals, and the tale of the Pied Piper describes him as carrying valerian roots on his belt.

Hops This plant is used as a calmative to help alleviate nervousness and produce sleep. It is also antibacterial and digestive aid. Its bitter taste is due to antibiotic bitter acids that help with the removal of toxins from the body.

Passion flower This has a mild sedative effect that aids sleep and relaxation.

Homeopathic *Arnica* 6X and *Ipachacuana* may be helpful in stress situations, as are the tinctures of Rescue Remedy and Emergency Essense.

GUT–BRAIN–IMMUNE SYSTEM CONNECTION

The intestines and immune system are closely interlinked in that 80 per cent of the body's immunoglobulins are produced in the gut membrane when sufficient B vitamins are present. This is one of the body's first ways to protect you from bugs and germs from the outside world. As already noted, the gut membrane is the largest immune organ in the body. If toxins were allowed to pass through the gut membrane, it would impair brain function. We know most about the effects of ammonia on the brain. It is usually cleaned out by liver enzymes but, in patients with liver disease, high levels of ammonia are left floating around and this can impair brain function, giving rise to personality changes, agitation and seizures. Research has uncovered a possible link between bacteria-derived toxins in the GI tract and neurological diseases such as schizophrenia and autism. It has been hypothesized that substances produced by anaerobic bacteria in the GI tract interfere with synaptophysin, an important brain protein required for the release of certain neurotransmitters.[23]

Phenylalanine is the precursor to cholecystokinin (CCK), a peptide that acts on the hypothalamus as an appetite suppressant, lessening the appetite.[24] CCK may induce satiety and terminate eating or feelings of hunger. It is thought that it may do this by altering gastrointestinal function (the stomach-emptying trigger). It is known that CCK effects on satiety depend upon intact vagal nerve fibres, which allow CCK to interact with the hypothalamus via CCK receptors on the vagal nerve.[25]

John Dwyer, a professor of immunology at Yale University in New Haven, Connecticut, states that the immune system and nervous system share the distinction of being homes for cells that remain intact from infancy to old age. The new discipline of psychoneuroimmunology has grown up around observations that link the function of the brain and the immune system. When we think of memory, we see that there has to be a core of cells in the body that are permanent, whereas other cells come and go. Indeed, there are cells in the ovary and testes that must be as old as time itself, carrying as they do the DNA and genes of past generations – a history of all our ancestors. Each cell carries DNA that encodes your ancestral memory. These long-term cells form the centre of every individual and allow the persistence of 'self' within every human being. These cells should be given our respect and their nutrition must be sound. To enhance fertility, these cells in the gonads should be treasured and protected at all cost. The only way we can do that is by eating well and avoiding pollutants wherever possible. The fundamental purpose of our body's chemistry is to allow a balance of glucose, essential fatty acids, proteins, vitamins and minerals to support the health and function of the cells.[26]

Cells within the brain remain undivided and unchanged, except for ageing, as do the lymphocytes of the immune system, whereas blood cells live for only three to four months. Both the cells of the brain and the lymphocytes hold memory. In the immune system, it is important to retain the memory of different viruses so that the B lymphocytes can fight again if a virus reinvades the body. That is how vaccinations work; they use the memory of the immune system to elicit a particular sense of say, measles, so that if the measles virus invades the body, the cells will 'remember' how to attack it and win.

The brain, and the nervous, immune and endocrine systems, and the gut are all intertwined. To regain full health, we have to treat all of these organs and systems at once. Treating one system in isolation will not be effective. We can see clearly that there is synergy, which is why getting the nutrition correct is crucial for regaining total health.

THE NUTRITIONAL APPROACH

We need to begin to look at correcting brain biochemical problems with nutrition. The majority of physicians are orientated to the toximolecular approach. A hearing before the Select Committee on Nutrition and Human Need of the Senate of the USA, held on 22 June 1977 included the following:

> Senator George McGovern: 'Achieving recognition of the relationship between nutrition and [mental] health is still very much a struggle. Established scientific thinking remains weighted against those few scientists and practitioners who are striving to understand the complex links between the food we consume and how we think and behave as individuals. For example, the newly appointed Mental Health Commission has no member with experience in this vital area. I find this oversight both surprising and distressing … If further research is undertaken along a nutritional line, we could find that a significant number of mental health problems could be cured by nutrition.'
>
> Dr Lesser: 'Tranquillisers came out of the 50s … they are drugs, and therefore patentable substances. In other words, a pharmaceutical house can receive an exclusive monopoly to produce that particular substance for, I believe, 10 years. This allows the company to make money off that drug. This money pays for research into the further use of drugs. It also pays to hire detail men to visit physicians who are treating patients, and every physician in this country is visited by detail men who tell him about the latest drug discoveries and for conference attendance … It also pays for the testing necessary in order to receive Federal Government approval to use those substances. Vitamins [all nutrients] are not patentable substances. Nutrients are available in nature and no one can patent them. The physicians in medical schools are taught to use drugs, not nutrients. Hours are spent teaching physicians how to prescribe various drugs to treat disease.'[27]

It is sad that the use of food and nutrition to correct an imbalance in brain biochemistry has still not yet come to the fore. But as we have just seen, this is because there is no money to be made from using nutritional supplements and counselling on diet, so medical professionals and pharmaceutical companies have no interest. Moses Maimonides, the great 12th century physician, stated that 'No illness which can be treated by diet should be treated by any other means.' If cell deficiencies develop, the concentration of nutrients needed for optimum health must be altered according to that individual's needs. The assumption is that, if each biochemically individual cell in our body is provided with the optimum nutrients necessary for its proper and healthy functioning, then the internal environment will be at its optimum for the individual, and chronic degenerative diseases will eventually be controlled.[28]

PAIN PATHWAYS IN THE BRAIN

There are two pain pathways in the body – the fast pain system and the slow pain system. Two classes of nerve fibres carry pain information from the skin and body tissues. Fast nerve fibres are small and work at 5–30 m/sec. They are protected by a myelin sheath, and conduct pain from the skin and mucous membranes. The slow nerve fibres have no myelin sheath and work at 0.5–2 m/sec, and serve all the skin and body tissues except brain nervous tissue.

Slow fibres contain a peptide known as substance P, which is thought to be a neurotransmitter that travels throughout the nervous system, spinal cord and brain regions. It is felt that this slow pain system is critical in learned fear and anxiety, and it appears to mediate aching, burning pain.[29] The endorphins and opiates have a powerful blocking action on the slow pain pathway.

However, the fast pain pathway is thought to be a more recent evolutionary development and, although it conveys information about pain to the brain, opiates and endorphins have little effect at dulling the pain from this fast pain pathway as there are no receptors for them. The fast pain pathway conveys sharp, prickling pain rapidly to the brain.[30] Chapter 4 goes into detail on the nutrients which support pain control in the body.

HORMONES, STRESS AND DEPRESSION

The catabolic hormones – adrenaline, noradrenaline, glucocorticoids, growth hormone and thyroxine – are raised at times of stress. Anabolic hormones – insulin, testosterone and oestrogen – decrease at times of stress.

A parallel of sorts can be drawn between the adrenal gland and the brain adrenaline circuit. Both systems yield an overall increase in the amount of adrenaline present throughout the brain. It is known that the adrenal gland secretes adrenaline and noradrenaline in response to stress- or arousal-producing events in the environment. However, we do not yet know the conditions that lead to increased activity of the brain adrenaline system (see p. 179 on stress and immunity).[31]

What we do know is that stress can make the symptoms of endometriosis worse. More research needs to be done on the levels of serotonin in the brain when the severe abdominal pain of endometriosis is affecting contractions of the uterus and intestinal smooth muscle. High levels of serotonin are known to induce powerful contractions of the smooth muscle of the gut. In times of arousal and stress, it could then increase blood flow in the brain. The balance of serotonin and endorphins, and their effects on intestinal cramps needs to be further researched.

Corticosteroid hormones are secreted by the adrenal glands during periods of stress. Short-term exposure to these hormones is fine, as it stimulates the 'fight or flight' response that can save us from dangerous episodes by giving us a boost of energy to run away. However, chronic exposure to corticosteroid when stress is prolonged is damaging to the immune system. It has also been seen to damage organ tissue and injure the arteries. Prolonged exposure to these hormones is linked to high blood pressure and raised blood sugar levels. They can block the growth of new bone cells. We age if this high exposure continues unabated, and become less able to cope during stressful times as the adrenals become exhausted as we get older. High levels of corticosteroid lower DHEA (dehydroepiandro-sterone) and shrink the thymus gland, thereby damaging the production of T lymphocytes.

Melatonin can reduce the negative effects of corticosteroids. Excessive corticosteroid levels are associated with depression. Indeed, if corticosteroid is administered orally, it may trigger the physiological effects of adrenal-released corticosteroid – patients show symptoms of depression, mania, nervousness, insomnia and schizophrenia. This effect of corticosteroid on mood is related to the prevention of serotonin synthesis from tryptophan in the brain. Cortisol inhibits the production of GnRH (gonadotrophin-releasing hormone), luteinizing hormone (LH), oestradiol and testosterone. In the condition known as Cushing's syndrome, high cortisol levels suppress reproductive function and reduce libido in both sexes. But prolonged exposure appears to upset LH regulation and therefore may upset ovulation.

Melatonin is secreted by the pineal gland, and promotes sleep and normalizes cholesterol levels. It also stimulates the parathyroid glands to ensure that bone mineralization is correctly regulated. It can also block oestrogen from binding with the oestrogen receptors on cells, as it regulates the synthesis of the steroid hormones from the ovaries. However, an excess of melatonin can cause infertility as it raises prolactin levels and series 2 prostaglandin levels. Research has shown it to lower libido and trigger mild depression. A deficiency, on the other hand, has been shown to create a state of premenstrual syndrome and insomnia. Caffeine, alcohol and tobacco reduce the availability of melatonin to the body.

DHEA comes from the adrenals and is the precursor hormone of testosterone, dihydrotestosterone, androstenedione, oestrone and oestradiol. It improves the body's handing of glucose in times of stress, and increases muscle strength and lean body mass. It has been suggested that there is an opposing action between DHEA and testosterone on insulin resistance. As DHEA levels decline with age, the secretion of insulin increases. Research by Mobbs suggests that insulin resistance may result in damage to the hypothalamus.

Follicle-stimulating hormone (FSH) is produced by the pituitary gland and is crucial in the maturation of the ova in the ovary. Stress can upset the pituitary gland and its pulsatile release may be changed. Normal levels are around 5–20mU/ml; at menopause, it rises to around 30–40mU/ml. High FSH is an indication of low fertility. A level less than 5mU/ml suggests that the girl has not yet reached puberty and one over 20mU/ml suggests that menopause may arrive in the next few years. It can fluctuate wildly during the perimenopause years. However, women with high FSH levels can still be fertile. Low oestrogen can elevate FSH, and IVF may raise FSH levels temporarily.

LH-releasing hormone is produced by the pituitary at around day 14–17. This causes the ovary to release the ova so that it can be sucked up into the Fallopian tubes ready for fertilization. It is hypersensitive to stress, and increases when testosterone and oestrogen are low. Normal levels are 7–14 mU/ml, which means that ovulation can occur. LH levels rise abruptly when menopause begins. Stress inhibits GnRH production and this in turn reduces LH release.

Thyroid hormone is essential for growth and metabolism. Synthetic chemicals like polychlorinated biphenyls (PCBs), phenols, thiols and excessive histamines are thought to impair thyroid function and cause brain damage. Thyroid hormones help to regulate body chemistry by assisting neurotransmitters in their mission to attach to cell membrane receptors. Anything that interferes with the process of normal neurotransmitter attachment to a membrane receptor inevitably alters brain chemistry. Animal studies have demonstrated that certain toxins may actually block normal thyroid hormone action by mimicking other hormones and so are transported to the brain in their stead. Because the brain is primed to accept hormonal messages, it may quite easily take up the wrong one if the molecule is similar in shape.[32] Poor thyroid function can lead to extreme fatigue, and all depressed patients should been screened for hypothyroidism, which is common in women with endometriosis.

Oxytocin is a sensory peptide produced in the posterior pituitary gland and is used during labour to produce contractions. It is believed to play a role in stimulating the 'bonding' response between mother and baby. It also stimulates milk production with prolactin. It has a half-life of three minutes, and is inactivated in the liver and kidneys.

The hormone CCK in the digestive tract increases oxytocin levels. It is thought from animal experiments that oxytocin also plays a role in feeding behaviour. At times of stress, people either overeat or lose all appetite. Oxytocin may facilitate sperm transport as it causes uterine contractions, and it may play a role in orgasm. Oestrogen increases the effects of oxytocin on smooth muscle in the uterus. Levels of oxytocin change in response to noradrenaline, dopamine, serotonin, acetylcholine, glutamate, CCK and beta-endorphins. Oxytocin release is regulated by signals resulting from touching of the breast, uterus and genitalia. The body increases the secretion of oxytocin in response to stress, pain, exercise, nausea and nicotine.

Vasopressin, another sensory peptide from the posterior pituitary gland, constricts blood vessels and increases peristalsis in the gut during digestion. It may also be responsible for muscle contractions of the uterus. It has a half-life of 5–18 minutes, and is inactivated in the liver and kidneys. Both oxytocin and vasopressin are antidiuretic hormones – they decrease the production of urine. Vasopressin is involved in reproductive behaviour, and is strongly associated with testosterone; it can facilitate aggressive behaviour and also slows the heart rate. Research suggests that it plays a role in the imprinting of memory. The body increases secretion of vasopressin in response to stress, pain, exercise, nausea and nicotine. High levels of vasopressin increase levels of testosterone, oestrogen, acetylcholine and dopamine. Low levels decrease levels of progesterone, dopamine, serotonin and endorphins.

Testosterone is produced by the adrenal glands and ovaries. It improves cognition, inhibits serotonin and prolactin, and facilitates dopamine, adrenaline and vasopressin. It has anti-depressant effects in both sexes. Meat in the diet increases testosterone whereas vegetarian diets lower its levels. It can trigger psychotic behaviour. It is very sensitive to the environment and stress can disrupt its production.

Progesterone can kill off the sex drive by its effect in lowering testosterone. (Provera is used to chemically castrate sex offenders.) It decreases pheromones, and can make a woman irritable and aggressive, yet paradoxically, may have a sedative effect. Normal levels in menstruating women are 10 ng/ml in the mid to late luteal phase of the cycle. It is virtually absent during the follicular phase. It thickens the endometrium. If conception does not occur, then levels fall, which brings about the disintegration of the endometrium and the menstrual flow. As stress can disrupt LH levels so that the ova do not ovulate, the knock-on effect is low progesterone levels so that a normal corpus luteum cannot form. Progesterone maintains the pregnancy, and decreases testosterone and dopamine while increasing opioids and fluid retention. It can behave like a depressant and cause fatigue when levels are high.

Oestrogen comes from the fat cells, adrenals and ovaries. Levels vary throughout each menstrual cycle. Normal levels are 30–150ng/ml in the early follicular and late luteal phases, rising to 100–500ng/ml in the late follicular phase just before ovulation. In perimenopause, it is greater than 20ng/ml and, in menopause, it can range from 40–200 ng/ml. It maintains the menstrual cycle and promotes endometrial thickening. It is responsible for the thickening of endometrial implant tissue. Low oestrogen can trigger feelings of dizziness, palpitations, irritability, anxiety and depression, and increase insomnia and headaches. As oestrogen diminishes, so does oxytocin. Liver disease can increase oestrogen production, as can sexual intercourse. High oestrogen increases the risk of blood clotting by 200 per cent (to three per 1,000) among women using it in OCPs and HRT. As blood clots can cause a stroke, HRT increases the risk of stroke and heart attacks, as shown by the Women's Health Initiative.[33]

Prolactin, secreted by the pituitary gland, surges during stressful experiences. High levels may decrease testosterone and dopamine, and it dulls alertness and sensation.

Adrenaline causes a stress response. Adrenaline is synthesized from tyrosine to dopa, then to dopamine and noradrenaline and, finally, adrenaline. Adrenaline and insulin are antagonistic hormones – adrenaline raises blood sugar while insulin reduces it.

Serotonin can make you demure or aggressive. High levels lower sex drive and make people more violent and mean, whereas orgasms are easier with low serotonin, and people are also more at peace and sensitive. It transmits signals in the brain from one nerve ending to another. It has a relationship with oestrogen, but reduces testosterone, and facilitates the production of opioids and progesterone. Stress can upset serotonin levels.

Dopamine is the neurotransmitter that gives pleasure and increases sex drive. When its levels are low, we feel no joy or pleasure; we do not get excited or show enthusiasm. Testosterone increases dopamine levels. It can improve energy and alertness. When dopamine peaks, then oxytocin is lowered. It plays a role in human attachments to the person you love. Low levels in depressed states dull the senses so that people are unable to form attachments.

Pheromones are chemical substances produced by an animal which cause a specific reaction in another. They act on the brain and nerves via an organ in the nose. Research using male sweat on Q-tips placed under the noses of irregularly menstruating women three times a day for a couple of months triggered menstruation to become regular. Exatolide in male sweat cannot be detected by women who have had their ovaries removed. Stress may disrupt this effect as we perspire more when stressed.

Stress reduction is a vital factor in normalizing hormone levels. The onus is on every woman to reduce stress wherever possible in order to maintain fertility. As hormone levels and neurotransmitters are responsible for mood and wellbeing, it is crucial that sound nutrition, fresh air, natural daylight, and sleep and relaxation feature high in your life. This will keep the central nervous system happy and maintain normal hormone levels.

ENDOMETRIOSIS, STRESS EXHAUSTION AND DESPAIR

Many women with endometriosis symptoms complain of extreme tiredness that prevents them from living the lives they want most of all. Hypothyroidism is related to exhaustion, so this should be checked. Research by a supplement company, carried out with GPs, showed that over the past two years, there has been a 50 per cent increase in people who complain of extreme exhaustion. Exhaustion is a sign of a serious underlying problem that needs to be diagnosed and treated. Women with endometriosis describe this as feeling drained, sapped of all energy, like walking through treacle. All forms of exercise are exhausting, and leave you short of breath and in despair.

The main reasons for exhaustion are thyroid problems, anaemia, depression, chronic fatigue, low blood sugar and insomnia. Heaviness in the arms and legs, and being unable to breathe are indicative of exhaustion. Other signs are being unable to concentrate at work, feeling disorientated and faint for days on end, and waking early every morning unrefreshed by sleep so that you drag yourself through each day. You may have to give up working fulltime to recover your inner strength, as do many burned-out celebrities who go on retreats. A wise doctor will work with you through all the possible reasons for your exhaustion; a thoughtless one will just suggest anti-depressants. Although you feel ill, you must be assertive enough to insist that the correct tests be done: thyroid function, adrenal function, iron deficiency, ME, low blood sugar balance (fasting glucose), hyperinsulinism and melatonin levels. The reasons may be interlinked.

Emotional trauma can lead to adrenal failure, where you may just pass out as the whole endocrine system goes into crisis. Bereavement, loss of a loved one, being made redundant at work, chronic illness and acute pain may also lead to fainting spells. Starting a new job the day after you are rejected or trying to work at your normal rate through this period can be draining, and you may need to be easier on yourself. Often, with acute adrenal failure the body never really recovers as reserves are used up forever; at any point in the future, the slightest stress may cause you to implode. The symptoms of adrenal failure are excessive fatigue, fainting spells, muscle weakness, depression, insomnia, allergies, headaches and swollen lymph nodes under the arms and in the groin.

The adrenal glands contain the highest levels of vitamin C of any organ in the body. It is a precursor of the production of adrenaline and noradrenaline, neurotransmitters which regulate the nervous system. Vitamin B5 (pantothenic acid or calcium pantothenate) is also crucial in this pathway. Other nutrients for adrenal support at times of extreme stress are the essential fatty acids, zinc, magnesium and vitamin B6. Foods such as caffeine, sugar and alcohol act as stressors to the adrenal glands so are best avoided at such times. Herbs such as Siberian ginseng and liquorice contain substances which also support adrenal function. (Liquorice is oestrogenic in large doses so it is best to keep its consumption at moderate levels.)

LAUGHTER IN THE HEALING PROCESS

> Nothing was ever achieved without enthusiasm.
>
> *Ralph Waldo Emerson*

They always say that laughter is the best medicine, and new research shows that it does improve immune system function. Joy and laughter should be taught in all medical schools! Research looked at 26 women with rheumatoid arthritis and 31 controls. They were given humorous stories to read for an hour. Measurements taken showed that there was a decrease in negative mood and pain. Serum cortisol levels fell from 11.5mcg/dl to 8.3mcg/dl. There was a decrease in serum IL-6 from 34pg/ml to 10.6pg/ml. Induced laughter evoked significant improvement in objective facial manifestation of mood along with significant decreases in the patients' subjective sense of pain. There was also significant improvement in several hormonal and immunological markers of the disease.[34] Perhaps watching comedies, listening to jokes and reading funny stories may be helpful in recovery.

Trina H of Bedfordshire

After a number of doctors failed to diagnose my condition and after my repeated pleas for help, I finally found a doctor who would listen to me, after I had collapsed at work. She predicted endometriosis or a chocolate cyst. After scans and a laparoscopy, I was diagnosed with both! This led to laser surgery and the removal of half my left ovary. This was followed by one year of hormonal treatment, which led to bloating and emotional turmoil. One year later, I luckily fell pregnant. I eventually had two children, born close together as advised. I breastfed both children for as long as possible to stop my cycle returning. My endo returned within nine months of giving up breastfeeding.

I consulted my gynaecologist, who told me my options were either hormonal treatment or laser treatment every nine to twelve months. I was recommended to see a classical homeopath, who relieved and controlled my pain and symptoms considerably, but not fully.

After reading an article on nutrition by Dian and after my first consultation with her, I was given more satisfaction and answers than from anyone previously. I followed her advice and cut out bovine dairy and reduced wheat. I adjusted my diet to include more fish, and fresh, organic vegetables and fruits. I also took the recommended supplements.

After one month, I feel like a new person. My cycle has become regular, my energy has returned and my pain is virtually gone. I cannot believe that I suffered for seven years before finding the nutritional path.

PSYCHIATRIC HELP

Many women with endometriosis have been informed that they are clinically depressed, which usually means suicidally depressed. Yet most of the women are basically just feeling very low and are not contemplating suicide. Things have to be pretty extreme to feel so low – like the sudden loss of a loved one on top of the pain from the disease. Counselling may help some people, but not others, although in extreme cases, a visit to a psychiatrist may be the only way to regain sanity after a period of mental illness. In these extreme cases, anti-depressants are prescribed.

One in 20 Americans suffers from clinical depression and requires medical psychiatric treatment. It is the leading public health problem in the USA, with 15 per cent of these sufferers committing suicide as a result.[35] This is a chronic disease of the brain that is completely different from what we call 'despair depression' in this book. With endometriosis, it is more a case of mental anguish with life's normal ups and downs. The loss of joy in life can push people to a very low point, and it may be very difficult to find joy in the midst of endometriosis pain.

CLUES TO BRAIN DEFICIENCIES

OMEGA-3 ESSENTIAL FATTY ACIDS

Low cholesterol has been seen from research to trigger symptoms of depression. This may be due to a low intake of essential cis fatty acids which affects hormone production and leaves the brain's neural pathways deficient in essential fatty acids, or it may be due to the intake of hydrogenated omega-6 fatty acids from margarines and cooking oils, causing imbalances in brain chemistry.

These were thought to be important for heart health, but have since proved to be problematical. The Framingham Heart Study found that patients with low cholesterol (below 4.2mg/dl) had low heart disease, but they had a higher rate of suicide than the general population. Fish oils, however, could lower cholesterol yet maintain a sense of wellness in the patient. Work by Michael Crawford and Sir Alister Hardy suggests that, in the distant past, humans' link to the sea and consumption of fish oils aided the development of the higher brain function we see today. These crucial omega-3 fatty acids appear to be vital to brain function because they are an essential part of the cell membranes in the brain. The quality of the fats in this membrane ensures that the neurotransmitters pass normally along their message routes. The bad fats impede their journey so that the wrong message is passed or is simply blocked.

Research suggests that decreasing these omega-3 fatty acids impairs brain function. If you are vegetarian or vegan, then the use of flaxseed (linseed) oil is a suitable replacement. Omega-3 oils are important for the fatty acid phosphatidylserine that research has shown can reduce depression, and improve mood and memory. This is used by cells to metabolize glucose for energy, thus allowing them to release and bind with neurotransmitters. It also acts as a barrier to prevent antioxidants from causing damage. The brain synthesizes certain fatty acids into hormones, cell membranes and parts of the immune cells. Without the omega-3 fatty acids, the neuro-transmitters serotonin and noradrenaline cannot bind to their receptors. Thus, the brain cannot work efficiently if it is deficient in these oils.[36]

B VITAMIN COMPLEX

Many researchers, including those in the field of psychiatry, have looked for the links between vitamin deficiencies and depressive states. The entire family of B vitamins is involved in the brain– immune connection. This includes thiamine (B1), riboflavin (B2), niacin (B3), pyridoxine (B6), cobalamin (B12), folic acid, pantothenic acid (B5), biotin, choline and inositol. They all work together to help protect nerve endings against oxidation, and are thought to enhance memory and aid insulation of nerve cells by myelin. B vitamin deficiency can show up as memory loss and emotional lability.

Studies have shown that riboflavin (B2), pyridoxine (B6), folic acid and vitamin C are linked to depression, and the classical symptoms of deficiency of these vitamins and others of the B family are seen in patients with depression. Folic acid deficiency impairs the synthesis of BH4, a chemical needed by the brain to synthesize dopamine and serotonin. The Harvard Medical School has found that patients with depression are deficient in B2, B6 and B12.

Another B vitamin called inositol is able to cross the cell membrane and trigger reactions within the cell. In depressed patients, inositol is low in the cerebrospinal fluid. Inositol has been shown to aid patients where the usual anti-depressants were of no help.[37] Choline also contributes to restructuring of the brain as it helps in the formation of neuronal connections. It is part of the neurotransmitter acetylcholine, and aids memory and recall. As phosphatidylcholine, it is able to cross the brain–blood barrier.

CALCIUM AND MAGNESIUM

Magnesium plays a role in the energy production within brain cells as it activates adenosine triphosphate (ATP), the energy exchanged between cells. It is also important in the production of serotonin. It strengthens the cell membrane and protects them from the effects of excessive excitatory neurotransmitters. Calcium is vital to brain chemistry as it boosts the potential of nerve and muscle cells to aid the electrical impulses throughout the brain, thus improving cell communication.

ZINC

As 20 enzymes in the brain are dependent upon zinc, this mineral plays an important role within the brain. There is a connection between zinc deficiency and fatty acid levels. Zinc is essential for the body to produce an enzyme used to convert fats into DHA.

CHROMIUM

Dramatic changes in blood sugar levels may be caused by insulin resistance or metabolic changes. The brain is dependent upon glucose as an energy source. If glucose levels become wildly erratic, it may lead to behavioural changes and depression. The University of Pittsburgh has demonstrated, using positron emission tomography (PET) scanning, that people with depression have a reduced ability to metabolize glucose in various areas of their brain. A five-hour glucose test showed that depressed patients had higher glucose readings and different insulin responses than non-depressed individuals. Refined sugars are not natural to the body. Indeed, early humans could only obtain sugar from a beehive, or from maple or silver birch trees. It may be important for those with depression to avoid all refined sugar products and to use complex carbohydrates in their diet.[38]

BRAIN DISRUPTORS

SUGAR AND ASPARTAME

The brain, as we have seen, requires a continual supply of glucose to fuel up the cells. Low blood sugar levels due to hypoglycaemia may cause neurological symptoms, such as dizziness, tremor, double-vision, confusion, incorrect speech and depression. Perception and coordination may also be affected. Many patients have reported an aggravation of symptoms while using products containing aspartamine (aspartic acid). It is important to check if consuming aspartamine in fizzy drinks worsens any symptoms. Large doses of phenylalanine may stimulate prolactin secretion, research carried out at Northport, New York, has shown.

Aspartame may precipitate or aggravate hypoglycaemia in several ways. It is known that phenylalanine can stimulate the release of insulin, which could provoke a bout of hypoglycaenia. When women are trying to lose weight and therefore use more aspartame products, it may further reduce their blood sugar level. There are important relationships between the blood sugar level, insulin concentrations and aspartame. Insulin-induced hypoglycaemia caused a sharp increase in brain aspartate concentrations in experimental studies.[39] The best way to provide the brain with an even level of glucose is by eating complex carbohydrates which break down slowly.

MONOSODIUM GLUTAMATE (MSG) AND HYDROLYSED VEGETABLE PROTEIN

MSG can stimulate a wide range of abnormal endocrine responses from the hypothalamus. The release of hormones by the hypothalamus and pituitary controls the release of hormones from the endocrine glands throughout the body – such as the thyroid gland, adrenals, ovaries and testes. Researchers found decreased levels of growth hormone, prolactin and LH in animals exposed to MSG.

We know that 44 per cent of the British population never cook and use only processed foods for their meals. Many of these foodstuffs use flavour enhancers like MSG (E621) and aspartame (NutraSweet). When given to pregnant animals, MSG was found to have the same effect. Glutamate crosses the barrier of the placenta and enters the fetal bloodstream. Animals exposed to MSG were short in size, often overweight and had difficulty with reproduction.

Obesity may be due to early exposure to excitotoxins as it does not appear to be linked to food intake, and the weight cannot be dieted away. MSG and aspartame have been shown to cause an early onset of puberty in female rats. Other research has also shown that small doses of MSG can stimulate the hypothalamus to secrete large amounts of LH, which controls reproduction and the onset of puberty. MSG appears to cause immature neurons in the hypothalamus to become reorganized such that they disrupt the secretion of vital reproductive steroid hormones.[40]

Research from the neurosurgical department of the University of Mississippi found that MSG caused the ovaries to shrink, leading to reproductive problems. Large doses have also been seen to lower thyroid hormone levels and increase cortisone levels.

Clearly, for women with reproductive problems and those who are attempting pregnancy or are pregnant, it may be prudent to avoid MSG, aspartame and other excitotoxin-containing foods. Most salad dressings contain MSG, as do packet foods labelled 'natural flavouring', 'spices' or 'hydrolysed vegetable protein'. This additive can bring out the 'beefy' taste of foods while others highlight creamy flavours. MSG contains three powerful brain cell toxins – glutamate, aspartate and cysteic acid – as well as some carcinogens. Chips, sauces, rice dishes and gravies are often extremely high in MSG and other excitotoxin taste-enhancers. It is always best to avoid these unnecessary additives whenever possible, using processed foods only as occasional necessities in a busy life-style. Canned drinks may also contain aspartame. Environmental exposure on a daily basis to such substances may not be a good idea for women with endometriosis. Antioxidants such as vitamin E appear to afford some protection against damage. Magnesium is also protective, so eat more broccoli and spinach.

BASIC NUTRIENTS FOR BRAIN HEALTH

To correct brain biochemistry, we need to put theory into practice or, as one book title terms it, 'food for thought'. It is a matter of choosing wisely the foods that support brain cell and neurotransmitter function. These are designated 'therapeutic neuroimmunomodulators'.[41] As we already know, eating well by choosing the freshest, nutrient-rich foods is the most beneficial way to obtain the best building bricks. The use of nutritional supplements in the short term to support the nervous system while the diet is being adjusted may be helpful for two or three months.

FOOD CHOICE GUIDE

1   Eat the freshest vegetables, fruits, nuts and seeds every day.
2   Choose 'rainbow-coloured' meals to improve nutrient intake.
3   Eat complex carbohydrates in the form of wholegrain cereals and other plant foods (wheat excluded).
4   Keep fat to 25 per cent of your total daily intake and choose cold-pressed oils such as fish oil, flaxseed oil, nuts and seeds.
5   Reduce saturated fat intake (reduce dairy foods and red meat).
6   Eat a daily portion of 3oz (75g) of protein foods (game, lean meat, fish, eggs, nuts, seeds, peas, beans, lentils, broccoli, cauliflower), and goat's and ewe's milk dairy.
7   Follow a short-term nutritional supplement programme of multivitamins, an antioxidant, and a multimineral supplement containing calcium, magnesium, copper, zinc, iron, manganese, iodine and selenium plus an essential fatty acid.[42]

Zena B of London

I was in despair after a miscarriage, but since reading your book, may life has changed. I am now happy to report that I am pregnant after following the dietary advice and supplement programme. I feel better than I have done for years. You have given me my life back. Thank you.

STRESS

Once stress takes hold and the adrenal glands begin to work overtime to produce adrenaline, we use up supplies of magnesium, zinc and B vitamins at an alarming rate. The adrenals require a constant supply of vitamin C, B5 and essential fatty acids. As the nervous system becomes involved, so are calcium, magnesium and B vitamins required. The digestive system may shut down as we are thrown into the 'fight or flight' syndrome. (Do we fight that grizzly bear or run like the clappers?) Either way, our body is preparing us for action. The blood thickens in case we are attacked so that it will clot quickly, and the digestive system shuts off to allow us to run faster and use energy elsewhere. The liver throws more sugar into the blood to ensure that we have enough fuel to take us away from danger fast. But the body is only meant to be in this state for short periods of time, so when the stress is prolonged, everything begins to go wrong. Being nutritionally sound helps to bolster us against this effect. A selection of the following may also be useful:

Vitamin C	Pantothenic acid (vitamin B5)
Magnesium malate	Calcium gluconate
Zinc citrate	Chromium polynicotinate
L-Tyrosine	Bach Flower Rescue Remedy
Lime blossom tea	Multivitamins/minerals
Probiotics/acidophilus	Digestive enzymes
Manganese	Choline and inositol

(for depression see p. 337)

SUMMARY

1 Choose your food wisely. Eat from fresh as often as possible.

2 Avoid packet foods, using them only for emergencies.

3 Eat foods rich in essential fatty acids, B vitamins, calcium, magnesium, zinc and chromium.

4 Reduce sugar in the diet.

5 Avoid foods containing MSG, aspartame and hydrolysed vegetable protein.

6 Laughter is the best medicine. Remember all the happy times with your true love.

7 Do a good deed every day to make you smile.

8 Use basic supplements: a multivitamin, a multimineral and essential fatty acids to support the nervous system. If you are in a state of despair, try a mixed amino acid supplement for a month.

9 In cases of extreme fatigue, take one 500mg L-tyrosine tablet in the morning to lift energy production. Do this infrequently as small doses on occasion are more likely to be effective.

10 DLPA (D,L-Phenylalanine) may alleviate depression and reduce pain that is intractable.

> It is not the place, not the condition, but the mind alone that can make anyone happy or miserable.
>
> *Sir Roger L'Estrange, 1616–1701*

9 Strengthening the immune system

> The obscure we eventually see. The completely obvious, it seems, takes longer.
>
> *Edward R Murrow*

Something major is going wrong with the immune system in endometriosis, and it may be that subclinical deficiencies of nutrients are not allowing the body to work at optimum efficiency.

HOW THE IMMUNE SYSTEM WORKS

The immune system exists to protect us from danger. Outside our body are bacteria, viruses and parasites which can do us harm. The immune system consists of the liver, spleen, lymph glands (which filter cells), bone marrow and the thymus gland (which is located behind the breastbone). These are the chief organs which produce the white blood cell army (*see* figure 9.1). There are other tissues which are supportive of the immune system – the pituitary gland, adrenal glands, tonsils, adenoids, appendix and Peyer's patches in the lower part of the digestive tract.

The white blood cells behave like an army; they are the forces at the ready to do battle with an enemy invasion of the body. The lymphatic system is composed of the glands and lymph vessels, which are similar to the blood vessels, except the lymph is not pumped by the heart; it is moved by the body's movements. The vessels act as the main highway through the body on which the white blood cells can travel in the lymph (a yellow oil-based medium) to sites which are being threatened, the lymph glands. If the immune system begins fighting infections in the lymph glands, the glands enlarge (in the neck, groin and under the arms).

Research shows that 'over 2,000 immune cells per second are produced in our long (marrow) bones in the body'.[1] That figure, of course, presumes the body is healthy, fit and well fed. Such rapid growth and development deserves to be well supplied with the nutrients from your diet.

There are many different types of cell to suit all types of attack. They all originate from basic stem cells, primarily in bone marrow, which requires folic acid, vitamin B12, zinc, vitamin B6, iron and amino acids in abundance. If these are in short supply, the body cannot fight infections or remove cell debris (like endometriotic implants) efficiently. However, 80 per cent of the immunoglobulins (one of the major immune defence systems of the body) are made in the small intestine, therefore the gut

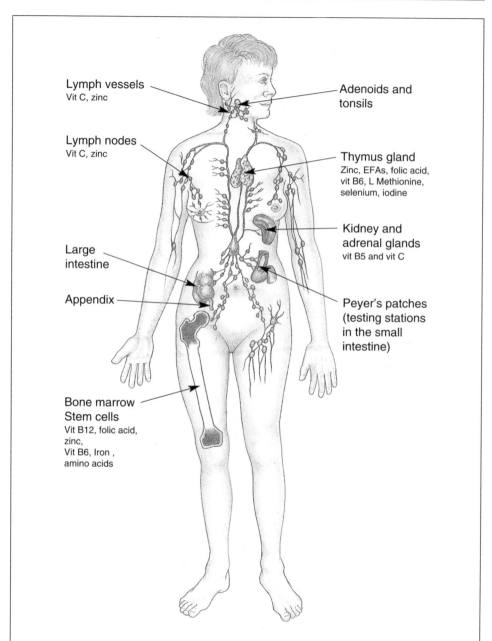

Lymph vessels
Vit C, zinc

Adenoids and
tonsils

Lymph nodes
Vit C, zinc

Thymus gland
Zinc, EFAs, folic acid,
vit B6, L Methionine,
selenium, iodine

Kidney and
adrenal glands
vit B5 and vit C

Large
intestine

Appendix

Peyer's patches
(testing stations
in the small
intestine)

Bone marrow
Stem cells
Vit B12, folic acid,
zinc,
Vit B6, Iron ,
amino acids

Figure 9.1
The lymphatic system, showing the major tissues which are associated with the
immune system.

membranes also need to be in the peak of health.[2] The gut as an area of immunity cannot be dismissed lightly. If your gut is ill, you will be ill.

Why are some people better endowed with stronger immune systems than others? Archibald Garrod in 1908 gave a lecture on inborn errors of metabolism at Yale University, USA, that is still pertinent today. He stated:

> 'The existence of chemical individuality follows of necessity from that of chemical specificity, but we should expect the differences between individuals to be still more subtle and difficult of detection. Indications of their existence are seen, even in man, in the various tints of skin, hair and eyes, and in the quantitative differences in those portions of the end-products of metabolism which are endogenous and are not affected by diet. Even those idiosyncrasies with regard to drugs and articles of food which are summed up in the proverbial saying that what is one man's meat is another man's poison, presumably have a chemical basis.'[3]

Lynn S of Yorkshire

Dietary changes as restrictive as the anticandida diet are extremely difficult to adhere to if the therapy is started when the patient is at a low ebb. I could not cope with the withdrawal symptoms as I had recently had major surgery and felt too ill to start immediately. The dreadful aching in all my muscles as well as extreme fatigue meant that I was bedridden.

I tried again when I felt better able to cope. I feel building up the immune system by diet and good food and supplements is better used as a preventive measure because, once endometriosis is established, comfort eating comes into play.

CASE STUDY

RECOGNIZING AN ALIEN INVASION

The immune system, as our first line of defence against infection and allergies, must be able to rapidly recognize 'alien' material like bacteria and viruses. In this way, as soon as our body is invaded, it can assemble the immune army of white blood cells and antibodies to rapidly destroy the 'alien' invaders. Inherent in this is the body's unique ability to recognize 'self' and 'non-self' material. As you may expect, this is accomplished very early on in our lives.

During our development as a fetus, the thymus gland in the chest and the other immunological tissues in the body compute and register all of the molecules that are present in the body as 'self tissue'. This stops our own immune system from attacking our own healthy cells.

However, there is a paradox with endometriosis. These cells are natural to the body, so they are not perceived as a threat. Or are they? Much of the pain from endometriotic implants could be from the release of strong chemicals as the macrophages try to remove these misplaced cells. There is only one other disease in the body where our own cells grow in the wrong places, and that is rare. This is splenosis and it only occurs when spleen cells are splattered after an accident. (The spleen is the only organ where endometriosis never appears to grow. It is the only part of the lymphatic system which filters blood.) All other body cells seem to behave themselves and stay where nature intended. If we can answer the question as to why endometrial cells roam, we may be halfway to finding the cure.

After birth, any alien molecules, like the molecules that make up the outer covering of a bacterium, are considered as 'non-self'. This is a miraculous system that is usually quite efficient at protecting us from 'alien' molecules which get into our bloodstream or lungs, or enter our bodies through breaks in the skin. However, there are some weaknesses in the system, one being that those tissues that are outside the body are not considered as part of the 'self' group. For instance, the sperm which are contained in tiny tubes within the testes are treated by the body as if they are outside the body, and are therefore recognized as 'non-self'. If you inject a man's sperm into himself, he will mount an immune attack against his own sperm!

This may happen in women with endometriosis. The endometrium which lies in the centre of the uterus can be viewed as being on the outside of the body because it is open to the outside through the vagina, and the immune system may not consider it to be part of the 'self' group. When the endometriotic implants develop in the abdomen, the body responds with an immunological attack on the implants because it sees them as cells from outside the body – 'aliens'. Since the implants are the same as the normal endometrium, the antibodies we make then also begin to attack the endometrium within the uterus. When this happens, it may well interfere with conception and the reproductive process.[4]

This immunological attack may actually be beneficial, in that women who do not have endometriosis may be devoid of the disease because their immune system constantly cleans up the endometriotic implants that form after each menstrual period. Women with an impaired immune system may not be able to clean up their abdomen of the endometriotic implants and thus they develop endometriosis.[5] How well we clean up inside the peritoneal cavity is dependent upon the nutrients which the white blood cells need for their function as 'rubbish disposal men'. If the white cells cannot do their job, then we fall ill.

Further research emphasizes the connection between endometriosis and an impaired immune system: 'Women with endometriosis have impaired ability of this disposal system, which is presumably mediated by either macrophages or peritoneal lymphocytes, or both. Alternately, it is possible that there are differences in the capacity of endometrial tissues to be destroyed even in immunocompetent environments.'[6] It is possible that the endometriotic implants outside the womb behave in a different way to the endometrium inside the womb. The mystery deepens. It may be painful to us and cause a great deal of misery, but the behaviour of this endometriotic tissue is intriguing. If we can find out why it behaves in this way, we may be closer to finding the cure.

It is felt that endometriosis may be an autoimmune disease (this is explained later on in this chapter). There is certainly immune dysfunction from many different perspectives (too many macrophages and too few natural killer cells) and whatever is happening also has a profound effect upon the reproductive system. The body tries to dispose of 'alien' endometriotic implant cells by phagocytosis (when white blood cells, the macrophages, come along and gobble up all invaders), but some mechanism goes wrong and some of the endometriosis is left behind. Women and researchers need to find out why. Then we will have the answer, the cure.

THE IMMUNE ARMY

The white cells behave like an army, holding the forces ready for when they are called out to do battle with an enemy. Each part of this immune army has its own unique functions, but like any successful army they all have to work as a team. All the parts help each other and support what the others are trying to do. There are two main 'battalions', the cell-mediated and humoral systems. There are different levels of immunity; some happens inside cells, some occurs outside cells on receptors nearby. Plasma proteins act as another phase of immunity and circulating hormones give rise to a fourth level. It is useful for us to understand how our immune system works in order to help it improve its task of cleaning up endometriotic implant debris.

CELL-MEDIATED IMMUNITY

Cell-mediated immunity (*see* figure 9.2) involves many free-floating cells, both red and white, found in the blood. Zinc is very important in this system, and antibodies require B vitamins in order to produce T lymphocytes, which destroy 'alien' bacterial and viral infections. They 'eat up' all the 'aliens' captured by the immune army cells.

Red blood cells

Red blood cells deliver oxygen to all the tissues in the body, and they are always on the alert, watching for 'aliens'. If they find them, they arrest them and escort them to the white blood cells for destruction. Red blood cells require folic acid, iron, vitamins B12, B6, A and C, and zinc, calcium and magnesium, manganese, good quality oils and copper.

White blood cells

White blood cells are the main fighting force. They include:

1 Macrophages
2 Polymorphs
3 T lymphocytes
4 B lymphocytes
5 Mast cells

These all have different ways to attack 'alien cells' which threaten danger. They require vitamins C and E and zinc for their production: 'One gram of vitamin C enhances the action of macrophages and stimulates the T cells and the B cells. (Aspirin is anti-vitamin C.) The macrophages which engulf "aliens" only work if they contain at least 20μ of vitamin C per 100 million cells.'[7]

Macrophages

These are like 'Pac-men' in a computer game. They go around the body gobbling up cell debris or stay inside cells (as monocytes) eating up the garbage (phagocytic behaviour). In other words, they collect all the refuse and keep our internal organs clean. They have receptors on their surface which are able to recognize dead cells and 'aliens'. Macrophages also make enzymes which can clot blood and aid fat transport. They need ample calcium in order to absorb antigens, which are used to create lyzyme (the 'bleach' the macrophages use to digest the aliens). When we have a fever, we rapidly use up calcium supplies, so the diet needs to be complete, and then macrophages work much faster and are more effective. Selenium also increases the ability of phagocytes to clear away 'alien' cells and tumour material. Vitamin B also has a vital role: 'Vitamin B6 is needed by macrophages to work efficiently. If B6 is deficient these immune cells cannot clean up body debris inside the body cavity.'[8] By contrast, the effects of sugar have been shown to be detrimental: 'Dr Yudkin's research showed that sugar-rich foods interfere with the way in which phagocytic white blood cells clean up "alien" invaders. Refined sugar was shown to depress immune function. Recent research has shown that this effect lasts for up to four hours after sugar is eaten.'[9] Macrophages also produce interferon and prostaglandins.

Polymorphs

Polymorphs are rather like *The Terminator* – they exterminate everything in sight. They work in kamikaze fashion; they engulf the 'aliens' and then release 'bleach-like bombs' at danger sites, thus killing themselves as well as the 'aliens'. Vitamin A is needed for the enzyme lysozyme in these bleaches.

T lymphocytes

T lymphocytes behave as homing missiles; they cruise around to survey areas and carry deadly chemicals on board ready to bomb the threat. Choline has been shown to increase lymphocyte production 3–4 times and helps the liver detoxify harmful chemicals. T lymphocytes lie in wait, watching for 'alien' invaders, and are ready to set off the alarm at any time if they are well nourished. They produce interferons.

There are four types of T lymphocytes that watch out for viral infections:

1   *T helper cells* – look after all the other immune cells and try to safeguard the immune system from making mistakes. They have the power to stop or start the warfare, and are very powerful in switching the immune system off or on. They also protect us from both viral and fungal infections.

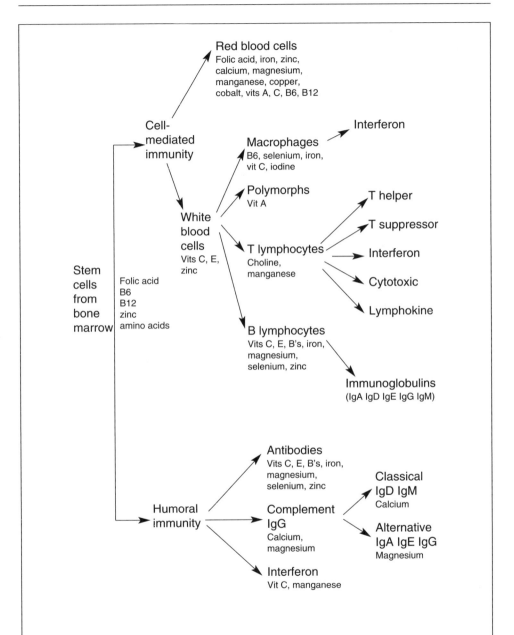

Figure 9.2
The immune system is separated into two main areas, the cell-mediated and the humoral. This diagram shows which nutrients each area relies on in order to work effectively.

2 *T suppressor cells* – have the power to switch the immune system off only. They cannot switch it on. Once the threat of infection is over, they turn the attack off. There should be a ratio of 1.8 T helper cells to 1 T suppressor cell.

3 *Cytotoxic T cells* – behave like rockets and are very destructive. They seek out viruses hiding inside cells and hunt 'aliens'. They contain very powerful enzymes which are capable of breaking up and destroying infected cells.

4 *Lymphokine-producing T cells* carry 'killer missiles' to destroy aliens which travel between cells.

B lymphocytes

B lymphocytes are very specific white blood cells which watch out for bacterial infections. They interrogate the 'alien' to discover its exact size and shape, and make a perfectly fitting straitjacket to hold it safe. B lymphocytes are able to form a production line making matching straitjackets to fit every 'alien' around. These are known as antibodies or immunoglobulins (Ig). Antibodies are able to arrest and hold the 'alien' until a macrophage can come along and gobble it up. B lymphocytes have memories, so if the same infection strikes again, they can go into production to make the right antibodies before the infection overtakes us. If we do get an infection twice, our immune system is functioning under par, and needs a boost. There are five antibodies in the blood all the time which are described in the section on 'humoral immunity'.

Mast cells

Mast cells are found all around the peritoneal cavity. They release histamines, serotonin (a neurotransmitter) and prostaglandins, which cause inflammation, increase blood flow, and may trigger acute food reactions. Prostaglandins can cause or dampen down inflammatory reactions and they modify one another's actions so they need to be in balance. They are constantly being made and destroyed.

HUMORAL IMMUNITY

Humoral immunity involves immunoglobulins (Ig), produced by B lymphocytes, which form antibodies against 'alien' bacterial protein material.

Antibodies

Antibodies are produced by B lymphocytes and they reinforce the humoral immune system response to danger. There are five types and they are labelled as IgA, IgD, IgE, IgG and IgM. Antibody production requires vitamin C, iron, magnesium, B vitamin complex, vitamin E, zinc and selenium. The different types of antibody have different roles: 'The IgE antibody, for example, is responsible for allergic reactions such as hay fever, asthma, eczema and arthritis. IgE is attracted to mast cells involved in allergic responses',[10] and 'IgG is required by cells active in destroying cancers and autoimmune diseases. It has the ability to activate the complement system of immunity.'[11] Research has shown that 'there was a trend to higher immunoglobulin

IgG levels in women with endometriosis, than in controls. Women with endometriosis have significantly higher levels of antiglandular antibodies than cord blood or male controls.'[12] It has been suggested that 'IgG defends us against agents which invade tissues, which is why it is prevalent in endometriosis.'[13] IgG is involved in food intolerances.

IgA occurs in mucous membranes, and in all body orifices open to the atmosphere, e.g. the mouth, nose, ears, vagina, bladder, anus, etc. It appears to malfunction in people with food intolerances and allergies. IgD is present in only very small amounts and its function is presently unclear. It is found in semen and on the outside of lymphocytes. IgM is synthesized by immature B lymphocytes; it is the predominant type of immunoglobulin produced in blood plasma after initial contact with an 'alien' in food and bacteria. This is the largest mucus-like molecule found in the spaces between the blood vessels that line the throat, nose and vagina. It is also the first antibody produced in newborn babies.

Interferon

Interferon affects both mind and body. Macrophages and T lymphocytes produce interferon, which is taken up by cells for their protection. Interferon shuts down the mitochondria (energy production powerhouse) in each cell to stop viruses using them for their replication. Interferon is dependent on manganese, choline and vitamin C. It has antiviral properties which prevent the virus from multiplying within the cells. As cells are damaged, they lose their ability to produce interferon. Damage can come from the external environment: 'There is a problem with the use of insecticides on crops as they inactivate choline-containing enzymes, which prevent the uptake of manganese by the plants. Overuse of insecticides can then lead to manganese deficiency in humans.'[14] Therefore our ability to produce interferon is reduced by pesticides. This implies that macrophages and T lymphocytes will not be as effective if the body has absorbed pesticides from foods.

Complement

Complement reinforces the humoral response and it acts in a cascade, rather like a tiered fountain. Once the cascade is set in motion, the complement cell dies. Complement production requires vitamin C. Complement works in two ways:

1   The classical pathway is activated by IgM and IgD and requires calcium.
2   The alternate pathway is activated by IgG, IgA and IgE and requires magnesium.

Complement destroys the 'aliens' by bursting cells using phagocytosis and inflammation – it 'blows up' dangerous 'alien' cells. Complement acts rather like the second unexpected, but spectacular, SAS-type assault on the battlefield. It provides specific immunity to complete the work begun by the T cells and B cells.

Antibiotics (which the body produces naturally) require vitamin C, as does the production of complement and macrophage ability to digest alien debris.

• C A S S E T U D Y •

Anon

Although I have unfortunately never achieved a pregnancy, I feel it is very important to continue eating a healthy diet. My ME did improve but has never entirely gone away. However, the right supplements combined with a healthy diet went a long way to help improve my immune system and I have had better general health ever since.

AUTOIMMUNE DISEASES

Autoimmune diseases involve a self-destructive element because 'in autoimmune disorders the immune cells make a big mistake and see their own "self tissue" cells as a danger'.[15] Autoimmunity is where the immune cells produced by the body begin to attack the body's own cells as well as 'alien' viruses, bacteria and parasites. This is, of course, bad news as healthy tissue can be harmed. Some researchers think that endometriosis is an autoimmune disease similar in nature to rheumatoid arthritis and systemic lupus erythematosus.

There is a strong connection between the immune system and nutrition, food allergies and intolerances, digestion and autoimmune diseases. Diseases such as type II adult onset diabetes, thyroiditis, systemic lupus and multiple sclerosis are thought to be autoimmune.

The three common features of autoimmune disorders can be described as follows:

1 The inside of cells becomes too acid.
2 The electron transport system malfunctions.
3 Nutrients which support the immune system are depleted.[16]

Endometriosis fulfils the majority of classical characteristics of autoimmune diseases:

1 Polyclonal B-cell activation
2 T-cell immunological abnormalities
3 B-cell immunological abnormalities
4 Multiorgan involvement
5 Tissue damage
6 Female preponderance
7 Familial occurrence
8 Possible genetic basis
9 Altered apoptosis (cell death)
10 Environmental factors
11 Increased alignment with other autoimmune diseases.[17]

If we are subclinically nutritionally deficient because we do not eat well or because our digestive tract has been compromised in some way, then the uptake of vitamins and minerals will be low and this may have a knock-on effect on the immune system. Therefore, for a disease like endometriosis we need to eat a healthy, balanced diet full of nutrients, and ensure our digestive tracts are working at maximum capacity.

Reducing our stress load, and allowing some time for ourselves (at least 20 minutes of relaxation each day) plus gentle exercise can benefit the immune system. The body heals faster when it is at rest. There are chemical dangers in the environment over which we have no control, and our bodies need to be strong in order to combat them, but other mechanisms could be at work.

NUTRITION AND THE IMMUNE SYSTEM

> If you are waiting for your ship to come in, start working days,
> nights and weekends building the dock.
>
> *Paul Micall*

Trying to build up our immune system may be the best way for healing to occur. Research suggest a connection between endometriosis and the immune system: 'The hypothesis that the peritoneal "disposal system" may malfunction whilst trying to eliminate misplaced endometrial cells has been advanced to explain the development of endometriosis.'[18] The immune system is affected by the state of the reproductive system, as they use many of the same nutrients. The rogue endometriotic implants should be removed and destroyed by the immune system's white blood cells before they take hold on the organs. But if the immune system has been compromised by poor diet, pollution or harmful drugs, it may be too weak to remove this rogue tissue.

Vitamin B6 is vital for the body macrophages so that body debris can be cleared away. If this is in short supply along with low intake of vitamin C, iron, magnesium, selenium, zinc and other antioxidants (vitamins A and E), trouble is brewing. Debris from old menstrual flow may accumulate, but cannot be cleared away efficiently. As we have seen, 'a deficiency in vitamin B6 causes a decrease in the way the phagocytic cells hold the alien tissue captive so that we cannot clean up inside as efficiently as we should'.[19]

Vitamin B6 and folic acid together have beneficial effects on immune function. If there is a good supply of folic acid, zinc, methionine (an amino acid) and vitamin B6, the thymus gland in the chest is larger and produces more white blood cells. However, the size of the thymus changes naturally in the course of our lives: 'The thymus is a mysterious gland as it is large until puberty and then begins to shrink in adulthood, though is still recognizable.'[20] Folic acid allows cells to divide and therefore is essential for efficient immune system function, but folic acid has to be in balance with other B vitamins and zinc to work effectively. If women are zinc- and B vitamin-deficient, folic acid will not be effective.

IMMUNE PARALLELS BETWEEN ENDOMETRIOSIS AND CANDIDA

Research by German and Russian scientists has focused on the proven immune abnormalities in endometriosis, which run parallel to the changes in immune function provoked by the yeast *Candida albicans*. *Candida albicans* induces production of interleukin (IL)-1, tumour necrosis factor-alpha and IL-6. It has also been seen to activate macrophages and prostaglandin F2 (PGF2) production. Activation of *C. albicans* appears to inhibit phagocytosis. The yeast is associated with allergic reactions to it and is highly allergenic, and may be a factor in some atopic diseases. It can bind to mammalian hormones, including oestrogen, progesterone and cortisone. Indeed, antibodies to *C. albicans* are influenced by progesterone and oestradiol. Oestradiol was shown to stimulate the transition of the yeast cells to the invasive hyphal form. *Candida* has been seen to bind to the oestrogen mimic bisphenol A (a plasticizer). Women with endometriosis often test positive for allergy to *C. albicans*, luteinizing hormone, oestrogen, chemicals and food proteins. The International Endometriosis Association, head-quartered in the USA, has produced a paper on immunotherapy for endometriosis.[21] More details are given in chapter 10 and in Appendix B (p. 343).

ENDOMETRIOSIS AND THE IMMUNE SYSTEM

The precise details of the relationship between endometriosis and the immune system need clarifying, as the following observations suggests: 'Endometriosis involves the implantation and survival of endometrial tissue on peritoneal surfaces in the pelvis. The process is stimulated by sex steroid hormones (oestrogen and progesterone); other factors which determine the fate of endometrial tissue outside the uterus are unknown.'[22] Research shows that certain chemicals (cytokines, which may be produced by macrophages) are implicated in cell proliferation and inflammatory reactions: 'The volume of peritoneal fluid and its content of the inflammatory cells called macrophages have been shown to be significantly increased in patients with endometriosis, particularly in mild forms of the disease.'[23] This secretion of cytokines from macrophages may be the trigger for the cell proliferation seen in endometriosis, and may be responsible for the inflammatory response. Macrophages also produce interferons and prostaglandins, inducing inflammation and affecting the energy output of cells. Could this be why women with endometriosis feel tired all the time?

Menstrual debris is found in the peritoneal cavity of 90 per cent of women with endometriosis with open Fallopian tubes,[24] yet only 50 per cent of all women have active endometriosis. Therefore in 40 per cent of women their immune system is working effectively to clear away the menstrual debris and prevent it seeding itself onto other organs. It is suggested that the women with endometriosis do not have effective immune systems, possibly due to faulty nutrient uptake or an enzyme deficiency.

Research suggests that peritoneal fluid in patients with mild endometriosis supports cell proliferation owing to chemical signalling from the immune army as it attacks the site. Moreover, 'new research shows that endometrial tissue may be producing its own supply of oestrogen which would also trigger cell proliferation. Levels of IL-1 and tumour necrosis factor (types of cytokine) are increased in women with endometriosis'.[25] This points to inflammatory and hormone secretions from the endometriosis may be increasing the staying power of the rogue tissue. Normal endometrial tissue is natural to the body, so some immune signals try to maintain it within the womb. When endometriotic implants are outside the womb, other immune cells see it as growing in the wrong place and try to remove it. This is the dichotomy of endometriosis.

Johannes Evers, a prominent gynaecologist and researcher, suggests that one reason for the development of endometriosis may be that the endometrial deposits are so viable that the peritoneal macrophages do not recognize them as rubbish and do not try to remove them, allowing them to implant: 'Normal menstrual debris which enters the peritoneal cavity should be cleared away by the macrophages, but it appears that their capacity may be limited by some factor, either the quantity is too large or the disposal is inefficient and this leads to the cells staying around and implanting.'[26]

Peritoneal fluid volume and its components depend on follicular activity, corpus luteum vascularity and hormone production. The volume of peritoneal fluid in women with unexplained infertility was higher than that in controls. The fluid contains macrophages, mesothelial cells, lymphocytes, eosinophils and mast cells. The macrophages produce cytokines, whch cause an inflammatory response. Recent studies suggest that the endometrial implants and cysts also produce cytokines. They express IL-6 mRNA and IL-6 proteins. Peritoneal fluid from patients with endometriosis has frequently been shown to be toxic to the preimplantation embryo. Correcting the immune system would be a key to finding a cure.[27]

FERTILITY AND THE IMMUNE SYSTEM

The female genital tract is considered part of the mucosal immune system. The Fallopian tubes, endocervix and vagina contain plasma cells that produce IgA and the J-chain molecule needed for effective IgA secretion. The immunoglobulin found in uterine and cervical secretions, however, is IgG.

The immune system plays a major role in the normal physiology of human reproduction and high levels of cytokines have been implicated in fertilization, preimplantation embryo development, implantation, and placental and fetal growth. Abnormalities in this system are linked to reproductive failure.[28]

Endometriosis, as we have seen, upsets immune system function in such a way that the normal levels of immune cells in peritoneal fluid becomes disrupted; a compelling body of evidence suggests a cellular immunological basis for endometriosis-associated infertility.[29] All these factors in the fluid around the womb and ovaries, and others within the cervix and uterus may be harmful to the incoming sperm or to the conceptus as it travels in the Fallopian tube and tries to implant into the endometrium. What women with endometriosis and subfertility require is a quiet immune system in which no harm befalls the sperm or embryo. The principles of nutritional medicine aim to reduce the burden on the immune system by using nutritional supplements in the short term to support the immune system, and to look for any food allergies or intolerances which may be putting the immune system into a constant state of red alert. Removing a particular allergen from the diet or environment may be appropriate in some cases.

Future therapeutic strategies to reduce the immune inflammatory reaction associated with endometriosis should target pathological proteins. Drugs such as pentoxifylline, a phosphodiesterase inhibitor, have been suggested to improve fertility by targeting and switching off the immune system.[30] However, this drug is not approved by the FDA in the treatment of endometriosis as yet. Losing the power of the immune system's protection from disease could be problematical in the long term, so clinical studies investigating ways to reduce local inflammatory reactions in the peritoneum are needed. Cold-pressed cis fatty acids aid the reduction of inflammation, and evening primrose, linseed and fish oils have been documented to reduce the size of endometriotic implants.

Is endometriosis growing where it should not owing to faulty macrophages? Are they deficient in vitamin B6, iron, calcium or selenium, so they can't work effectively? We need research to look at this question. It could be that more macrophages are in the peritoneal cavity as they are too ineffective in smaller numbers if these nutrients are poorly supplied. Both cell-mediated (T lymphocytes) and humoral (B lymphocytes) immunological defence mechanisms are involved in cleaning away debris from the peritoneal cavity. Antibodies to the endometrium, cell membranes and to the heart cells have been demonstrated in patients with endometriosis, indicating that the immune system is activated as a result of endometriosis.[31]

If there is some mechanism which prevents the white immune cell army from working at its optimum level, this may be due to a lack of nutrients, or it may be due to the effect of pesticides, such as dioxins, which are known immunotoxicants (poison to the immune system). This immune army needs feeding just like any other army. Without the necessary nutrients in plentiful supply, the cells will fail to complete their tasks efficiently. And if they are fed junk and pesticides, they will fail to protect you.

ALTERNATIVE HYPOTHESIS

There are other immune interactions which could be going wrong. These problems may be similar to the autoimmune effects which cause endometriosis.

MICROORGANISMS AND VIRUSES

Let us look at the microorganism that causes syphilis. An antigen (a substance that the body sees as 'alien' and therefore a potential danger) called cardiolipin on the surface of that microorganism identifies it as the same as some of the heart muscle cells. When the immune system sees the syphilis microorganism is causing damage it attacks it, but in doing so it also attacks the heart muscle (which has the same cardiolipin identity). Could a similar process be happening in endometriosis? Is some external microorganism causing a problem? Some researchers wonder if endometriosis is caused by a type of virus, which triggers a cascade within the body cells.

Autoimmune ovarian disease is found in various endocrine syndromes. Several possible causes of immune activation are thought to occur as a result of tissue damage. 'Assessment of antibodies present in 40 patients with premature ovarian failure showed that, relative to controls, there was a significant increase in antibodies against thyroglobulin, nuclear antigens, heart disease and gluten, and increased levels of IgM. Decreased levels of complement were also described.'[32]

Gluten, the elastic protein in wheat, is also implicated in thyroid failure. Research at the ImmunoLaboratories in Florida is looking at the links between gluten and thyroid problems and it is thought that the gliadin portion of the gluten is the same as a protein in the thyroid: 'If the body builds up an intolerance to gluten then the immune cells will automatically begin to attack other similar tissue types, even though they are our own cells.'[33] It may be that both thyroid and ovarian cells come under fire. Much more research is needed in this area to show if it is of significance with endometriosis and infertility, but it is a very interesting hypothesis.

Research has shown that subclinical autoimmune disease may be involved with reproductive failure: 'Forty-four per cent of women who miscarried were seen to have antibodies implicated with anti-cardiolipin. It has also been speculated that two thyroid auto-antibodies are involved with reproductive failure. Thyroid auto-antibodies have been used as guides to point to women at risk from miscarriage.'[34] Research suggesting a link between coeliac disease (gluten intolerance) and auto-antibodies to the thyroid warrants further investigation, as 'adults tend to present with these problems in their 30s and 40s, tiredness, mouth ulcers, malaise, fertility problems and malabsorption being the main problems'.[35] All women with unexplained infertility should request very basic tests for auto-antibodies to the thyroid, coeliac disease (gluten sensitivity) and genito-urinary infections.

EFFECTS OF STRESS ON THE IMMUNE SYSTEM

Prolonged or extreme stress can be very harmful to the immune army, sapping its strength when it most needs help.

The hormone cortisol (from the adrenal glands) is an immuno-suppressant which reduces the levels of T helper cells; increases the levels of T suppressor cells; inhibits production of natural killer cells and interferon; decreases secretion of IL-1 and IL-2; blocks the production of lymphocytes; shrinks the thymus gland; and reduces progesterone levels.

Studies show that 'cortisol secretion occurs usually for six hours around waking time, it prepares the body for action and in doing so suppresses sleep, growth, reproduction and libido. It also reduces production of GnRH, LH from the pituitary gland, oestradiol and testosterone from the gonads'.[36] Corticosteroids are stress hormones which are released from the adrenal gland when toxins, infections, emotions, pain and disease strike. Stress raises cortisol levels in the adrenals, and this hormone competes with progesterone production and lowers it, which in turn alters oestrogen levels. Ongoing stress is very damaging in any illness, but particularly in endometriosis as oestrogen levels must be balanced with progesterone. If the stress 'fight or flight' reaction is continuous, the adrenal glands would always be on red alert, constantly producing high levels of adrenaline and cortisol. This would have a knock-on effect on all the other endocrine glands, such as the pituitary, ovaries and testes. The pituitary gland in the brain coordinates immune activity in the head and neck areas, so stress also depletes the immune system, and it also causes blood to thicken in case of injury so that it will clot easily. Adrenal stress triggers an aching neck and shoulders.

Stress affects the reproductive system in many ways. Insulin, progesterone, testosterone and oestrogens decrease at times of stress, whereas corticosteroids, catecholamines, thyroxine and growth hormone output is increased when the body is under stress. Because the corticosteroids inhibit release of GnRH from the hypothalamus and LH from the pituitary, this has an effect on the reproductive, digestive and immune systems. Corticosteroids increase sympathetic nervous system activity, which is implicated in a decrease in natural killer cell function. They also decrease the secretion of gastric juices and halt gastrointestinal mobility – peristalsis shuts down and the bowel begins to malfunction.

Try to understand how these three systems (reproduction, digestion and immunity) are interlinked and entwined. Nutrients and stress reduction are parts of our jigsaw, parts of the key to keep systems strong. Even the nervous system will be affected because neurons have receptors for LH. So, stress damages the reproductive, nervous, immune and the digestive systems in one fell swoop. Stress reduction techniques described in chapter 6 can help to minimize the damage.

OTHER DANGERS FOR THE IMMUNE SYSTEM

Fluoride

Fluoride breaks off a portion of the Y-shaped antibody, breaking the antibody into two and making it ineffective; 'fluoride causes immune system weakness and reproductive problems'.[37] Perhaps women with endometriosis should avoid products containing fluorides to help strengthen their immune systems. This includes certain toothpastes, mouthwashes, medications, aerosols, pesticides, herbicides, foods processed with fluoridated water, shampoo and deodorants. Look for those which are fluoride-free.

IMMUNE SYSTEM SUPPLEMENTS

The immune system is our battleground against disease. We usually expect it to protect us against outside agents which try to do us harm, such as viruses, bacteria and gut parasites. When it starts attacking 'self tissue', something drastic is going wrong. As many of the white blood cells rely on nutrients to supply their needs, what we eat is important in helping us to maintain the immune system's function. We should take in adequate amounts of:

- Selenium (yeast-free)
- Vitamins A, C and E
- Echinacea (take in three-week blocks only)
- Coenzyme Q10
- Zinc
- Magnesium
- B-complex vitamins

SUMMARY

The immune system controls the ways in which the body copes with attacks from bacteria, viruses, cell debris and infiltrating tissue such as endometriosis. You can help to support your immune system to function by eating foods which are nutrient-rich. This gives the immune cells a fighting chance at eradicating misplaced tissue such as endometriotic implants.

1 Endometriosis may be due to immune dysfunction. Women who have endometriosis may have impaired immune systems which may not be able to clean up debris in the abdominal cavity.

2 A strong immune system is dependent upon a varied nutrient and phytochemical intake.

3 Make sure that your foods are rich in the antioxidant nutrients as they are protective – the mineral selenium and vitamins A, C and E.

4 Sugar-rich foods interfere with the way in which white blood cells clean up cell debris, so reduce your intake of sweet foods.

5 If you have unexplained infertility or if your endometriosis seems to be blocking your fertility, request tests for auto-antibodies to the thyroid, coeliac disease (IgE and IgG gluten-sensitivity blood samples) and genitourinary infections, as well as for steroid hormone levels.

6 Reduce your stress levels wherever possible. Make a list of all the things which stress you and think hard about ways in which some of them could be eliminated.

7 Avoid products containing fluoride, such as toothpastes, shampoos and deodorants, as they can inhibit antibody function.

8 If you are from an atopic family, with a history of asthma, eczema, hayfever and/or arthritis, avoid bovine dairy foods. If you have constant pain and bloating, and feel tired all the time, avoid wheat. If your body is reacting to these foods, it may calm your immune system if they are excluded (see chapter 10).

10 Digestion and the reproductive system

> Throughout prehistoric times and historic times, supplies of food and resultant eating patterns have been powerful factors influencing human development and the human condition.
>
> *Stamler, 1994*

> Such is the idea that poor nutritional standards may be blocking human-kind's path to future health.
>
> *Dian Mills, 1996*

You are what you eat. Rather – you are what your body can digest. That is far more important. You could be eating an amazing diet and yet not digest and absorb the nutrients effectively.

Does the food you eat really make that much difference to your health? Does your digestive system obtain the maximum amount of nutrients from the foods you eat every day? Are the foods you eat rich in nutrients? Many processed foods are high in calories but lack essential nutrients, therefore it is vital that you eat fresh foods daily. It is very important to have an efficient digestive tract, removing nutrients from foods, processing them and sending them into the bloodstream. These nutrients affect the way each cell functions, trigger production of hormones and enzymes and keep the body healthy.

A key to the whole reproductive system working normally is the regular supply of nutrients, and that is dependent upon the health of your intestines. Without absorption of nutrients, fertility begins to fail. Hormone production becomes erratic, affecting the function of the hypothalamus, pituitary gland, ovary and womb lining. Ensuring that your digestion is working at its best should be your number one concern.

In this chapter we are going to look at factors that help and factors that hinder the digestive system's ability to absorb nutrients from even the most superb of diets. Your digestive tract health is vital to the state of your hormone profile; it really is the body's first line of defence against disease.

Nutrition is not an alternative approach like herbal medicine and homeopathy; it is essential to life. Eating is something we all do every day. It sustains us, it can keep us healthy – or it can make us unhealthy.

Table 10.1
A comparison of foods 1939 and 1991[1]

Food	Potassium 1939	Potassium 1991	% change	Calcium 1939	Calcium 1991	% change
Old raw carrots	225	170	-24%	48	25	-48%
Boiled cauliflower	152	120	-21%	22	17	-23%
Celery	279	320	15%	52	41	-21%
Old potatoes	568	360	-37%	8	5	-38%
Swede	138	170	23%	56	53	-5%
Lettuce	208	220	6%	26	28	8%
Onions	137	160	17%	31	25	-19%
Tomatoes	288	250	-13%	13	6	-54%
Mushrooms	467	320	-31%	3	6	100%
Cucumber	141	140	-1%	23	18	-22%
Chicory	182	170	-7%	18	21	17%
Kellogg's All Bran	955	1000	5%	82	69	-16%
Hovis	243	200	-18%	28	120	329%
Kellogg's Cornflakes	114	100	-12%	7	15	114%
Cheddar	116	77	-34%	810	720	-11%
Whole milk	160	140	-12%	120	115	-4%
Butter	15	–	–	15	–	–
Eggs (chicken)	138	130	-6%	56	57	2%
Boiled chicken	381	300	-21%	11	11	0%
Beef roast/lean	337	350	4%	6	6	0%

We all try our best to eat the mythical 'well-balanced diet'. A new assessment of the mineral content of fruits and vegetables shows that vital minerals can be 30–40 per cent lower in 1991, compared with 1939 (see table 10.1). So even if we eat as well as people did in 1939, we still cannot take in the same amounts of mineral without eating more, and unfortunately most people eat far less fruit and vegetables today than was consumed in the early twentieth century. Professor Tim Lange, of the Centre for Food Policy, believes that plant breeders are developing disease-resistant crops at the expense of low mineral uptake – thus changing the content of what we are eating.[2]

Thomas McKeown has argued that 'the major changes in health status in the twentieth century have been due to improved personal hygiene, better housing and healthier diets rather than to curative medicine'.[3] This is real preventive medicine.

Magnesium 1939	Magnesium 1991	% change	Iron 1939	Iron 1991	% change	Phosphorus 1939	Phosphorus 1991	% change
12	3	-75%	0.6	0.3	-50%	21	15	-29%
7	12	71%	0.5	0.4	-20%	33	52	58%
10	5	-50%	0.6	0.4	-33%	31	21	-32%
25	17	-32%	0.7	0.4	-43%	40	37	-8%
11	9	-18%	0.4	0.1	-75%	19	40	111%
10	6	-40%	0.7	0.7	0%	30	28	-7%
8	4	-50%	0.3	0.3	0%	30	30	0%
11	7	-36%	0.4	0.5	25%	21	24	14%
13	9	-31%	1	0.6	-40%	136	80	-41%
9	8	-11%	0.3	0.3	0%	24	49	104%
13	6	-54%	0.7	0.4	-43%	21	27	29%
420	210	-50%	10	12	20%	–	–	–
80	56	-30%	3	3.7	23%	257	190	-26%
17	14	-18%	2.8	6.7	139%	58	50	-14%
47	25	-47%	0.6	0.3	-50%	545	490	-10%
14	11	-21%	0.08	0.06	-25%	95	92	-3%
24	–	–	0.16	–	–	24	–	–
12	12	0%	2.5	1.9	-24%	218	200	-8%
26	25	-4%	2.1	1.2	-43%	270	190	-30%
25	23	-8%	4.4	2.6	-41%	264	200	-24%

LIFESTYLE AND THE PSYCHOLOGY OF EATING

We all want to enjoy the food we eat. That is a part of the pleasure of eating. The whole world over, people invite others into their homes and offer them a meal. Friendships are made, deals are struck, and families come together over the meal table. Mediterranean cultures are especially skilled at creating relaxing and enjoyable mealtimes. Preparing and sharing of food is a statement of caring for our fellow friends. Cooking is creative and people gain great pleasure in the giving of good food. We should all learn to take time out to enjoy the food we eat and share it with friends.

The following guidelines may help to improve your digestion:

1 Relax for 10 minutes before you eat to allow the digestive enzymes to begin working.
2 Sit down while you eat; never stand or rush around with a sandwich in your hand.
3 Chew slowly in order to mix salivary amylase, the carbohydrate-digesting enzyme in the mouth, into the food.
4 Avoid too many distractions during mealtimes. Talking with friends is one thing, but if you are watching TV and trying to read the newspaper as well, you will not get the best enjoyment from your meals.
5 Take time to enjoy what you are eating, savour the flavours, and try to avoid 'snatch and grab'-type meals.
6 Prepare food just before you are going to eat it, and cook it as quickly as possible in order to preserve the maximum vitamin content. Steaming, grilling or stir-frying are the best ways to preserve nutrients.

To understand the quantities of foods required for mealtimes, the following old adage is still useful: eat like a king for breakfast, a prince for lunch and a pauper for dinner. This will allow the body to absorb the maximum nutrients needed at the beginning of the day to sustain energy in the hours to come.

PATTERNS OF HEALTHY EATING

Man has drastically altered his diet over the past 50 years, and our digestive systems have not yet fully adapted to these changes. At first man was a scavenger, eating whatever came his way each day, and because he was nomadic; no stores of food were kept save those he could carry. Food (nuts, seeds, berries, fruits, wild vegetables, wild grass seeds, meat and fish, and occasionally honey) was eaten fresh when it was available, and in times of famine only the strong survived. Then around 6000 BC man learned to cultivate crops and herd animals, so the diet changed. More cereal grains were eaten and as hamlets were established, food was stored. Nowadays few of us grow our own food. Instead we rely on farmers and multinational organizations to produce the food for our meals. Apparently, '44 per cent of people rarely cook; they merely rely on processed foods, developed to have a long shelf-life'.[4] Studies show that '35 per cent of household food bills are spent on ready-cooked meals'.[5] The idea of eating really fresh, 'just picked', vibrant food has diminished.

We are thought to have been omnivores, implying that we ate a wide variety of foods in our recent past, and this is what our digestive systems still expect. Nowadays, however, we tend to have a very restricted diet and most people do not eat a wide variety of foods. The gut and liver have to deal with many new chemicals that are added to our foods in order to 'enhance' their taste and to give them a longer 'shelf-life': 'the average person eats an alarming 3–12 pounds of additives each year'.[6] If the liver is overtaxed with chemicals, it will need detoxifying before you can heal. Many cultures follow detox measures – Swedes have their saunas; American Indians have their sweat lodges; Arabs have Turkish baths; Eastern Europeans have mud baths, and

Muslims their cleansing Ramadan fasts. All these activities draw toxins from the body to help it to remain healthy.

We need to look at the foods we eat and make sure that we choose well, as that will help our ailing digestion. The shops are full of foods which look tempting, but do they contain the nutrients our bodies require in order to keep us healthy? Wholemeal flour contains 22 nutrients. White flour has had 98 per cent of its vitamin B6, 91 per cent of the manganese, 84 per cent of magnesium and 87 per cent of its fibre, and most of its chromium removed by processing. Refined foods have a lot of nutrients removed by processing, and unfortunately many foods have additives, pesticides, antibiotics and hormones within them. Our digestive enzymes and body cells are not designed to deal with such a cocktail of these compounds, and some sensitive people can have extreme reactions over time as their livers, digestive and immune systems weaken in the face of chemical onslaught.

THE DIGESTIVE TRACT BARRIER

Remember that your digestive tract is a 26-foot-long (780cm) tube, open at each end, so its contents are not really internal but are external to the rest of the body. It consists of the mouth, oesophagus, stomach, liver, pancreas, gallbladder and small intestine and large intestine (*see* figure 10.1). All these organs have a strong mucous membrane which acts as a barrier between the outside world and the bloodstream. This membrane protects us from harmful substances in the outside world. Only the nutrients, amino acids, glucose, fatty acids, glycerol, and phytochemicals should cross this mucosal barrier into the bloodstream. Larger molecules pass through, from the mouth to the anus, and are expelled as waste without causing harm; therefore 'this mucosal barrier has to be extremely resilient. Its surface is 300m^2 (almost the size of a tennis court), which makes it the largest surface area in the body which is in contact with external substances'.[7]

THE DIGESTION AND IMMUNE SYSTEM LINK

Tissue called 'Peyer's patches' on our gut wall, sample and test all the substances we pour into our body. If they sense a dangerous 'alien' they call up the immune army by secreting IgA antibodies. IgA antibodies are part of the lymphatic system, the immune system. They are on watch all the time (like sheepdogs) for any dangers: 'The IgA binds to the antigen (alien bug) and makes it much bigger so it is more difficult for it to pass through the gut wall.'[8] The dimensions of the gastrointestinal tract reflect the importance of its role: 'Gut association lymphoid tissue (GALT) is distributed throughout the GI tract. GALT consists mainly of Peyer's patches and the total mucosal surface area of the adult human GI tract is up to 300m^2, making it the largest body area to interact with the environment – tennis-court size! This huge surface area has to be very effective at absorption and yet exclude all infectious agents, allergenic material and toxic substances from entering the bloodstream via the villi. The GALT makes the gastrointestinal tract the largest lymphoid or immune organ in the human

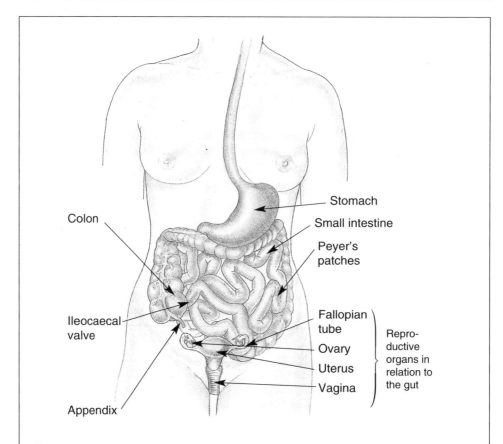

Figure 10.1
The digestive system is open to the outside at either end and therefore has to form a strong barrier internally to protect us from invaders such as harmful bacteria. It does this through the good gut flora and the integrity of its mucous membrane. The GI tract consists of the mouth, oesophagus, stomach, liver, pancreas, gallbladder, small intestine and large intestine. The gut mucosal barrier requires zinc, beta-carotene, biotin, butyric acid, pantothenic acid, vitamins A, C and E, and essential fatty acids and L-glutamine for its health. Herbs like slippery elm can help protect it when it becomes inflamed.

body. It has been estimated that there are approximately 10^{10} immunoglobulin-producing cells per metre of small bowel – accounting for approximately 80 per cent of all immunoglobulin-producing cells in the body.'[9] This vitally important membrane is our first line of immune defence and needs looking after, and 'adhesion of the good bifido bacteria, the lactobacilli, to this mucosal lining may be a critical factor in stimulating the immune system'.[10]

We all have four pounds of gut flora living in the intestines of each one of us and by keeping this healthy and balanced we may improve our general health. The health of the digestive system can profoundly affect your immune and reproductive system, your fertility and perception of pain. It is in your interest to keep both systems in tiptop health.

FOOD INTOLERANCES

Some normal foods, such as wheat and milk, may suddenly begin to be a problem if they have not been digested correctly. The body becomes intolerant if large molecules pass through the mucosal barrier. Some of our white blood cells are thought to have a memory of three months, so avoiding a problem food for three months may solve the problem. You can then start to reintroduce the food gradually. But why do food intolerance problems arise?

1 If the gut membrane becomes compromised in susceptible people by such irritants as excess gluten from wheat, food additives, pesticides, drugs or filaments from yeast overgrowth, the protective mucous membrane may be breached.
2 If the gut flora are upset by an onslaught of antibiotics or hormonal preparations (such as the contraceptive pill or HRT), or even severe prolonged stress, they may become unbalanced.
3 If the liver and pancreas enzymes are not fully functional.
4 If the stomach's hydrochloric acid supply is too low.
5 If gut parasites or food-poisoning bacteria or yeasts invade this space.
6 If the small villi (projections in the gut wall) are damaged by wheat bran or gluten, absorption of nutrients may fail.

Once large molecules are able to pass through damaged gut membranes into the blood, the body's immune army reacts, as it perceives danger. You may begin to feel 'sick all over' from the toxins released into the body via the blood – known as auto-intoxification. It can also happen if the ileocaecal valve between the small and large intestine becomes faulty and allows backward flow of bacteria into the small intestine. Systemic kinesiology treatment (*see* pp. 136, 399) may help to correct this.

Ailish P of London

I have suffered from the debilitating condition of endometriosis since the age of 14. Over the years, the pain and symptoms became worse until eventually the condition was diagnosed when I was 24. By the age of 31, and several hormone treatments and operations later, the disease was still affecting my life.

I suffered from a lack of energy, poor concentration, bloating, bad skin and gums and, for several days of each month, severe abdominal and back pain. Throughout the month, I had severe pain on defecation and alternated between having diarrhoea and constipation.

CASE STUDY

I realized that medical treatment was not really working and decided to try an alternative approach. Nutritional supplements and a healthy diet which excluded wheat seem to be the answer to my problem. I am now pain-free, have normal bowel habits, have much more energy and feel so much better – less anxious and depressed about the whole condition. It is hard to exclude wheat from one's diet as it is contained in so many foods. However, the benefits I have gained from this diet far outweigh the fact that I cannot have a hot buttery slice of toast in the mornings! It is far better to feel so well and switch to alternative foods – now toast does not seem very attractive any more.

FACTORS WHICH INFLUENCE NUTRIENT INTAKE

DIGESTION AND ABSORPTION

Eating fresh and healthy food is not much help if the digestive tract is not working efficiently. Even if we eat organic food all the time, a damaged digestive system does not effectively break down the foods into nutrients, and, if there is any damage to the mucous membranes or liver, or if the pancreatic enzymes are poorly secreted, our absorption of nutrients will be impaired. According to one study, 69 per cent of the population studied showed signs of at least one gastrointestinal disorder over the previous three months. In the USA alone it is a common reason for people to seek medical advice and annual costs are $41 million (£25.6 million). Surveys show that 'constipation affects four million Americans each year. Physicians write more than a million prescriptions for constipation annually, and we [Americans] spend $725 million a year on laxatives.'[11]

Any disorder of the gut and its membrane (stomach upsets, indigestion, bad breath, abdominal pain, irritable bowel syndrome, diarrhoea, constipation, piles, anal irritation) implies that some degree of malabsorption may be present. This leads to poor uptake of nutrients no matter how healthy a diet is eaten.

> Every tissue in the body is fed by the bloodstream which is supplied by the bowel. When the bowel is dirty, the blood is dirty and so are the organs and tissues. It is the bowel that must be cared for first.
>
> *Lindsey Duncan, CN*

Illness is not always recognized as a subclinical nutrient deficiency; often treatment entails suppressing symptoms by drug treatments instead of addressing shortfalls in the diet. Doctors who take an interest in nutrients and foods which promote health are a rare breed. However, good nutrition is central to our wellbeing. The Office of Population and Census Statistics (OPCS) in 1991 reported that 'there were 28 deaths in 1989 and 32 deaths in 1990 due to avitaminosis (vitamin deficiency)'.[12] But many more people fall ill due to long-term subclinical deficiencies which deplete the effective way the body should be working. Low nutrient intake or poor absorption can reduce our ability to fight diseases, virus and bacteria. The link between many of the diseases of Western civilization and poor digestion is not yet fully recognized in orthodox medicine. The health of the digestive tract and the integrity of the mucous membranes which line the tract are vital to your health. This has to be the first line of your defence against endometriosis.

FACTORS THAT ARE IMPORTANT FOR HEALTHY DIGESTION

For the digestive tract to work efficiently and support the immune and reproductive systems, four factors have to come together:

1 Transit time is the time it takes for food to be processed in the digestive tract and to pass through the body.
2 Liver function tests; can look at how efficient the liver is at producing the enzymes required for good digestion and for degrading oestrogens so that they can be passed harmlessly from the body.
3 Healthy gut flora are vital to our general health as the intestinal flora provide us with B vitamins and vitamin K and provide immune protection.
4 Fibre if regularly eaten, is vital for excretion of toxins and waste products from normal metabolism (see pp. 196, 212, 282).

TRANSIT TIME

Transit time is the time in which the food you eat is digested, absorbed and then excreted from the body. This is very important to your state of health. You can easily check your transit time by eating some sweetcorn kernels and watching how long it takes for them to reappear in your stools. Transit time for a healthy gut is 12–24 hours. Faster than that and the body will not have time to obtain sufficient nutrients from your food. Much slower than that and the waste fermenting inside your body can begin to putrefy the food and cause build-up of chemical compounds (some of which are carcinogenic).

If you have ever been constipated you may remember feeling toxic and bloated, until the laxatives did their job. Fibre holds water and this keeps the stools soft. If the waste is kept for too long inside the bowel, the water is reabsorbed and constipation results. Both vitamin C and magnesium can soften stools and they can be used to help alleviate constipation. But if constipation is due to a food intolerance, the culprit food needs to be found and eliminated. Constipation is triggered in some people by wheat, eggs, bananas or dairy foods. Drink at least three glasses of water each day and take three brisk 20-minute walks each week to help stimulate peristalsis waves along the intestinal walls. This helps you expel waste and prevents the build-up of harmful toxins. Exercise in general helps to stimulate peristalsis in the gut and also endorphin production in the brain (which helps reduce pain levels). Diarrhoea, on the other hand, is saying 'get this stuff out of here fast'. Something is irritating the gut membranes and it needs to be expelled as it is bad for the body. Listen to what your body is trying to tell you.

LIVER FUNCTION

The liver is a vast chemical factory which deals with everything the body takes in, and renders it safe. Liver enzymes have the ability to biotransform dangerous substances and make them harmless. The liver enzymes need a constant supply of B vitamins (found in green leafy vegetables), as well as vitamin A; L-taurine, L-methionine, L-carnitine and L-glycine (amino acids); vitamin E; vitamin B6; and lecithin (choline and inositol).

The foods which contain nutrients and phytochemicals beneficial to the liver are lemons, carrots, beetroot, cucumber, tomatoes, artichokes, chicory, celery, radishes, leeks, onions, cabbage, spring dandelion leaves, parsley, cold-pressed olive oil, apricots and grapefruit. For one day every three months you could eat a liver-cleansing diet of these foods in a salad. A glass of weak tea with lemon, hot water with lemon or organic carrot juice helps the liver work efficiently at detoxifying chemicals. You can also use lemon juice and olive oil as a salad dressing. Herb teas, such as thyme, rosemary, chamomile and meadowsweet, also aid liver function.

Foods which congest the liver are dairy foods, eggs, alcohol, meat, manufactured hydrogenated vegetable trans oils, sugar and tobacco. Obviously chemical food additives should be avoided wherever possible. Coffee and tea are best avoided in a liver-cleansing diet. Detoxifying the liver must be done gradually. As we detoxify, the toxic substances enter the bloodstream and they may make you feel unwell for a few days as 'die-off' symptoms (flu-like symptoms or headaches) may occur as the body begins to cleanse itself, but that means that you are getting on top of the problem. Drinking a lot of fresh water helps to flush out the system.

The road to wellness can sometimes seem like two steps back for every one step forward, but if you understand what is happening and why, it is easier to cope. As these are only the symptoms of a passing phase, they should be an encouraging sign that the right track is being followed. So whenever you undertake a detox diet, always take your time. The body does not need any more shocks to its system, endometriosis has been enough. If we have been ill for a long time it would be nice to take a 'magic bullet' tablet and get well overnight. Nutrition is not like that; it requires some perseverance to allow the body to heal in its own time. If it has taken several years for the body to become ill, be patient as healing may take 3–6 months. Reading the many comments from women who have followed this path of liver cleansing, you can see that it can be a fast or more gradual process, due to our inherent uniqueness and our biochemical individuality. We all react differently to different treatments.

GOOD GUT FLORA

> Surely no man can live without friends.
>
> *Aristotle*

About 2kg/4lb of friendly bacteria live in our intestines. We provide them with food and warmth and, in return, they help us digest foods, and they support immunoglobulin production. The good bifido bacteria make vitamins B and K. This is symbiosis – you scratch my back and I'll scratch yours. Drawing upon research findings, it is estimated that there are '100 trillion organisms in our intestinal tract – 400–500 different species with an active metabolic action equivalent to the liver'.[13] There is so much vibrant life inside us, which acts to protect us from harm if you look after it carefully.

The gastrointestinal tract acts as a strong barrier between us and the outside world. Think of the good gut flora as our protective atmosphere. Just as the atmosphere around planet Earth helps to protect it from radiation and meteorites, all these good bacteria are shielding and screening us from the dangers of parasites, viruses and bacteria lurking in food and water.

Three pounds of bifidobacteria and one pound of *Bacteroides* bacteria live inside us. The bifidobacteria are the 'good' guys who produce B-complex vitamins and vitamin K. The bacteroides bacteria are required to break down protein foods; in doing so they produce gases. Drugs such as antibiotics upset this balance. Antibiotics are 'anti-life' and kill off all bacteria whether good or bad, whereas probiotics, such as acidophilus, are 'for-life' and help to restore the levels of bifido-bacteria to normal. It is important to keep the ratio of three bifido-bacteria to one bacteroides bacterium in balance, by eating live yoghurt or acidophilus after antibiotic or hormonal drug treatments, or if you are suffering from severe stress. If there is an excess of bacteroides, too much gas will be produced; if there is too little bifidobacteria, insufficient levels of vitamin B-complex will be produced to keep the gut membranes healthy.

We have often been taught that bacteria are all bad, but here within us, we have some of the best bacteria one could ever wish for; they keep us in the peak of health if we look after them. The use of drugs (such as antibiotics, the oral contraceptive pill, HRT or other hormone drugs, indigestion tablets, non-steroidal anti-inflammatory drugs [NSAIDs]), sensitivity to gluten in wheat, even severe ongoing stress, take their toll.

In some cases, long-term antibiotic therapy may induce liver problems.[14] Antibiotics frequently produce profound changes in the composition of the human intestinal microflora, permitting the overgrowth of resistant endogenous bacteria or colonization by organisms acquired from the outside environment.[15] Once antibiotics have killed both the good and bad bacteria in the gut, they will have broken down the body's natural barrier of protection against infection. Pathogenic organisms may then gain a foothold and proliferate, and their overgrowth may produce serious infections in the host as the precious living gut flora system is left defective. If the gut is injured, we are very likely to develop ill health. Agents of disease are able to pass through a damaged gut, and may enter the bloodstream and infect any organ in the body. Good gut flora keep us alive.

If you bloat a lot and experience abdominal pain, you probably need to take some digestive enzymes and acidophilus to replace the flora which are out of balance and to improve your digestion and speed up your healing process. This bloated condition is known as dysbiosis and it may also arise when the diet is high in animal fat and low in fibre.

The digestive enzymes help to rest the liver for a short time and they aid the breakdown of foods into nutrients. A nutritionist can guide you as to which supplements may speed up the healing of the gut membranes, for example, slippery elm, N-acetyl glucosamine, L- glutamine, essential fatty acids, butyric acid, vitamin A or zinc.

Digestive enzymes

A healthy liver and pancreas produce enzymes which help break down foods into nutrients ready for digestion (*see* table 10.2). In fact, we begin producing enzymes even before we start eating. The thought of a tasty meal starts enzyme production, so that our digestive system is ready to receive food by the time we begin to eat, although American-style grazing and fast food has altered this pattern, and snacks often arrive in the stomach before it is ready to begin digestion. Stress also upsets enzyme secretion so that we cannot digest food when we are upset.

Poorly digested food can cause a build-up of gas in the intestines. Flatulence is a sign that you are either not producing sufficient digestive enzymes or that the gut flora is unbalanced, leading to malabsorption. The worst foods for producing gas are beans, onions, eggs, meat, cabbage and sprouts. Drinking one small glass of fluid with a meal may help. Vitamins C and B6 can improve absorption of nutrients from the gut into the bloodstream, as they act as carrier molecules to take nutrients from the gut and into the bloodstream.

Digestive enzyme tablets (available from healthfood stores or by mail order) are made from animal and/or vegetable sources and can be taken with meals to aid digestion and absorption if you have liver or pancreas problems. They consist of:

1 Amylase to digest carbohydrates
2 Lipase to digest fats
3 Protease to digest proteins.

If you are unable to digest fats, this upsets their potential to manufacture steroid hormones, the good anti-inflammatory prostaglandins which aid the body to heal wounds, reduce pain, increase immune potential and enhance fertility. Blurred vision and left-hand-side rib pain are signs of pancreatic insufficiency. A sluggish liver can produce various symptoms such as fibrocystic breasts, food intolerance, acne, fatigue, nausea, greasy fatty stools, intolerance of fatty foods, itchy skin, rashes, a bitter taste in

Organ	Enzyme	Food	Digested particle
Mouth	Salivary amylase	Carbohydrate	Simple sugars Glucose, fructose, galactose
Small intestine	Pancreatic amylase	Carbohydrate	Glucose, fructose, galactose
Stomach	Pepsinogen	Proteins	Amino acids
Small intestine			
Pancreas	Trypsin	Proteins	Amino acids
Pancreas	Chymotrypsin	Proteins	Amino acids
Pancreas	Carboxypeptidase	Proteins	Amino acids
Intestinal membranes	Aminopetidase	Proteins	Amino acids
Pancreas	Lipase	Fats and oils	40+ fatty acids Glycerol

Table 10.2
Taking digestive enzymes for a short time if the digestive system is malfunctioning may enhance the body's digestion of these vital nutrients while the body is trying to heal.

the mouth and PMS. Choose reputable digestive enzyme tablets containing lipase, amylase, protease, bromelain (a digestive enzyme found in pineapples) and papain (found in papaya), and avoid those enzymes derived from animal glands and especially from a bovine source.

Probiotics

Probiotics may be required if the body's natural bacteria have been compromised in some way. Probiotics are live microbial supplements, taken in either capsule or food form (such as live yoghurt and kefir), which help to replenish the bifidobacteria and increase the number of naturally resident bacteria to benefit the host's health. Research shows that 'the main positive effects associated with probiotics include cholesterol and/or triglyceride reduction, antitumour properties, increased vitamin production and stimulation of the immune system'.[16]

Research also suggests that improving the gut flora is critical to improving health. It is suggested 'that the adhesion of lactobacilli to mucosal epithelial cells may be a critical factor in immune stimulation'.[17] Choice of a good probiotic is very important, as some of the cheaper ones are less effective. Look for dairy-free formulations which contain *Lactobacillus acidophilus* and *Bifidobacterium bifidum*, and where each capsule delivers four million live bacteria. These products must be pure and must persist when in the GI tract. A nutritionist will guide you as to the best products available.

Fructo-oligosaccharides (FOS) or prebiotics

Fructo-oligosaccharides (FOS) are comprised of sugars linked together in a way which stops the body digesting them, and the bifidobacteria use FOS for their own growth. The Japanese regularly use FOS in over 500 of their foods. Research revealed that feeding 15mg of FOS per day to healthy volunteers caused bifido bacteria to become more predominant in faeces, showing that their intestinal environment was healthy. Ninety-five per cent FOS encourages the growth of beneficial bacteria and reduces the growth of unfriendly bacteria, and they may also help relieve constipation. FOS are found naturally in honey, barley, rye, garlic, asparagus, onions, bananas and artichokes, but in insufficient quantities to be of benefit. Studies show that 'chlorine in the water supply has a damaging effect on our good bacteria, so FOS are of help in maintaining the correct environment in our gut'.[18] Water filters could be used to remove chlorine.

Fibre

Fibre is a cellulose form of carbohydrate which the body cannot break down and it therefore passes through the GI tract more or less unchanged; however, in doing so it absorbs toxins, cholesterols and oestrogens, holds water to keep the stools soft, and stimulates peristalsis contractions in the gut membrane, which helps to expel waste matter from the body.

Fibre also delays the absorption of glucose and improves glucose tolerance, thereby keeping blood levels normal and preventing mood swings, and the presence of fibre promotes 'good' bifido bacteria in the intestines. It improves faeces transit time and reduces the muscle strain that can lead to piles. Fibre keeps us 'regular'; a healthy stool should be brown and float because it is high in fibre. If stools sink this is a sign that not enough fibre is being eaten.

There are different types of fibre, some of which are insoluble (bran) and some which are soluble (pectins in fruits and gums, and alginates from seaweeds). Sources of fibre include cereal grains, fruits, vegetables, nuts and seeds. However, many people experience digestive problems with cereal grains, and may be better off consuming fruits and vegetables. Wheat bran can make some people constipated, so choose oat bran products instead.

Importantly, as fibre absorbs degraded oestrogens and helps to eliminate them from the body, it prevents them from stimulating more endometriosis to grow. Therefore, eat lots of good sources of fibre, such as fruits and vegetables, nuts, seeds and cereals, to help to protect yourself against the high oestrogen levels that may trigger endometriotic implants. The role of fibre will be discussed in greater detail later in this chapter (see p. 212). We should all eat around 30mg of fibre per day.

Lisa C of Sussex

My menstrual cycle has always been a cause for concern to the extent that I had gone for as long as of 12 months without menstruating. In early 1994, my symptoms peaked, after three months' antibiotic treatment for a throat infection. I suffered months of recurrent thrush, cystitis and bacterial vaginosis. My periods became extremely heavy and very painful. I either suffered from constipation or diarrhoea, especially before menstruating. I felt cold all the time, my hair thinned and I had all the classic PMT symptoms and developed a rash on my upper body. I began to experience acid indigestion after each meal.

After numerous exploratory operations, it was established that I had endometriosis, irritable bowel syndrome and hiatus hernia. The nutritionist advised me to change my diet and exclude many foods that could be aggravating my condition. I excluded all foods containing the following: sugar/honey, salt, preservatives/additives, chocolate, coffee, tea, alcohol, dairy foods and yeasts. I adopted what is known as a wholefood diet, eating all foods from fresh to help the healing process. A daily salad, green leafy vegetables, red/orange-coloured vegetables, one or two pieces of fruit (not citrus), wholegrains (such as rice, oats, rye and corn), three organic eggs a week, 10 almonds per day, some live soya yoghurt, chicken, fresh fish, seeds, pineapple juice and plenty of fresh water. In addition to these dietary changes, I began to take supplements daily: an acidophilus, a multivitamin/mineral, digestive enzymes, vitamin C, magnesium and vitamin A drops, and I followed a gentle colonic cleanse with herbs.

Slowly my symptoms began to ease. My periods became lighter and considerably less painful. My hair began to thicken and look healthier. My skin rash completely disappeared and I now rarely suffer vaginal infections. Although there are a few foods I still cannot tolerate when I try to reintroduce them, I am now able to reintroduce many into my daily diet. I still have a few bowel and indigestion problems, but I would say they have improved by over 50 per cent. Fourteen months after beginning this programme, I am expecting my first child in 20 weeks' time. I believe that this would not have been possible so soon if I had not adopted this wholefood diet and supplement programme.

FACTORS HARMFUL TO DIGESTION AND ABSORPTION

Having looked at three areas which support the health of the digestive tract, we will now turn our attention to the five areas which are detrimental and can cause great harm to our health. These are a leaky gut, chronic candidiasis, malabsorption, food intolerances, and the harm caused by environmental oestrogens (as well as the build-up of natural oestrogens if the diet is low in fibre and high in fat).

1 LEAKY GUT DYSFUNCTION SYNDROME

Julie A of Kent

The one important factor I learned was to listen to your body. It soon tells you what it needs and what it does not want. How you feel after drinking or eating certain foods tells you a lot. The worst part was excluding dairy foods and wheat for three months. That was really hard, but it does open your eyes to the effects of food on your body, and I felt much better for it and am now able to eat normally again with no problems. I certainly learned a lot. Healthy eating is a great way to achieve normal weight.

C
A
S
E   S
T
U
D
Y

In leaky gut dysfunction syndrome, damage to the mucous membrane wall of the intestine allows food particles to be absorbed into the bloodstream before their digestion is complete. The gut wall can become leaky through damage to the membrane by drugs, gluten sensitivity or *Candida albicans* overgrowth. Unfortunately, the immune cells in the blood think that the undigested food particle is 'alien' and dangerous, and therefore they attack it. Often, these particles are the protein parts of foods, such as gluten in wheat or casein in dairy foods, as small chains of five amino acids joined together like popper beads. Normal food molecules are recognized by the immune system cells as normal and are left alone to be absorbed, but larger, partially digested molecules (exorphins) are seen as 'alien' and may be attacked by immune cells in the bloodstream. If this happens, susceptible people develop food intolerances to normal foods. These toxins enter the bloodstream, leaving you feeling sick all over. The liver can become overloaded and digestive enzyme production may be affected.

Once we have antibodies to foods, they can attach themselves to a lung space or a joint and cause inflammatory reactions. This is how autoimmune diseases begin. These exorphins (exogenous morphine-like molecules) are similar to endorphins, the natural painkillers produced by the brain: 'If they manage to get through the liver, experiments suggest they may affect mood, inducing a sense of comfort and craving for yet more of that food.'[19] This would explain why we crave the foods which are doing us the most harm. Deficiencies of protein-digesting enzymes would affect the way in which the body deals with exorphins.

It is reported that 'research at the National Institutes for Health in the USA has shown that these larger food particles may get into the bloodstream where they are able to bind to receptors for endorphins'.[20] Yet more research is needed in this area to see how this affects body chemistry.

An article on research into the intestinal absorption of macromolecules reports: 'Normally proteins would be broken down by digestion into amino acids but if they are still large peptide (protein) molecules, an attack can be mounted. Generally the mucosal barrier allows substances less than 0.4mm in diameter to be absorbed into the body, while preventing larger molecules from entering.'[21] Beads of amino acid chains will get across the barrier if the mucosa has been breached by candidiasis. *Candida albicans* hyphae (long thin filaments) could penetrate the membrane and cause the gut to 'leak' large molecules into the bloodstream to which the immune system reacts.

As 'increased permeability is a highly sensitive measure of disruption of the normal mucosal barrier function of the small intestine, it is therefore not surprising that many potential toxic agents cause increased permeability – NSAIDs, alcohol, cytotoxic drugs, bile salts, detergents, gold compounds, chelators, ischaemia and dietary idiosyncrasies'.[22] Stress and hormonal preparations can have similar effects. Research by Dr K. L. Reichelt has shown the relationships between peptides, digestive function and permeability, and food antigens and neurochemistry in brain dysfunction.[23]

Mary Lou Ballweg, of the International Endometriosis Association, reports: 'Rarely, lumps of endometriosis implants grow inside the bowel, causing obstructions (lumps the size of a grapefruit have been removed having the texture of black rubber). Out of 5,000 endometriosis patients, 10 per cent have significant bowel involvement.'[24] We need to look more closely at the relationship between common symptoms of irritable bowel and endometriosis, as it could relate to smooth muscle diseases.

Misdiagnosis for several years can lead to long-term antibiotic or NSAID use for conditions such as IBS, PID or cystitis. Digestive processes can easily be disrupted by a cocktail of pharmaceutical drugs. As GnRH agonists and the contraceptive pill are prescribed for endometriosis, the poor gut membrane and flora may be compromised and become less effective. The side effects of many drugs are legion and women often have other medications prescribed by their GP. It is not uncommon to find that, alongside GnRH agonists, women are also taking eight to ten other drugs to ward off side effects – such as antihistamines, antispasmodics, antibiotics, anti-depressants, headache medication, painkillers (sometimes as many as four types) and even antiepileptic drugs. Each has its own list of side effects in the *British National Formulary*.

A review of this area is long overdue as it is unknown what long-term effects this mixed cocktail has in the gut. Consultants prescribing the GnRH and contraceptive pill are often oblivious to the additional medications prescribed by GPs. Most drugs list as side effects gastro-intestinal disturbances and liver or kidney effects. Once the delicate digestive balance is compromised, the immune system also works less effectively and, thus, a vicious downward spiral is begun.

Recovering digestive health after surgery for endometriosis

Surgery for endometriosis may require considerable preparation of the bowels prior to the operation. If laser or other surgery is to involve the bowel, there is a real danger of developing peritonitis afterwards if the bowel is perforated. The bowel can be completely emptied prior to surgery by removing fibre from the diet completely for a few days, followed by laxatives and, finally, drinking large quantities (around five litres) of saline/electrolyte solution. This programme will effectively empty and wash out the whole intestinal tract. Then, if the bowel is perforated during surgery – either deliberately to remove adhesions or accidentally – there will be an absolute minimum leakage of bacteria into the peritoneum.

Although this is all very well, afterwards, there is hell to pay! The recovery period after an operation is not the ideal time to have your immunity compromised due to poor digestion. Nature will appreciate a helping hand in recovering your normal digestive balance. Your intestines contain 4lb of good bacteria that support your immune system, provide B vitamins and vitamin K to improve your digestion. Once these are flushed out, your digestion will suffer unless they are replaced within three weeks.

There are five main thrusts to this campaign:

1   Eat great food – lots of fresh (preferably raw) fruit and vegetables.
2   Take frequent small meals so as not to overload your digestion and avoid fatty or spicy foods which are dificult to digest.
3   Supplement with digestive enzymes at each meal (taken with a cold drink).
4   Reestablish your 'friendly' bacteria by supplementing with probiotics such as *Lactobacillus acidophilus*, *Bifidobacterium bifidum* and *L. bulgaricus*. (These are available from BioCare, a Birmingham company that also does a five-day course of mixed digestive bacteria in powder form designed for use after colonic cleansing – exactly what has occurred. Probiotics are also widely available in healthfood shops – only look for those kept in a fridge. All of these should be taken with a cold drink; *see* p. 397.)
5   Soothe the gut lining by supplementing with herbal digestive aids such as slippery elm and marshmallow, and take aloe vera juice, which is restorative and tastes rather nice! (ESI Laboratories make an aloe vera preparation with added digestive aids, available from good healthfood shops. You can safely take these at twice the recommended dose for one week.)

If you have had to do the full gut-emptying routine before your operation, it will probably take four or five days before you pass your first stool and, in the days prior to this, you will experience the most astonishing rumblings imaginable. Don't forget that the gas used in laparoscopic surgery is slow to disperse – it all has to be absorbed and excreted by your body. Some of this gas will make its way into your intestine, with subsequent bloating and gassiness.

Two homeopathic remedies may be useful here: *Carbo Veg*, good for helping you deal with the gas, and *Nux Vomica*, good for settling things down. If *Nux Vomica* suits you, it can be amazingly effective at quieting those loud and persistent rumbles. The 30c potency of each should suffice, taken as often as necessary (suck the pills in a clean mouth between meals and drinks), and stop when improvement is evident, but take it again if symptoms return. If these remedies don't seem to work for you, stop taking them. (Never use coffee and mints when using homeopathic remedies since, being diuretics, they will nullify the tablets' action.)

You need to be prepared because you will certainly not feel like going shopping the day after your operation, so stock up on supplements and remedies beforehand. Remember to have your fridge full of healthy fruits and vegetables to speed up your healing. Vitamins C and E and zinc speed up healing of scar tissue.

Good luck!

2 CHRONIC CANDIDIASIS

An overgrowth of the single-cell yeast *Candida albicans* in the gut flora has also been associated with endometriosis and leaky gut syndrome. Candidiasis is very difficult to diagnose, as the yeast occurs naturally in all of us.

Liz R of Croydon

*I followed an anti-*Candida*-style diet from September to December 1993. Before following the diet, my symptoms were hypoglycaemia, tingling and numbness in my arms and legs, and anxiety attacks. I was taking the drug Fluanxol for these symptoms, which my doctor felt were stress-related. I had read a lot about* Candida, *and my symptoms were much worse after eating sweet foods and refined carbohydrates. I thought that was the problem so gave the diet a try. On the diet the symptoms initially got worse, but then, when I stopped the Fluanxol, I had no symptoms. I assume the diet cured me.*

•
C
A
S
E

S
T
U
D
Y
•

How can a tiny organism cause health problems? *Candida albicans* is a one-celled yeast. We all have this yeast within our digestive tract, normally living in harmony with us. Only when it grows out of proportion can it become a problem.

Symptoms from disrupted intestinal flora can include constipation and diarrhoea, or both, headaches, chronic fatigue, depression, dizziness, bloating, poor concentration, vaginal irritation, sugar and bread cravings, mood swings, PMS, digestive problems and blurred vision. You know best how you feel. If you are experiencing these symptoms, this may be an area to explore.

The harmonious relationship between yeast and gut flora

Three things can play havoc with the delicate balance of intestinal flora, weakening the immune system so that it is less able to cope with yeast overgrowth:

1   A diet high in saturated and trans fats and refined sugars
2   Prolonged use of antibiotics, the contraceptive pill and HRT, or exposure to toxic substances
3   Prolonged stress.

Candida albicans is a very aggressive yeast and, if it sees a space for growth, it will proliferate. It can change from a one-celled yeast into a 'hyphal' form, spreading in long filaments (hyphae) which may puncture minute holes in the intestine wall, causing a 'leaky gut' (*see* p. 198).

Carol B of Suffolk

*The anti-*Candida *diet has brought about a remarkable improvement in my condition. I am 42 and suffered from distressing symptoms (including anaemia) for at least five years before being referred to a gynaecologist 15 months ago. A laparoscopy revealed really quite bad endometriosis. But hormone treatments (Danazol, Provera, Primolut) were unsuccessful. I was attempting to come to terms with the prospect of radical surgery when a lessening of symptoms occurred during a weight-reducing diet. I subsequently purchased the* Candida albicans *book by Leon Chaitow, and felt that prolonged stress could have been responsible for the manifestation of yeasts. I embarked upon the recommended diet, taking supplements. The first change was the absence of pain, which had been very severe and accompanied by nausea and diarrhoea, and I was able to abandon the six-hourly use of Ponstan. After several months the flow has also lessened, and I now have no flooding or large clots, and the most recent improvement would seem to be the absence of midcycle bleeding.*

• C A S E S T U D Y •

Candida also has the potential to upset the hormone balance: '*Candida* has receptor sites in its cell membranes which accept hormones; if progesterone binds to *Candida*, it fails to reach its destination.'[25] Acetaldehyde (a breakdown product of alcohol produced by *Candida* from sugar) reacts with the neurotransmitter dopamine to cause emotional disturbances like anxiety, spaced-out feelings and depression. Aldehydes cause suppression of T-cell function, increased susceptibility to infection and an inability of the immune system to respond efficiently to infections or allergens.[26, 27] *Candida albicans* yeast needs to be contained at a low rate in the gut, but overgrowth upsets your wellbeing.

Penelope S of London

My diet includes omitting as much yeast as possible (i.e. bread, cakes, pickles, etc.), limiting refined sugar intake, no coffee, only Earl Grey tea or herbal teas. I have a list of 'mould' foods to avoid, e.g. mushrooms, and I eat no milk or milk products, except live yoghurt and cottage cheeses or feta cheese. I follow this as much as possible and have found that lapses, such as coffee, cause the niggly pains to restart. I sometimes live on the threshold of cystitis which is kept under control with Cynoloen and feel that my endometriosis is closely related to candidiasis.

• C A S E S T U D Y •

Redressing the balance

Treatments are best undertaken with a nutritionist's guidance, and some environmental medicine practitioners may be able to offer advice. The first area of attack is to reduce the *Candida albicans* yeast to normal proportions via the following four steps:

Diet. It is important to reduce the foods which are 'feeding' the yeast. *Candida albicans* thrives on sugars (sucrose, glucose, fructose, dextrose, maltose, honey, molasses). Therefore, refined sugars, yeasts, fermented foods, dried fruits, dairy foods (other than *live* yoghurts) should be removed from the diet for two or three months. This diet can seem daunting, but with the right guidance, it is easy to find a vast range of alternative foods to provide the nutrient intake you require. Some diets recommend no fruit for the first two to four weeks to cut out the fruit sugar, fructose. After that, you can eat one piece of fruit a day.

For the first month, you can eat plenty of fresh vegetables, pulses (legumes), wholegrain cereals, meat and fish, nuts and seeds, which provide substantial meals. Avoiding snack-type foods is important. The body craves nutrients from fresh meals; it needs solid wholefood meals, but many people replace wholesome dinners with sugar- and wheat-based snacks that are nutritionally unsound. The following foods have anti-yeast properties and should be used frequently: garlic, onions, cabbage, broccoli, Brussels sprouts, kale, watercress, mustard cress, cauliflower, turnips, cinnamon, olive oil, and aloe vera juice. Pau d'arco tea from South America also has an anti-*Candida* effect.

Antifungal treatment. If the overgrowth is chronic and allergies abound with intolerances to ordinary foods, then diet alone cannot help. You will need antifungal agents to help reduce the candidiasis. These are available from the doctor as Nystatin, Diflucan or Betacanzale, or from healthfood shops as caprylic acid. Garlic is also excellent at reducing yeast overgrowth, with the aid of pau d'arco tea and aloe vera juice. Occasionally, chronic candidiasis can produce headache and flu-like symptoms. This is because toxins are released into the bloodstream as it dies off. If this happens, reduce the antifungal treatment and drink lots of water for two days to help cleanse the system. Then you can add the antifungal agents back into your regime. Two to three months of treatment may bring vast improvement to your health.

Beneficial probiotic bacteria. To replenish and repopulate the intestinal flora, *Lactobaccillus acidophilus* and bifidobacteria can be taken. Two very good forms (bioacidophilus and acidophilus plus) are acid-stable and capable of surviving the gastric secretions of the stomach. Repopulation of the digestive tract with these good bacteria is important for the maintenance of B vitamin production, especially after taking antibiotics, oral contraceptives and HRT. Take a B-complex-containing supplement while taking such drugs.

Nutritional supplements. While the diet is being adjusted and food exclusions are undertaken, short-term supplementation with vitamin and mineral tablets, digestive enzymes and acidophilus will help to ensure that all essential nutrients are being absorbed. The supplement must be yeast-, sugar-, dairy- and gluten-free. (See Appendix B for details on anti-*Candida* diets and the rules to follow for the next four to six months.)

Sally G of Tyne and Wear

You had been advising me for quite a while to go onto a Candida-*style diet to help my endo. To be honest, at the time (about four years ago) I had just turned 18, been diagnosed with endo and didn't believe that nutrition would help. I first cut out wheat and yeast products and much to my surprise there was a huge improvement in pain. I've then gradually eliminated foods from my diet such as processed foods and refined white sugar and have increased my nutritional supplements and fresh foods. I wish I had done it earlier.*

I find that out of all the supplements I benefit the most from Efamol Marine which helps to decrease inflammation, hence reducing pain (plus the added bonus that it is great for the skin!). I've had three laparoscopies and, on my second and third, my surgeon expressed how surprised she was that there was such little inflammation present (although the endo had spread). It is hard for most people to stick to a 'nutritional path', but when it works, you know it's been worth it. You have to listen to your body, take regular exercise (even just gentle) and eat well. I am a great fan of complementary therapy. My favourite is reflexology, which I just love. It is relaxing and alleviates digestive and menstrual problems.

Everyone is different, and different things work for different people. I've had three colonics very close together and, in my experience, it was a bad move. A year later I still suffer a lot of pain in my colon. I would think very carefully before using such aggressive therapy again.

CASE STUDY

3 MALABSORPTION

By now we have established that 'you are really only what your body can digest and absorb'. What you eat is vital to your health, but if the digestive tract is on the blink then it does not matter if we live on organic wholefoods as those nutrients will not be effectively absorbed and the body may still become subclinically deficient.

If you suffer from bloating, stomach upsets, abdominal pain, poor digestion of fats, diarrhoea or constipation, anal irritation or bad breath, these need sorting out before you can get better. Consider reducing your sugar intake as 'even excess sugar can cause proliferation of E. coli bacteria which trigger infections in the intestines'.[28] Refined sugars can disrupt the balance of gut flora. If you take indigestion tablets, diuretics or laxatives, this will reduce absorption of vital minerals even further.

Many long-term steroid treatments may disable the gut flora which would normally produce B vitamins which aid in oestrogen degradation. Maintaining this vitamin B production is crucial for all women with endometriosis. Malabsorption may be improved by following a healing programme. The use of the herb slippery elm, probiotics and digestive enzymes during drug treatments may help to correct some of the symptoms.

4 FOOD ALLERGY AND INTOLERANCES

'A little of what you fancy does you good' is a saying which food-intolerant people should be wary of. To believe that ordinary foods can make you ill is sometimes hard to swallow! A true allergy is an immune response to a foreign substance (antigen). It is usually an IgE overreaction which, in extreme cases, may prove fatal, for example, in peanut and fish allergies, where the body goes into anaphylactic shock. In a classical allergy, there are rarely any food cravings, and very small amounts of the allergen can trigger a full-blown reaction.

A food intolerance, however, to 'normal' foods may be 'masked', as a weakened immune system tries to defend us from attack but reacts with ailments/distress signals – this is often an IgG response. The IgG response may involve many different reactions. It often involves several foods, and reactions may be delayed for up to four days after the allergen in the food has been eaten. Frequently eaten foods trigger the response and there is often a food craving involved.

Studies suggest a link between food intolerances and endometriosis: 'American research points to a higher incidence of allergic-related symptoms in endometriosis sufferers.'[29] Many women with endometriosis often appear to have food allergy or intolerance problems to very ordinary foods and chemicals. To relieve the pain from endometriosis and to try and get pregnant, women have taken many different drugs, which may have affected the bifidobacteria which inhabit the small intestine. In some cases, drugs and foodstuffs can also damage the mucous membrane lining of the intestines.

More and more people are becoming sensitive to ordinary foods: 'Food sensitivity or intolerance is more common than true food allergies, around 24 million American adults are affected by the foods they consume.'[30, 31] This may be due to environmental pollutants, chemicals within food, changes brought about by genetic engineering, poor gut mucosa or a weakness inherited from the family. But the result is usually the same – damaged intestinal lining and reactions within the immune system which trigger reactions in other body systems.

Some families are 'atopic' – that is, they have a history of illnesses such as asthma, eczema, hay fever and arthritis: 'The risk of being predisposed to an allergen is 50 per cent if one parent has an allergy. It rises to 75 per cent where both parents are involved. However, a third of atopic people are born into families where no intolerances have been recognized. The most usual symptoms are recurrent headaches, regular bouts of indigestion or persistent fatigue.'[32]

Which foods make you feel drained of energy and which foods revitalize you? The most common food intolerances are to cow's milk products (cheese, butter, yoghurt, cream), food preservatives and colourings, wheat (cakes, biscuits, pastries, pastas), chocolate, eggs, citrus fruits, and foods containing salicylates (including apples, cherries, grapes, peaches, aubergine, broccoli, tea and coffee).

Wheat intolerance

Most British foods now use wheat as their staple base. In South America it may be corn, in Japan soya, in India rice. It can be easy to eat an excess of wheat over one day, with wheat bran and toast for breakfast, sandwiches for lunch, pizza or pasta for dinner, and various cakes and cookies throughout the day. Wheat, barley, rye, oats and spelt are known as gluten grains because they contain a stretchy protein called gluten, which can inflame the lining of the gut membrane in sensitive people.

The non-gluten grains (rice, corn, buckwheat, quinoa, sago, tapioca, arrowroot and millet) can be used instead, although millet, corn and rice may also affect extremely sensitive people. Healthfood shops, nutrition cooperatives, Lifestyle and the Gluten-free Bakery (*see* p. 398) have lots of wonderful alternatives.

Wheat was not always the staple food of Western cultures. In Britain, flour from lupins, broad beans, acorns and bullrush roots was used as staples until Norman times. None of these flours contained gluten, so unleavened breads were the norm. The first wheatgrains, emmer and einkorn, were very low in gluten, but the poor had no access to them. Modern types of bread wheat were introduced in the post-Roman period.

Wheat was genetically modified in the early 1970s. The head of the wheat was made to contain more seeds. This made the plant top-heavy and the crop fell over. So a hormone was added to thicken the stalk. Then a fungus grew on the stems because they grew so close together, leading to another hormone being added to destroy the fungus. It may be that these two hormones, when absorbed in excess, upset the hormone profiles of women with endometriosis. Research is needed to look into these possible effects.

Sometimes, eating one type of food too often can bring on intolerance. If you feel you are wheat-intolerant, avoid wheat for 30 days and use the alternatives, such as rye crispbreads, oatcakes, ricecakes, corn pasta, corn tortilla and tacos, buckwheat pasta, millet flakes, quinoa, potato-based pizza, pastry made from ground almonds and brown rice flour. The majority of women with endometriosis have found that excluding wheat helps to reduce much of the bowel pain they experienced. Wheat can be constipating and may trigger irritable bowel symptoms in susceptible people. We need more research to investigate this phenomenon (*see* p. 278).

Barbara H of Cheshire

During the nutrition trial, it was pointed out that I was eating a lot of wheat products. This probably stemmed from earlier attempts to lose weight via the F-plan diet, and a general belief that large quantities of fibre via bran and brown-bread products was beneficial. Actually, I think now that the wheat products were doing me harm.

Some years after the nutrition trial, I had a period of very bad health following some surgery for other health problems (and was taking antibiotics for flu). [Excess use of

CASE STUDY

antibiotics can adversely affect health as antibiotics may damage the protective gut flora, which can lead to the onset of many diseases.] I had now developed what was recognized as food intolerance, mainly to wheat-based products and dairy foods. With nutritional advice, I was able to cut out the foods that were making me ill. I also lost a stone in weight.

The supporting nutritional supplements helped me at a time when I was suffering from a lot of pain from endometriosis and very low energy levels. I therefore continued to take nutritional supplements for five years on and off. However, I have improved all the endometriosis symptoms. I now take a low dose multivitamin/mineral every day.

Dairy intolerance

Dairy foods are mucus-forming and may affect people who come from an atopic family (a family with a history of asthma, eczema, psoriasis, hay fever or arthritis). By excluding dairy foods for one month, you can see whether your symptoms improve. A generation ago, the average dairy cow yielded eight quarts of milk per day, ate mainly grass and produced only one part per 100,000,000 of antibiotics to a pint. Today a typical cow yields 50 quarts per day, may be fed meal made from bone and blood (from cattle, pig and chicken carcasses) and produces an average of 52 different residues of antibiotics, plus blood and pus, in milk.[33]

Alternatives to dairy foods include soya milk substitutes, rice and oat milks, tofu, soft soya cheeses, hummus (chickpeas), avocado and fish pâtés, and nut butters (*see* p. 270 for a list of calcium-rich foods other than dairy products). Bovine dairy foods may trigger diarrhoea and IBS in some people. Try using goat's or ewe's milk, yoghurts or cheeses instead (*see* p. 280).

Lisa C of London

CASE STUDY

In the past 2½–3 years, I have been suffering from a whole range of symptoms including dysmenorrhoea, amenorrhoea, digestive and bowel complaints, skin rashes and depression, and the list goes on. After numerous examinations and operations, it was established that I have acute irritable bowel syndrome, endometriosis and hiatus hernia. I was virtually told that there was no permanent cure, and the various drugs I had been prescribed had only worsened my symptoms. I have been seeing a nutritionist for seven months and following a strict dairy exclusion diet supported by supplements. However, I have been eating more wholefoods than ever before. My symptoms have improved by about 70 per cent and, with a little more help, one day I hope to have the old me back again.

Food exclusion diets

To show intolerance to particular foods, nutritionists may ask their clients to remove that food from the normal diet for one month and then to reintroduce it, and watch for any symptoms which may arise over a 24-hour period. When the excluded food is reintroduced, there may be reactions such as headaches, flu-like symptoms, constipation, diarrhoea, extreme fatigue or blurred vision, or a sense of mental grogginess. If there is a reaction, that food is best avoided for three months before being reintroduced very slowly into the diet.

There are expensive tests which can be done, but they are not always 100 per cent accurate. Food exclusion diets cost nothing but perseverance and often highlight intolerances.

Natalie C of London

I eliminated cheese and caffeine. At laparoscopy, nothing was detected and I am expecting a baby at Easter.

• S
C T
A U
S D
E Y
•

Some people comply with the exclusion, but many do not. This can be due to such factors as cost, availability of alternatives, or being 'conservative' about food and therefore unwilling to change even if it means better health. Or they may not understand the full implication of the damage that is being inflicted on their gut membranes and immune cells when that food is eaten. It is very important to 'rest' these immune cells by excluding 'harmful' proteins in foods as this will allow the immune system to heal.

While on an exclusion diet, you can eat all the alternative foods to provide nutrients and take a multivitamin/mineral supplement. If necessary, rare foods not usually in your diet can be eaten to increase the nutrient intake. There is less likelihood of an allergy or intolerance to foods you have not eaten before, such as starfruit, kumquats, salsify, kale or celeriac.

Understanding why you need an exclusion diet is half the battle. Food molecules to which we are allergic can weaken the immune system. The white blood cells react to large molecules, the 'exorphins'. An over- or under-reactive immune system can affect the reproductive system (*see* chapter 9).

Leading health writer Leon Chaitow reports: 'Alterations in gut flora are felt to be linked to autoimmune disorders. Research at King's College London has looked at the body's way of ridding itself of undesirable bacteria by attacking its own tissues instead.'[34] If you feel that a certain food does not agree with you, see how you feel when you remove it from your diet.

The important thing to recognize is that if a food has become a problem, then something has to be done. It may mean avoiding that food for a few months and, if that is all it takes to get well and feel healthy, then surely it is worth a try.

Immune responses to food intolerances

The body struggles to deal with what it sees as 'alien' molecules. Once they have been 'captured', they are generally devoured or, occasionally, sent along to the joints (often used as a dumping ground for waste), which can cause aching joints. Orthopaedic surgeons know this dumped material as 'plica'. The incidence and amount of plica has increased over the past 10 years.

Food allergy and infertility – Coeliac disease, hypothyroid and infertility

Coeliac disease is a condition where the small intestine fails to digest and absorb food due to a sensitivity to wheat gluten (gliadin). Hypothyroidism occurs when the thyroid gland in the neck becomes sluggish. In adults the symptoms are sensitivity to cold, constipation, coarse skin, slow pulse, mental and physical slowing, and the outer third of the eyebrows can be lost. Infertility is a condition where both male and female can find it difficult to achieve conception (*see* chapter 5). In this section we will look at the links between these three conditions.

Research has linked coeliac disease and thyroid disease with possible thyroid auto-antibodies and infertility: 'Fourteen per cent of women with coeliac disease were found to have thyroid disorders.'[35] Recent research has estimated the numbers of women affected by hypothyroidism in the UK: 'Hypothyroidism is prevalent in 1.4 per cent of women. The commonest cause is autoimmune failure and the measurement of thyroid auto-antibodies confirms the diagnosis.'[36] These figures lead to the suggestion that 'testing for thyroid disease seems to be warranted in all women and men with unexplained infertility'.[37] This suggestion would appear to be supported by tests that are already in place: 'Autoimmune diseases, such as those involving the thyroid, are thought to be involved in infertility. Indeed thyroid auto-antibodies are used to predict women at risk for miscarriage.'[38] As two-thirds of all pregnancy loss occurs before the pregnancy is recognized, testing for thyroid auto-antibodies would help to catch those women in need of support. The human placenta produces the hormones human chorionic gonadotrophin (hCG) and human chorionic thyrotrophin which may interact with thyroid auto-antibodies. More research is needed in this important area. How many women with fertility problems are screened for thyroid auto-antibodies as a matter of course?

When symptoms of coeliac disease were removed by excluding wheat gluten from the diet, many infertile patients became pregnant. It is very important for doctors to check for coeliac disease in patients presenting with unexplained infertility and endometriosis. Many of the painful abdominal symptoms experienced in endometriosis could also be caused by gluten or wheat intolerance. The incidence of coeliac disease in Europe has been estimated as follows: 'The prevalence of coeliac disease varies from one person in every 2,500 in the UK, to one in 3,000 in the USA, one in 10,000 in Denmark and one in 300 in the West of Ireland.'[39] However, new research suggests these figures may be an underestimate.

Other research suggests that the longer women with coeliac disease are left untreated, the greater the risk of developing autoimmune thyroid disease and infertility. Tests for both conditions should be done automatically when infertility is present. Studies show that 'in males gliadin (the active portion of gluten) reduces semen quality in susceptible people. Deficiencies in zinc, folic acid, B12 and iron have been implicated in coeliac disease. Successful conception was reported after gluten exclusion in patients with infertility.'[40] It is thought this is a subclinical disease which subtly alters immune system function, and also causes malabsorption of vitamins and minerals from the digestive tract due to the damage inflicted on villi by the gluten.

It has been found that 'untreated hypothyroidism and hyperthyroidism can both give rise to very similar changes in the gut mucosal damage, as can coeliac disease, which makes diagnosis difficult'.[41] Research from the seventies highlights the connection between the health of the digestive system and general wellbeing: 'All those tested had IgA antigliaden antibodies, showing that they were wheat intolerant. Failure to recognize either of these conditions, the researchers felt, could lead to a lack of response to treatment. Oral gliadin has been shown by research to affect neurotransmitters, dopamine and noradrenaline, in the brain.'[42] Get your doctor to check for both hypothyroid and coeliac disease as a matter of course. Long-term undiagnosed coeliac disease can also lead to short-term lactose intolerance (intolerance to dairy foods). This should also be assessed.

Barbara W of London

After three years of trying for a baby, and with four failed IVF attempts behind me and a diagnosis of endometriosis, I had almost given up hope of ever becoming a mother. My marriage was in tatters, I was badly depressed and couldn't bear to look at a baby in the street, let alone the babies of my friends. I was desperate. I decided half-heartedly to have what was probably a final attempt at IVF, but at the last minute it was called off as my hormone levels were too high. The news devastated me and I came to the conclusion that I couldn't stand the IVF emotional treadmill any more.

With one last heave of my depleted energy I decided to work on my diet and visited Dian. She told me about the possible link between wheat gluten and infertility, and told me about a client with endometriosis who had phoned in pregnant after following a gluten-free diet. I took that story away with me and it inspired me to begin a strict wheat- and dairy-free diet, making sure I used all the alternatives.

A few weeks later, I discovered to my shock and amazement that I was pregnant – naturally! I am still struggling to believe that, after all this time, such a miracle could have happened, and I still have months ahead before I can be sure that this pregnancy will work out. But I hope that this story gives others the hope I needed to keep going.

CASE STUDY

Coeliac disease would appear to be affecting greater numbers of people: 'During the 1980s and 1990s it has become apparent that coeliac disease is under-diagnosed and that the clinical features have changed in both children and adults. The shift has been towards milder symptoms, such as indigestion in adults and recurrent abdominal pain in children. The prevalence of coeliac disease from recent screening studies has been found to be as high as one in 100 to one in 300. Infertility or miscarriages have been described in women and reversible infertility in men.'[43] This change in prevalence may be due to wheat being genetically engineered or diets containing excess hidden wheat: 'In Ireland the highest reported figure (of coeliac disease) in a random sample of the general population has been found to be one in 122 people.'[44] Research shows a definite link between coeliac disease and infertility which the medical profession and IVF units seem to ignore and never test for when infertility is unexplained. However, the evidence for a connection is powerful: 'Coeliac disease is associated with infertility in both men and women. Subclinical coeliac disease in women may be an unexpected cause of delayed menarche, amenorrhoea, premature menopause, recurrent abortions and low pregnancy rate. Many individuals without apparent symptoms who are found to have coeliac disease remark on a new-founded vitality and sense of wellbeing when started on a gluten-free diet.'[45]

Removing as many problems as possible from an ailing immune system will enhance its strength and improve fertility, as health begins to be renewed. In susceptible people, the gliadin in wheat causes tremendous damage to the gut mucosa and is seen to be toxic to human tissue cells in culture. We need to encourage more testing and research in this area of infertility. The GP can do a simple blood test for gluten sensitivity in both IgE true allergy and IgG food intolerance.

Undernutrition has always been suspected when fertility is impaired. During wars and in famine areas, it has been noted that fertility was reduced at times when the food supply was cut off. This is due to atrophy of the reproductive organs. If the gut mucosa are badly damaged, then nutrients will not be absorbed.

Nutrients which strengthen the gut mucosa

To improve the function of the gut mucosa the nutrients zinc, beta-carotene, biotin, butyric acid, pantothenic acid (vitamin B5), vitamins A, C and E, essential fatty acids and L-glutamine are known to be important. Slippery elm can have a soothing effect as it builds up a protective layer of mucus on the membrane, allowing healing to take place. Often the mucosa may be inflamed from the substances which irritate it. The body then acts in one of two ways: it either rushes to expel the offending food, causing diarrhoea; or it seizes up altogether and we experience constipation. Either way, we are left with a malabsorption problem.

5 NATURAL AND ENVIRONMENTAL OESTROGENS

Natural oestrogens of body origin

Natural oestrogens are made from cholesterol in the ovaries, testes and the adrenal glands in response to signals from the pituitary. They can also be made by every fat cell in the body. From these sites they are secreted into the blood and are carried to the cells of the breasts and reproductive organs. Oestrogens send chemical signals or messages to help other cells respond to the body's internal environment, and oestrogens are responsible for cell growth in the breast, uterus, bone, liver and cardiovascular system. However, some environmental synthetic chemicals, such as pesticides, insecticides and herbicides, appear to mimic the role of oestrogens in the body.

Natural oestrogens come in many types and vary greatly from one another, for example, 'oestradiol is 12 times more potent than oestrone and 80 times more potent than oestriol'.[46] Carlton Fredericks states that 'control of natural oestrogen is a nutritional process which is disturbed by too much sugar, too little protein and is incapacitated almost completely by lack of vitamin B-complex'.[47] Indeed, it is our digestive system, in particular the bile from the gall bladder and the liver, which aids the excretion of oestrogen from the body. This is very important to all women who have endometriosis. You can help control oestrogen in your body through your diet and gentle exercise.

Fibre and oestrogen excretion

Excretion of oestrogens bound to fibre is another key to our management of endometriosis: 'Dietary fibre increases excretion of excess oestrogens from the body.'[48] The Western diet rich in animal and trans fats elevates the levels of sex hormones produced in the body. Fats and fat cells store oestrogenic pesticides and cause a build-up of free radicals which can damage cell membranes, so a low-fat diet is advisable. Avoiding the bad saturated animal fats and trans oils, and eating mainly the good cold-pressed cis oils is vital to health as we saw in chapter 4.

You can take action to aid excretion of oestrogens:

1 The best fibre to eat is found in unrefined wholegrain cereals, nuts, seeds, berries and the pulse/legume vegetables (peas, beans and lentils), although the cellulose in soluble vegetable fibres are more effective in triggering the normal processes of breakdown in the colon than fibre from grains/cereals such as oats. Fibre also binds the oestrogens and inhibits their reabsorption: 'Some fibres such as the lignins found in rye, other grains and seeds are changed by gut flora to form antioestrogen compounds, enterolactone and enterodiol, which are protective against cancers.'[49] There is a direct effect of the quality of plant fibre consumed: 'Good quality fibre encourages a hormone known as serum hormone-binding globulin (SHBG) which can be used as a marker for steroid hormone abnormalities. SHBG is a unique transport system for oestrogen, because while the oestrogen is bound to the SHBG it cannot exert any biological effect within the body.'[50] If the diet is low in fibre, then the oestrogens can have a biological effect. The other soluble fibre we referred to earlier as FOS also aids oestrogen clearance.

2 The bifidobacteria also encourage oestrogen clearance by inhibiting an enzyme known as beta-glucoronidase. This hormone normally encourages the deactivated safe oestrogen to become reactivated, so that it can be sent back into circulation (not a good idea with endometriosis).

3 At least four vegetables, two fruits and a handful of nuts and seeds should be eaten each day with some wholegrain cereal. These will also speed up the transit time of

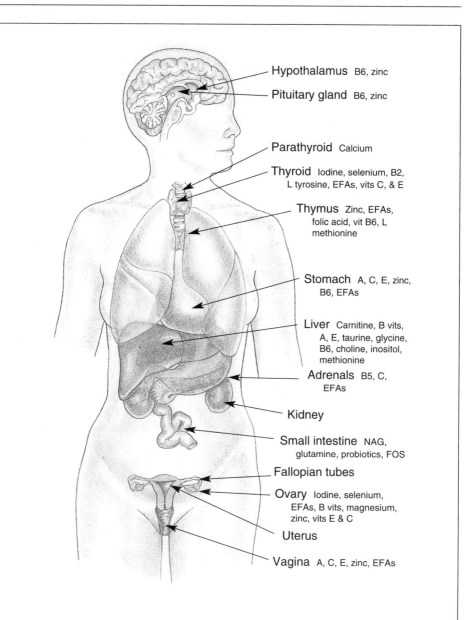

Figure 10.2
The endocrine system is responsible for balancing all hormones in the body (see also figure 2.1). Here we can see the main nutrients known to be involved for each organ. These are all dependent upon the nutrients eaten and absorbed by a healthy digestive tract.

food through the digestive tract. The best vegetables to eat are those from the cruciferous family, all rich in B-complex vitamins and magnesium: cabbage, Brussels sprouts, broccoli, cauliflower, kale, turnip, swede, radish, horseradish, mustard and cress: 'These contain three unique compounds – indoles, dithiolthiones and isothiocyanates, which influence certain enzymes that rev up the body's degradation system [...] oestrogen is "metabolized" and ultimately excreted from the body.'[51]

4   'Other protective factors may be the phytoestrogens from a moderate soya intake and a high natural level of selenium in foods';[52] for those suffering with endometriosis, it is in our own interest to keep circulating oestrogen levels moderate. Therefore, by eating green leafy vegetables, a little soya protein and selenium-rich seafoods, we are helping our body to protect itself. So, Granny was right when she told us to eat up our greens!

5   The clearance system for oestrogens, cholesterol and toxins is the liver. The steroid hormones are metabolized (broken down) in the liver. The bile from the gallbladder stores these inactive hormones and excretes them bound to fibre in the stools. Choline and inositol make up lecithin, which helps the liver deal with fats. The herb silymarin and zinc methionine may also assist in liver cleansing (*see* p. 192).

As other scientists have demonstrated, 'we know from research that the form of oestrogen known as oestradiol causes tissue proliferation'[53] and that 'uncontrolled levels of oestrogen, if the body goes into oestrogen dominance, have been indicated for contributing to the serious problem of endometriosis and breast cancers'.[54] When this oestradiol form of oestrogen reaches the liver, enzymes which use B vitamins as cofactors, change this sex hormone into the less harmful oestriol. A healthy liver with a plentiful supply of B vitamins can degrade oestradiol into oestriol which is important for optimum wellbeing: 'If the sum of oestrone and the oestradiol is greater than the oestriol in a 24-hour urine sample, women may be at greater risk of illness related to oestrogen excess.'[55, 56] Your doctor can check your oestrogen levels with a simple blood or saliva test.

Oestriol is the form in which oestrogen can be bound to fibre and excreted. Therefore the diet needs to have sufficient fibre and B vitamins to help the body deal with the constant breakdown of circulating oestrogen. If the diet is high in animal and trans fatty acids and low in fibre, the gut flora in the bowel behave differently and change the way they break down oestrogen. If the gut flora in the small intestine and the liver enzymes are in a poor state, the levels of oestradiol and oestrone in the blood may become higher than they should be and this can unbalance reproductive hormones.

Research shows that 'dietary fat may influence oestrogen metabolism due to the stimulation of animal fats upon the growth of colonic bacteria which are capable of synthesizing oestrogen as well as breaking the oestrogen–glucoronide linkages'.[57] Eating fish can be beneficial: 'A diet rich in fish oils (herring, mackerel, sardines, pilchards, salmon, trout, tuna) has been shown to help women suffering from high-circulating oestrogen levels and also help those with PMS who are oversensitive to the hormone prolactin.'[58] However, women must make sure that the fish they choose is from a clean source that is low in pesticides. Deficiency of B-complex vitamins may impair the function of liver enzymes in inactivating oestrogens. How environmental synthetic oestrogens behave when they reach the liver requires more research.

Unnatural oestrogens

Natural oestrogens made in the body have mimics – some occurring naturally in foods and others man-made – which confuse the normal hormonal messages.

1 Exogenous oestrogens or xeno-oestrogens, which our bodies metabolize from pesticides, are thought to be dangerous.
2 Phytoestrogens that occur naturally in foods such as soya are thought to be helpful during and after the menopause. In reproductive-age women, they should be eaten in moderation.
3 Endometriotic implants are thought to produce their own oestrogens directly into the abdominal cavity (*see* pp. 52, 78, 308).

Xeno-oestrogens

Unfortunately, some of the food we eat contains pesticides which have an oestrogenic effect (xeno-oestrogens).

Dioxins, PCBs and nonylphenols have oestrogenic effects in body cells. They produce chemicals which act exactly like oestrogens do in the body. These false oestrogens are bad news: 'Suspect chemicals include pesticides and phthalates (nonylphenols), a group of compounds which migrate from plastic wrappings and leak into the foods we eat, such as cheese, meats, cakes, sandwiches and confectionery.'[59] Research from around the world has shown that these compounds have a detrimental effect upon the reproductive systems of both humans and animals: 'USA production alone of synthetic organic chemicals (including pesticides) amount to 197.5 billion kilogrammes in 1992, with similar production in other countries. They ignore geographical boundaries and are found in rainwater, lakes, oceans and in the fat cells within our bodies.'[60] The effects of xeno-oestrogens are insidious: 'Biologists feel that these xeno-oestrogens can mimic the actions of natural signalling molecules such as oestrogens and also growth factors; i.e. a "natural" signal may be being sent by an "unnatural" signalling molecule. They do not alter genes themselves but may alter the way they [genes] are expressed.'[61]

In 1979 it was realized that diethylstilboestrol (DES), a synthetic man-made oestrogen used to prevent spontaneous abortion in pregnancy, caused a specific vaginal cancer in the daughters of women who had taken DES while pregnant. DES acts as a transplacental carcinogen – when given to the mother, it causes cancer in daughters and testicular problems in sons. Many daughters of DES mothers are also diagnosed with endometriosis. Therefore, worries about other synthetic oestrogen mimics which are awash in our environment are well-founded. We need to know what the long-term effects will be, and whether or not the increase in endometriosis and other reproductive disorders are linked to the use of pesticides.

Naturally occurring oestrogens are important in normal growth of organs. But these 'mimic' and synthetic xeno-oestrogens are soluble in all fats and oils, so they can cross cell membranes into the nucleus and can activate or repress gene expression; that is, they can change the cells' programming (even though they bind in a much weaker fashion than natural oestrogens). It is also known that the body's own metabolism can alter these chemicals, possibly to even more potent forms in the body: 'Metabolism can convert non-oestrogenic substances into ones with hormonal activity or they may just disrupt normal hormone levels. When one research group tested a combination of chemicals, their oestrogenicity jumped by 160 to 1,600 times their individual potency, probably due to synergy. So together they may be more potent than when alone.'[62] We need more research to look at exactly what these chemicals do to our oestrogen balance.

The Endometriosis Association, headquartered in the USA, discovered a group of monkeys in the University of Wisconsin Primate Center which had been treated with dioxins and developed spontaneous endometriosis: 'The disease pattern found in the monkeys was in direct correlation with the amount of dioxin they had been given. The 15-year study indicated that latent female reproductive abnormalities may be associated with dioxin exposure in rhesus monkeys.'[63]

Both humans and animals are exposed daily to a mixture of polyhalogenated aromatic hydrocarbons (PHAHs) via trace amounts present in food. Exposure to 2,3,7,8-tetrachlorodibenzo-*p*-dioxin (TCDD) is associated with a dose-dependent increase in the incidence and severity of endometriosis in the rhesus monkey. It has been postulated that increased concentrations of TCDD and dioxin-like chemicals in blood and tissues may disrupt endocrine and immune responses in susceptible humans and animals.[64]

Research has shown that rhesus monkeys are still affected by dioxins for up to 10 years after the initial exposure. If a similar effect applies to humans, it may be causing fertility problems due to the effects upon the immune and endocrine systems. This two-million-dollar research programme at Vanderbilt University in Tennessee is funded jointly by the Fairleigh S. Dickinson Jr Foundation, The Endometriosis Association and a grant from The National Institutes of Environmetal Health Sciences in Maryland, USA.

'It is now known that certain PCB congeners modulate or disrupt the activity of certain steroid and sex hormones, including oestradiol, vitamin A (retinoic acid), and thyroid hormones. The oestrogenic acivity of 3,3',4,4'-TCB was recently observed both *in vitro* and *in vivo*. Considering the critical roles of oestradiol, retinoic acid and immune cytokines in the regulation of normal uterine endometrial growth, immune–endocrine disruption by PCB congeners may have potential importance in the pathogenesis of endometriosis.'

In Belgium, Koninckx *et al.* (1994) noted that the incidence of endometriosis in women presenting at clinics with infertility is 60–80 per cent, and TCDD concentrations in breastmilk are among the highest in the world (WHO Environmental Series, 1992). This association between human endometriosis and PCBs was first suggested by Gerhard and Runnebaum in 1992. Other research showed that more infertile women with endometriosis had detectably high TCDD levels in serum than fertile women without the disease. Meanwhile, women with endometriosis should avoid fatty foods that may be high in PCBs and dioxin to reduce their exposure to these chemicals.

Man-made toxins used in lubricants, transformers and building materials bind to sediment and organic matter on the seabed and are eaten or absorbed into the fatty tissues of farmed fish. Feed for farmed salmon is created from material effectively vacuumed up off the ocean floor. Dioxins can be detected in all foods and cannot be removed from the diet. The highest concentrations are found in fatty foods such as meat, oily fish, eggs and diary products. These substances were linked in laboratory animals to severe effects on the uterus, learning difficulties, low sperm counts and malformations.[65]

The moral of all this is to reduce these foods in the diet. The Greenpeace website has much detailed information about the best fish liver oils to buy and lists those which are polluted.

Dioxins in food

Dioxins come to us from plants and animals through our foods. The higher up the food chain, the greater the dioxin contamination.

1   Eating from lower down the food chain may have a lesser effect – as with being a fish-eating vegetarian or lactovegetarian. The fats in meat and dairy foods may contain the highest levels of dioxins, so keep your intake of these very low.
2   Fish should be from a relatively clean source, not a polluted lake or river. Deep-sea oily fish are thought to be the least harmful.
3   Avoiding fruits and vegetables which have been sprayed is difficult, as buying organic vegetables may be neither easy nor affordable for most people. Besides, dioxins are everywhere, even on the skins of organic vegetables. However, it is extremely important that all fruits and vegetables be peeled to remove the chemicals. Just washing them will not work.
4   Processed foods, such as cakes and biscuits, may contain contaminated fats, so keep these to a bare minimum. If cooking is done at home, there can be more control over the use of pure ingredients. Lindane, often found in chocolate, is an oestrogenic pesticide that has been linked by research to breast cancer. For this reason, use organic chocolate for those special occasions.

We have to be aware but not anxious. Just do your best to avoid an excess intake of these harmful chemicals. Dioxins build up in our fat cells. Internationally, there is some debate over what are acceptable levels: 'The World Health Organization and the UK authorities accept a tolerance of 10 units of dioxin per day as acceptable while USA authorities set the minimum risk at 0.0064 units per day, stating that dioxins have a cancer risk.'[66] A pint of milk contains five times the quantity of PCBs contained in a single cod liver oil capsule, and a pat of butter contains three times the amount. Water should also be from purified sources. The way in which our liver enzymes deal with these man-made oestrogenic chemicals requires more research. The Women's Environmental Network can advise you on harmful chemical exposure, and the Lister Hospital in London can test for body levels of PCB and dioxin.

Weight loss and dioxins. If you are trying to lose weight, then do it slowly – 1kg (2lb) per week only. This is important as a sudden change in diet can result in too-rapid release of dioxins from fat cells, causing symptoms such as feeling toxic and exhausted. Such quick release also greatly stresses the liver. The use of the herb silymarin can gently cleanse the liver. Often a weight loss of 2kg (5lb) happens naturally over one month when on an exclusion diet, as food intolerance often causes fluid retention (oedema) in soft tissue. Researchers at the University of Los Angeles, USA, took 60 people off wheat for three months. At the end of this time, they were given one slice of bread. Twelve people put on 3.5kg (8lb) in weight overnight with fluid retention. Once the food is excluded again, the cells lose this fluid, the bloating disappears and body weight normalizes. The use of good quality cis oils can also help weight loss when used wisely: 'Researchers have observed that the more linoleic acid in the fat tissue, the less obese the person.'[67]

If you are pregnant or breastfeeding, take care as some dioxins stored in body fat cells can be transferred from mother to child. Try not to detox too rapidly and avoid a sudden candidiasis-type diet while you are very ill. It is better to wait until your immune system has become stronger and digestion has improved before embarking on a drastic detox diet.

Detoxing gently

The body has its own automatic detoxification systems to get rid of waste materials such as leftover hormones, neurotransmitters and ammonia. Some of this material comes from waste matter produced by body processes, but some is from germs which get into the system. As we have seen, the liver also deals with chemicals and biotransforms them into safe chemicals. This detoxification system uses pheno-sulphotransferases (PST), which prevent harmful build up of leftover waste and renders it safe.

'The biological process of detoxification involves synthesis as opposed to degradation. If you want to get rid of a molecule such as oestrogen, your chemistry usually sticks another molecule onto it, making it bigger but less toxic. Packaged in this way, the unwanted molecule is discharged from the body directly from the liver into the bile, which travels to the intestine and out of the system, or the liver puts the package into the bloodstream, where it travels out of the body in the urine via the kidneys. Some toxins, such as heavy metals, find their way out through hair and nails, and a small amount is through perspiration.'[68]

Thus, women with endometriosis should detox very gently to avoid overstressing the liver and kidneys. Signs that you may need a two- or three-week detox include bloating, weight gain and extreme fatigue or headaches. If the liver is overwhelmed by toxins, a toxic excess may always be slushing about in the bloodstream, causing the body systems to be sluggish. Often, once you begin to detox, you may feel much worse for a short time. This is okay for healthy women, but for those with endometriosis, this could make their disease worse, like walking on eggshells. Drinking lots of water (two litres each day) can help flush out the toxins. But if it all becomes too much, just try a detox diet one day a week until your health is robust enough to try it for one week.

Energy and clear skin are two of the prizes to be gained. Weight loss of up to half a stone is acceptable over a three-week period – any more than that may lead to problems. You could try one detox day every week and one detox weekend every three months to help maintain your health (*see* p. 192 for foods which aid liver function).

Detox rules
1   Eat fresh fruits and vegetables, nuts, seeds, legumes and wholegrain cereals other than wheat.
2   Drink eight tumblers of filtered or bottled spring or mineral water every day.
3   Eat when you are hungry from the allowed foods.
4   Eat half of the diet food raw and half lightly cooked.
5   Eat organic food if possible; if not, remove the peel.
6   Eat three regular meals each day and two healthy snacks.
7   Avoid junk food and caffeine in coffee, chocolate and cola.
8   Avoid wheat, cow's milk dairy foods, citrus and meat.
9   Avoid fermented foods, dried fruits, vinegars, mushrooms, and all yeasty foods and alcohol.
10   Make a plan of what you are going to eat for three days and stick to it.

Effects of high oestrogen levels

A condition known as oestrogen dominance (oestrogen out of balance with progesterone) is under review by researchers. This may be due to the effects of the exogenous oestrogens or hormone disrupters from the pesticides that surround us. Also, a very low-fibre and high-fat diet can compound these problems. We do not know what subtle effects an excess of phytoestrogens or xeno-oestrogens may be having on us.

High oestrogen levels:

1   can act as an abortive and may cause uterine cramping.
2   may also cause an imbalance in brain chemicals, with too many excitatory neurotransmitters and too few inhibitory ones, thus causing mood swings.
3   cause high copper levels, and low zinc and low prostaglandin series 1 levels. High copper levels have been implicated as a nervous stimulant, triggering mood swings, and may also inhibit essential energy-producing enzymes. High copper

levels also compete with iron, lowering it and causing heavy blood loss during menstruation, and have been linked in research to ovarian cysts.

4   stimulate serotonin, a neurotransmitter, to release aldosterone, a hormone, from the adrenal glands, which control the kidneys' water and salt retention. Excessive amounts of aldosterone cause bloating. It is therefore important to eat a low-salt, low-refined- sugar and low-refined-carbohydrate diet (white rice and white flour). The use of diuretics if you bloat just throws zinc and magnesium out of the body too rapidly and this will worsen all the other PMS symptoms. (Vitamin B6, zinc and magnesium are natural diuretics and will expel retained fluids, as do proanthocyanidins found in berries.)

5   correlate with low thyroxine levels, as these two hormones are antagonistic (act against each other). Hypothyroid symptoms can result – coarse skin, fatigue, constipation, feeling cold, weight gain and hair loss (especially the outer third of the eyebrows).[69]

6   stress raises cortisol levels in the adrenals and this hormone competes with progesterone production and lowers it, which in turn raises oestrogen levels. Low progesterone increases immune system reactions and makes miscarriages more likely. High progesterone lowers immune responses to make it easier for sperm to survive and function. Stress reduces the amount of B vitamins available to the body, so trying to reduce stress levels is a good idea. Taking a yeast-free B-vitamin complex is a good idea at such times, especially as vitamin B6 is the precursor of progesterone and works together with zinc, magnesium and L-carnitine. The herb blue cohosh taken five days before a period begins also aids the production of progesterone.

7   women who take an excess of antibiotics (for example, amoxycillin, penicillin, neomycin) change the amounts of oestrogen being recycled: 'The quantity of oestrogen found in the faeces is increased up to 60 times the normal levels. Looking at research, levels of aerobic and anaerobic bacteria drop to between 20–25 per cent of original levels during antibiotic treatment. In patients going for operations, only 9 per cent contracted infections when taking antibiotics compared to 35 per cent of those not receiving antibiotics.'[70] So the benefit of taking antibiotics is important, but the gut flora must be replenished within three weeks of the operation.

8   with oestrogen dominance, several symptoms may occur:
   • weight gain (extra fat may be deposited on the waist, hips and legs)
   • heavy and irregular periods
   • fibroids on the uterus
   • swollen breasts and formation of cysts
   • water retention (soft-tissue oedema)
   • more pronounced PMS symptoms
   • cravings for sweet foods
   • lack of sex drive.

If you have a number of these symptoms, then this book should help you find a way to correct the problem by normalizing hormone levels.

B vitamins are vital to the way the liver is able to break down oestrogens circulating in the blood (oestradiol, which is known to cause cell proliferation, is linked to endometriosis): 'Being able to break down oestradiol to oestriol, a hormone which is benign, is dependent upon the B vitamin levels in the liver.'[71] Therefore, your diet is very important in controlling oestrogen levels. Oestriol can be bound to fibre from the diet and excreted from the body, so your fibre intake is important. Only 30g of fibre per day are needed.

Healthy eating helps to control the processes which can lead to endometriosis. Choline and inositol (B-complex vitamins) are crucial for liver enzyme function and fat metabolism, so the diet should be rich in these B vitamins. Excess folic acid can increase oestrogen production, so care must be taken to keep it in balance with the other B vitamins.

Natural oestrogens of plant origin (phytoestrogens)

Phytoestrogens are naturally occurring oestrogens in plants such as soya, wheat, alfalfa, red clover and citrus fruits, and are found in tofu, tempeh, miso, liquorice, rye, rhubarb, anise, beansprouts, sunflower-seeds and linseeds (*see* table 10.3). Research suggests that these natural plant oestrogens (known as isoflavonoids and lignans) are protective and may help to lower or balance the oestrogens produced by the body cells: 'They are very similar to oestradiol but are not the same as oestrogen produced in women. It is felt from research that they act like weak oestrogens or may have an anti-oestrogenic effect to block excess uptake of natural body cell oestrogens. One isoflavonoid (genistein) does three amazing things in the bodies of postmenopausal women: it delays bone loss, it reduces blood cholesterol levels and it helps to keep oestrogen levels high in them.'[72] Little is known about effects on women of reproductive age.

More research is necessary to see what effect phytoestrogens have on the levels of oestrogens in endometriosis. If it acts as an anti-oestrogen and helps to normalize levels, it could be very helpful; whereas if it raises oestrogen levels it may be detrimental. When phytoestrogens act as antioestrogens they can lock into the body's oestrogen receptor sites, rather like the US Space Shuttle *Atlantis* is able to dock with

Carrots	Soya beans	Wheat + bran + germ
Rice + bran + polish	Oats	Barley
Potatoes	Apples	Cherries
Plums	Red clover	Mouldy corn
Citrus fruits	Ginseng	Alfalfa

Table 10.3
Foods containing oestrogenic factors

the Russian Space Station *Mir*. It is thought that they may therefore prevent the oestradiol (known to cause cell proliferation) from growing out of control, thus reducing the more potent oestrogens in the body from triggering other disease states.

Research done in America suggests that phytoestrogens may be protective against cancers of the breast, uterus and cervix. Indeed, 'in Japan breast cancer is low where the diet is high in soya products and fresh fish. Such a diet, which is higher in soya protein than in the West, indicates that Japanese women have lower oestrogen levels. Isoflavins present on soya beans have been seen to inhibit the growth of cancer cells.'[73] It is known that in cultures such as Japan where women eat an average of 100mg of indoles daily, there is a very low risk of breast cancer. In the West our average daily intake of indoles is a mere 20mg, which may be far too low.

Endometriosis may respond to the use of 'good' oestrogens in the diet in some women. Moderation may be the key. However, in Japan the incidence of endometriosis is extremely high, so it is unclear what is really happening with respect to phytoestrogens: how can they be protective against breast cancer in older Japanese women, but do not appear to lessen the levels of endometriosis in younger women? It is a mystery. Phytoestrogens in soya beans have been seen to act as contraceptives in excess. Exotic cats in Cincinnati zoo became infertile on a diet of 50 per cent soy protein. This effect has also been seen in other zoos. When the soya was replaced with chicken, fertility was restored. Use caution and moderation with foods containing phytoestrogens if you are attempting pregnancy.

However, it is felt that a combination of phytochemicals is the most beneficial, so that by eating a variety of natural fruits and vegetables we take in beneficial combinations of foods. For instance, the allylic sulphides found in garlic and onions and the limonene in citrus fruits work as enzyme activators and strengthen the body's immune system. Many phytochemicals have antioxidant properties, so they disarm the free radical molecules which rush around inside the body causing damage to cell membranes and cell DNA.

To obtain extra lignans, eat one to three teaspoonfuls of ground food-grade linseeds every day with breakfast, and drink water with the meal.

To obtain isoflavonoids, eat soya beans. The Japanese eat 100mg of soya beans per

Cottonseed	Safflower
Wheatgerm	Corn
Linseed	Peanut (*best avoided because of aflatoxins*)
Olive	Soya bean
Coconut	Linseed oil + glutamic acid = antipyridoxine (*need extra vitamin B6*)

Table 10.4
Oils which are oestrogenic. Use only one tablespoon per day of these good cis fatty acids. Buy only the cold-pressed, unrefined, unhydrogenated versions (linseed, olive, safflower and corn oils).

day; other Asians take in only 45mg per day from soya flour, tempeh, tofu or vegetable protein. Roasted soya beans contain 162mg isoflavonoid per 75g/3oz and tofu contains 62mg per 75g 3oz.

Meat and dairy foods raise fat levels in the body and therefore contribute to oestrogen production. A low-fibre diet with high animal fat can exaggerate oestrogen levels, so you should eat a selection of high-fibre foods. A balanced diet is essential; never eat too much of any one substance in a day and always ensure that the diet is rich in a variety of different foods.

Diana G of Shropshire

I put my improvement in health and endo symptoms down to a non-dairy diet, drinking bottled water, no coffee and keeping more or less to a candida-style diet – no grapes, mushrooms or yeast-based foods. I also find that not eating brown bread helps me (I'm all right with white). A positive state of mind and not to give up is essential.

CASE STUDY

A recent report from the UK Medical Research Council's Institute for Environment and Health concludes that 'though some epidemiological studies suggest that the consumption of foods containing phytoestrogens may have beneficial effects, almost no evidence exists to link these effects directly to oestrogens'.[74] Recent American research has shown that low doses of phytoestrogens at dietary levels can cause breast cancer cells to proliferate. While all this debate is ongoing about the true effects of phytoestrogens in normal healthy people, women of reproductive age with health problems related to imbalances of oestrogen need to be cautious in their use. Apply the rules of moderation and never eat in excess – and try to avoid snacking or comfort eating.

Making oestrogen safer with phytonutrition

By using the right type of phytonutrients (helpful chemicals in our food), the body can adapt to regulating hormone balance and correct cell behaviour. Cruciferous vegetables such as broccoli, cabbage, Brussels sprouts and cauliflower contain specific phytonutrients that can regulate the way in which the body metabolizes oestrogens. The active compounds are known as indoles and the most useful one is diindolylmethane. This compound helps the body to produce beneficial oestrogen breakdown. We know that an excess of oestrogen can lead to cancer, and the use of green leafy vegetables in the diet is a master key for promoting normal oestrogen activity and preventing oestrogen dominance.

Diindolylmethane causes 2-hydroxy and 2-methoxyestrogens to become active metabolites. These are 'good' oestrogens which act as antioxidants, and are able to remove damaged and cancerous cells from tissues in the body. If these two types of oestrogen are absent from the diet, then there could be an increased production of other damaging oestrogen metabolites.

Fish oils from deep-sea fish help in the production of the good oestrogens. The use of diindolylmethanes in the diet or as supplements blocks the aryl hydrocarbon receptor, which is then able to resist the xeno-oestrogens from pesticides and prevent them from damaging the body's cells. 2-Methoxy-oestradiol regulates cell growth and apoptosis (programmed cell death).

'Bad' oestrogens can damage cell membranes and allow oxidation, thereby promoting cancerous growths. These 'bad' oestrogens are 16-alpha-OH-oestrone and 4-OH-oestrone. A diet high in saturated and trans fatty acids will trigger metabolism to produce more of these 'bad' oestrogens. They are known to be involved with benign breast disease.

Diindolylmethane is not an oestrogen mimic like the soy isoflavones or genistein; it is not a phytoestrogen. However, it does aid the balance of oestrogen within the body by enhancing the activity of cytochrome enzymes and specific oestrogen receptor molecules. In this way, it helps to influence the way in which cells respond to oestrogens.

As endometriosis is driven by oestrogen factors, we should all heed our grandmother's advice to eat our green vegetables. Folk medicine throughout the ages has proved, with the aid of modern science, that foods have been used for the reasons most suited to the chemicals they contain. Diindolylmethane is formed from its precursor indole-3-carbinol (I3C). I3C is released in all cruciferous vegetables from the glucosinolates after enzyme action. Because this triggers production of the 2-hydroxyoestrogen metabolites, it means that the body is more able to protect itself from the harmful oestrogens. A serving of 500mg per day of vegetables contains 0.3mg/kg of diindolylmethane.[75]

OESTROGEN AND THYROID BALANCE IN ENDOMETRIOSIS

The thyroid gland and its hormonal products play a vital role in our overall wellbeing. The major hormone produced by the thyroid is thyroxine, which controls the basal metabolic activity of the body.

Thyroxine:

1 Speeds up most of the metabolic (chemical) reactions that take place in the cells of the body
2 Acts like a thermostat controlling the heating in a house. When the house needs to be warmed up, the thermostat goes up and the furnace burns more fuel to raise the temperature in the house
3 Increases the use of our dietary carbohydrates, proteins and fats by the body
4 Works with the other hormones of the body to enhance their biological actions.

Oestrogen is an antagonistic hormone to thyroxine,[76] so if we have oestrogen dominance, then thyroxine may be low. (This implies low intake of B vitamins, iodine, selenium and proteins alongside an excess intake of sugar.) 'Oestrogens do acutely inhibit the rate of hormone release from the thyroid in adults, but any effect appears to be transient.'[77] However, although this may be so in healthy individuals, in those who are ill with hormonal imbalances and endocrine dysfunction, there may be problems with balancing hormones correctly. This area requires much more research into the way this may affect endometriosis and subsequent fertility issues.

Thyroid hormone synthesis depends in large part on having an appropriate amount of iodine in the diet. Iodine is absorbed through the small intestine and transported directly to the thyroid, where it is used in the synthesis of hormones. Without iodine, the thyroid desperately tries to produce thyroid hormone, but without success, and the thyroid enlarges (goitre). A goitre can easily be seen as a lump in the region of the neck. Selenium is vital to enhance the uptake of iodine, so both should be taken together. In addition to iodine, a healthy thyroid requires cis fatty acids, proteins, vitamins and minerals. The thyroid gland also produces T3 (triiodothyronine) and T4 (thyroxine); these hormones all have to be finely balanced.

High or normal thyroid hormone is protective against cancer; low thyroid hormone invites it. Likewise, high oestrogen invites cancer while normal oestrogen discourages it.[78] Hormone levels need to be checked regularly in women with endometriosis, as many of the drug treatments have profound effects on normal pituitary and ovarian hormone levels that will take some months to correct after the course of drugs is completed.

HYPOTHYROIDISM

When a person has low amounts of thyroxine (hypothyroidism), the body slows up and constipation occurs. Someone with hypothyroidism feels the cold and is chilly when other people are not – the one wearing the layered look! This person feels tired and sluggish, and gains weight all too easily. Other signs are hair loss, skin thickening and a befuddled brain. But more important to the subject of this book, hypothyroidism leads to infertility. Some women with hypothyroidism may not menstruate. The absence of the menstrual cycle is called amenorrhoea. A normal menstrual cycle is dependent upon the presence of a properly functioning thyroid.

HYPERTHYROIDISM

Very high levels of these thyroid hormones cause diarrhoea, weight loss, an abnormal heart rate, hyperactivity, irritability and anxiety.

PITUITARY INVOLVEMENT

The pituitary gland produces thyroid-stimulating hormone (TSH). If the level of TSH is normal on tests, the patient is not hypothyroid. The level of TSH will change before thyroid hormone levels fall, so it is an extremely sensitive index for hypothyroidism.

Autoimmune diseases, such as those involving the thyroid, are thought to play a role in infertility. Indeed, thyroid auto-antibodies are used to predict those women at risk of miscarriage.[79] Fourteen per cent of women with coeliac disease were found to have thyroid disorders.[80] The relationship between thyroid function, endometriosis, subfertility and the use of oestrogenic hormones is intriguing. There appears to be a link between the hormonal balance of the thyroid, adrenal and endocrine glands, and the symptoms of endometriosis. Rare diseases of the ovaries may cause the thyroid to be overstimulated.[81]

THYROID TESTS

If you suspect that your thyroid is sluggish, check with your GP and ask to be tested for T3, T4, TSH and antibodies to the thyroid. It is especially important for women with endometriosis that all four tests be done, and not just the first two.

SOYA AND THYROXINE

Other findings from the USA National Center for Toxicological Research 'indicates that isoflavonoids could inhibit thyroid hormone synthesis, inducing goitre and even thyroid cancer,[82] which is why an excess of phytoestrogenic foods such as wheat and soya may give rise to fertility problems. Oestrogen will go up and thyroxine down. As oestrogen in excess is an abortive, the result could be an early miscarriage. All legumes should be consumed in moderation because of this effect on fertility.

Use the vegetables listed in table 10.5 freely, but do not eat them in excess. The B vitamins and magnesium they contain are necessary for your health. Cooking usually reduces the goitrogenic effect; eaten raw, they are effective at reducing thyroxine levels.

Cabbage	Broccoli	Cauliflower
Fool's parsley	Mint	Brussels sprouts
Mustard	Turnip	Cress
Radish	Horseradish	Spinach
Carrot	Peach	Pear

Table 10.5
Goitrogens: foods which suppress thyroid function

ACHIEVING HORMONE BALANCE

It is in the interest of every woman with endometriosis to keep her hormones well balanced, and this is governed by the foods which you choose to eat and the state of your digestive tract. Correcting the digestive tract function with specialist supplements and by eating healthily will be of benefit. Foods containing both phytoestrogens and goitergens need to be balanced, and most of us do that instinctively by not eating the same food all the time. We are meant to eat some foods from each food group every day, but at the same time we need to try to avoid or keep to a bare minimum those which may contain dioxins and other oestrogenic substances (such as chocolate, which may contain the pesticide lindane). By being sensible in our choice of foods we ingest a wide variety of different nutrients each day (in Japan they recommend eating 100 different foods each day). We can try to do our own best, to choose and buy wisely, for our enjoyment of food must not be stilted. It is very important that we enjoy the foods we eat, so a balance has to be struck.

If you are extremely ill and one or two foods appear to be upsetting you, remove them from your diet, but ensure that they are replaced by similar foods in order to maintain the nutrient level you need. It may be beneficial to try an exclusion or a rotation diet. We must all take care to listen to what our bodies are telling us by using our sixth sense. Become aware of exactly how different foods affect your health. The judicious use of supplements may help to speed up the healing process and heal the gut membrane.

THE MORAL OF THE STORY

You are what you eat only if your digestive system is able to obtain nutrients from the foods which you consume. You are only what you can absorb.

DIGESTIVE SYSTEM HEALTH

The first step is to heal the digestive tract.

Noel H of London

I would like to say to all the women out there who are reading this book that diet is an important factor in contributing to one's health. I eliminated dairy products, wheat, sugar, chocolate, anything with preservatives and colourings, tinned and packet microwaved junk food. I now include fresh fruits and vegetables, organic when possible, have cut down on red meat, substituting chicken and fish. I found it strange at first, because I hadn't realized what ingredients were in most foods as I hadn't looked before. I was amazed to see all the unnatural constituents.

It was difficult the first week, but gradually I enjoyed the change and now have a much healthier lifestyle. My bloated feeling has disappeared and my stomach cramps are almost non-existent, except when I am stressed or eat the wrong thing.

I do think that the new healthier diet is an acquired taste; as with most things, it takes time to find the right alternative foods. Instead of chocolate, I have carob bars and nuts.

CASE STUDY

Instead of dairy products, I enjoy goat's yoghurt and soya milk and cheeses. It has made such a dramatic difference in my life. It was a week before I noticed any change.

It was hard at first, but I wouldn't go back to the way I was because now I feel a totally new person. I know and feel that without this diet I would never be able to enjoy the everyday life of walking the dogs, travelling and having fun. After the initial change in food and once you begin to feel so different, it will be easier to continue with this and other things too – I found it an exciting experience. It takes slightly longer but it tastes fantastic.

Try it and see for yourself. It's brilliant.

To get an idea of exactly what we could be eating in processed foods, it is interesting to see what food additives are actually used in them. Some years ago the *Sunday Observer* ran a story about ice cream made naturally from eggs and cream in the home. It also listed all the ingredients in manufactured ice creams and explained their origins. The following list gives an idea of just what we may be eating in ice cream and other processed foods.

- Aldehyde C-17, for cherry flavouring, is a flammable liquid used in dyes, plastics and rubber. It is known to cause bladder cancer.
- Amyl acetate, for banana flavouring, is a paint solvent.
- Benzyl acetate, for strawberry flavours, is a nitrate solvent.
- Butraldehyde, for nutty flavours, is an ingredient in rubber cement.
- Diethyl glycol, used to emulsify eggs, is the same chemical which is used in antifreeze and paint remover.
- Ethyl acetate, used for pineapple flavouring, is used in the leather and textile industries. The vapours are believed to cause lung, heart and liver damage.
- Piperonal, used to give a vanilla flavour, is a chemical which was used to kill lice. The body stores this substance in its cells as it cannot be excreted. [83]

Looking at the above, our conclusion must be that it is always best to eat foods prepared from natural ingredients. Given the lack of available information, it is virtually impossible to surmise how damaging different combinations of food additives could be to the reproductive system.

Some short-term use of nutritional supplements may help correct imbalances in the digestive tract. Seek help from a qualified nutritionist.

If you suffer from stomach pains, diarrhoea, constipation, bloating, flatulence or anal irritation, you need to correct the digestive tract before health can be achieved. This is a key area to correct on the path to wellness. If you are malabsorbing nutrients, then no amount of good food or supplements can get you well. This area has to be healed first in order to allow nutrients to be absorbed so that they can help the reproductive system to function correctly.

Herbal teas (mint, fennel or ginger) are helpful, and a selection of the following may be beneficial over a two- or three-month period:

Herbal colonic cleansing
Probiotics such as acidophilus
Slippery elm
NAG
Caprylic acid

Prebiotics such as FOS
Digestive enzymes
Milk thistle (silymarin)
Butyric acid
Multivitamins/minerals

IRRITABLE BOWEL SYNDROME

Avoid all foods known to cause intolerance, particularly wheat and dairy products, and citrus fruits, but eat all the alternatives. Some sensitive people may need to exclude all gluten grains. Clearly, caffeine and sugars should also be avoided, and dietary fibre from fruits, vegetables and groundnuts should be increased gradually.

Probiotics: acidophilus
Slippery elm
Multivitamins/minerals

Digestive enzymes
Mint, fennel or ginger teas
Evening primrose and fish oils

BLOATING

Bloating is a problem in many women with endometriosis and may be due to an imbalance in the gut flora. If too many antibiotics or hormones have been taken, it can increase the amount of *Bacteroides* bacteria in the gut (those which produce gases). By taking probiotics, this balance may be restored and the bloating subside.

As the state of the gut flora can affect hormone levels, these have to be corrected for women to get well. A recent international congress held at the Royal Society of Medicine in the UK on gut flora looked at all these problems. Gynaecologists may not know about this excellent research work. Prebiotics, probiotics and digestive enzymes may be tried, and none have harmful side effects like those caused by many drugs.

Magnesium, zinc and vitamin B6 are natural diuretics as are proanthocyanidins (flavonoid family).

NAG
Digestive enzymes
Zinc citrate
Proanthocyanidins
FOS

Multivitamins/minerals
Acidophilus (dairy-free)
Magnesium malate
Vitamin B6 + B-complex (yeast-free)
TH207 (BioCare) or kelp tablets

SUMMARY

1   You are what your body can digest and absorb. It is important to eat nutrient-rich food and ignore calorie-laden junk.

2   Nutrition is essential to life. Your choice of food can make you ill or healthy. Analyse over four days exactly what you eat, then assess if you are giving your body the building blocks it needs to keep you healthy.

3   Your digestion is your first line of defence. Assess your digestion. If you suffer from heartburn, indigestion, stomach pains, gall bladder problems, flatulence and bloating, constipation or diarrhoea, something is wrong and it needs to be corrected before you can begin to get well. Introduce into your diet a digestive enzyme and acidophilus supplement to aid digestion and improve the gut flora. If you have been abroad where food and water are suspect, take some grapefruit seed extract which has antibacterial and antiparasitic effects.

4   The intestinal barrier's mucous membrane needs to be healthy. It is almost the size of a tennis court and protects us from external elements. It also makes 80 per cent of the immuno-globulin-producing cells in the body. By acting to protect this membrane and rebalance your gut flora, you are strengthening your immune system. To help the gut membrane use slippery elm, NAG, glutamine, essential fatty acids, butyric acid, vitamin A and zinc.

5   Cleanse the liver regularly every three months or so by eating foods such as lemons, carrots, beetroot, cucumber, tomatoes, artichokes, chicory, celery, radishes, leeks, onions, cabbage, spring dandelion leaves, parsley, apricots, cold-pressed olive oil and grapefruit. The liver is the organ that degrades oestrogen and it needs to be efficient in women with endometriosis.

6   Drink three glasses of water each day and take three brisk 20-minute walks each week if possible to help stimulate the intestines.

7   To test for food intolerance, cut out the suspect food from the diet for 30 days. Choose other foods as alternatives to ensure that your nutrient intake is maintained and take a multivitamin/mineral supplement to cover your change in diet. When you reintroduce the food, note any symptoms that you experience over the next 24 hours, such as a faster pulse rate, flu-like symptoms, headaches or joint pains.

8   Insist upon tests for hypothyroidism (T3, T4, TSH and auto-antibodies to the thyroid), gut fermentation, IgE and IgG, gluten sensitivity, fasting glucose levels,

liver enzyme function, and oestrogen and progesterone levels in the urine if you are suffering from fertility problems.

9   At least four vegetables, two fruits and some legumes plus a handful of nuts and seeds should be eaten each day along with some wholegrain cereal such as oats, rice, corn or rye. This will also speed up the transit time of food in the gut and provide the digestive tract with fibre, which can bind to oestrogen and cholesterol and escort them from the body.

10 Spending money to service your car and repair your home seems natural. Your body is more important. You might consider giving your body a detoxification diet and 'spring-clean'. The body is designed to last us some 90 years or more and it is vital to maintain its health. Give it the tools it needs to give you a healthy old age. Endometriosis symptoms can be relieved, but it takes effort and patience.

11 Nutrition for endometriosis and fertility

> If the patient has been to more than four physicians, nutrition is probably the answer.
>
> *Abraham Hoffer, MD, PhD*

Everything to do with nutrition is rather like the story of *Goldilocks and the Three Bears* in which Goldilocks settles for whatever is 'just right' for her. It implies that nothing should be eaten in excess, nothing should be eaten in deficient amounts, but that all food should be balanced: 'just right'. We hear so much about eating a 'balanced diet' that it all becomes a blur. After all, what is balanced for one person will not be correct for someone else, because of their differences in body build, health status and digestive and absorption capability. People rarely link what they eat with their state of health, although this is beginning to change. However, as we have seen in this book nutrients in food rule our state of health. But how does what you eat affect endometriosis and what should you eat to help reduce the symptoms of endometriosis?

What do we know so far? We know that endometriosis requires oestrogen in order to grow, and some women with endometriosis may have an oestrogen dominance, where oestrogen is out of balance with progesterone. We know that some pesticides may be a problem for us. Often the immune system does not function normally and remove the endometriotic implants as it should. We know too that the endometriotic implants are producing their own supplies of oestrogen and prostaglandins. There is inflammation around the implants which may cause extreme pain. There may be bowel and bladder involvement, some pain on intercourse, and women can suffer from a terrible leaden fatigue which prevents them from living the life they desire. Some women struggle terribly with a sense of loss if they are told they have subfertility problems. Periods, ovulation time, even just vacating the bowels can be excruciating agony. All in all, endometriosis causes a lot of trauma. Members of the medical profession often disbelieve the pains and other symptoms. Endometriosis is not as easy to treat as measles or a broken leg. It is a systemic disease, maybe an autoimmune disorder. When drugs and surgical treatment are used, they often just mask the symptoms and do not remove the cause. Women need to listen to the messages which their bodies give them. Illness is an imbalance and good nutrition can help to redress that imbalance. In previous chapters we have seen why and how nutrition can help to reduce the symptoms which we perceive as being triggered by endometriosis.

What you can do is try to help yourself. Living like a shadow of your former self is soul-destroying. You may wish to try the suggestions in this book. The nutrition path requires your co-operation. You have to make some changes to your life. You have to meet the needs of your body halfway. You have to feed it and you have to love it better, which takes time. You may have to work hard at this for up to six months. Inner strength may help you to reach this goal. Feeling well is a joy, particularly when you look back but now you can hardly remember what being well is like. Only you can make this decision. Become informed so that the choice can be made from the strength of knowledge. Read all the women's comments through this book again; they will help you and guide you. If they succeeded, then so could you. They were all ill, but they persevered because they believed that their bodies wanted to heal.

The main lessons to come from this book should be:

1　Eat as well as you can afford.
2　Buy the freshest food you can find.
3　Cook from fresh whenever possible or eat fresh food in salads daily once your digestion can tolerate raw vegetables.
4　Eat as wide a variety of foodstuffs as possible, remembering that 'variety is the spice of life'.

THE MYTHICAL 'BALANCED' DIET

This chapter should help you to understand the difference between natural and unnatural foods and how their nutrient content differs wildly; and how different nutrients and supplements may be used to help the body through periods of illness. Maybe you can revise your food choice and give preventive medicine a chance. As you can see from the comments of women who have trodden the nutrition path, eating for health is not a fallacy. The link between diet and health is strong. Once the body begins to be replenished with the nutrient-based building blocks it needs to make the necessary hormones and immune cells, then it can begin to fight off the endometriotic implants.

Poor diet and/or poor absorption equals poor health. We cannot expect a sick body to begin to heal until it has the tools it needs from within. You can assess the nutrient content of your diet with the help of this chapter. Getting all the nutrients your body requires from your food can be helpful, but giving the body a boost from short-term supplementation may help to speed up this process. Caroline Walker, the dietitian, wrote in 1984 'that the importance of positively good food, above all when preparing for pregnancy, is a message vital to the health of the child as well as the mother'.[1] You can fight endometriosis and subfertility by eating the best food available.

It is the *quality* of the foods eaten which can make all the difference in how our body cells function, including the cells in the reproductive system. By eating fresh, wholesome foods regularly you will give the body the fuel it needs to keep itself healthy. Fuel in this case includes the macronutrients (such as carbohydrates, proteins, fats and oils) and the micronutrients (the 52 known vitamins and minerals) plus the compounds known as phytochemicals. It is now recognized that dietary factors are closely linked with diseases. In fact, the World Health Organization states that 'over 30 per cent of all cancers are diet related'.[2] The American National Academy of Sciences 'estimates that 60 per cent of women's cancers are related to nutritional factors'.[3] Endometriosis mimics the way that cancer cells grow, so it may be that it will also respond well to diet.

The healthy choice should be the easy choice, but in our world of fast food and convenience meals, the healthy choice may be the hardest to make. It takes time and effort to eat well, and not resort to 'snatch and grab'-type meals. It takes conscious thought, 'Should I snack on fruit and nuts rather than cakes and cookies?' You should try to sit down and analyse all the foods you eat over the next four days. Write down absolutely everything you eat. It may be a surprise when you see the whole picture and analyse which vitamins and minerals are low in your diet. You will then be aware if you need to eat more of certain of the foods listed at the end of this chapter.

In 1991 research showed that 'older women were more likely to eat traditional foods like boiled potatoes, milk puddings, butter and preserves and bought more vegetables, while younger women ate out more and also ate convenience foods such as snacks and burgers more often'.[4] This calorie-laden food, as opposed to nutrient-rich food, leads to nutritional imbalances which have a domino effect on enzyme and hormone production. Despite the fact that so many of us eat junk food, most people today are aware of the importance of their diet: 'Seventy-one per cent of adults questioned believe that the most important thing that they do to protect their health involves eating.'[5] Choosing healthy food is the key we hold in our hands.

The word 'diet' has connotations of limp lettuce leaves and starvation, but this is not what is meant. A healthy diet is a choice of fresh, natural, vibrant foods eaten in the appropriate quantities. And that is all you have to do – just choose to eat fresh foods every day. Giving the body the vital vitamins and minerals it needs is not difficult, and chapters 12 and 14 look at how to do just that.

That is all there is to it – just buying and eating the best quality and freshest foods available. In chapter 10 we looked at how the digestive system was so important in the breakdown of oestradiol, the oestrogen which causes cell proliferation and is involved with uterine and breast cancers. Why do women with endometriosis need to be so concerned with the balance of oestrogen and progesterone? What are their effects? Table 11.1 shows the effects of oestrogen and progesterone.

As with everything in the body, there is an action and an opposite reaction. Oestrogen and progesterone have to be in balance with one another, as body systems always try to create a balance. Your choice of food matters as it affects hormone production. The choice of proteins and fats will determine the quality of hormones your body can produce. You can help your body to heal itself.

Nutrients are those substances within the foods which we physically ingest and are used in order to maintain body cells, to provide materials for growth and repair, to promote energy and hormone production, or are used in order to regulate these processes. Some substances in food, such as caffeine and alcohol, are not looked upon as nutrients as they have no role in body maintainance and, indeed, may hinder the

Oestrogen effects	Progesterone effects
Causes the womb lining to thicken	Causes the endometrium to shed
Body fat deposits increase	Body fat is used for energy
Triggers depression and headaches	Acts as an anti-depressant
Stimulates breast tissue	Protects breast tissue
Feeling less sexy	Normal feelings restored
Causes salt, sugar and fluid retention	Acts as a natural diuretic
Increases the risk of breast cancer	Helps prevent breast cancer
Counteracts thyroid hormone action	Aids thyroid hormone action
Causes copper levels to increase and zinc to decrease	Helps to balance copper and zinc levels
Reduces the supply of oxygen to all cells	Corrects the supply of oxygen to cells
Increases the risk of uterine cancer	Helps prevent uterine cancer
Increases the risk of blood clots	Normalizes the risk of blood clots
Prolongs menstrual bleed time	Normalizes menstrual bleed time
Acts as an abortive	Maintains the pregnancy
High corticosterone levels	Precursor of corticosterone production
Reduces bone building by restraining osteoclast function	Stimulates bone building by stimulating osteoclasts
Stimulates the nervous system	Calms the nervous system
Reduces the tone of blood vessels	No effects on blood vessels
Impairs blood sugar control	Normalizes blood sugar control

Table 11.1
Effects of oestrogen and progesterone

body's search for stability and health. They are stimulants that can cause internal stress, which is the last thing you need with endometriosis.

> Let food be your medicine and medicine be your food.
>
> *Hippocrates 460 BC*

Diane K of London

When my endometriosis started, various medical professionals told me that I was suffering from urine infections, pelvic inflammatory disease and a womb infection. I was placed on seemingly endless courses of antibiotics. When my symptoms continued, I was simply given stronger doses than before. The pains rapidly grew worse until my whole body was affected in some way: joints, hips, base of ribcage, chest, arms, legs, neck and back, as well as all the 'gynae' bits. My periods were out of control – leaping from 24 days to

CASE STUDY

31, the blood a dirty, rusty brown colour, and the flow so heavy that at times I could do nothing but sit on the loo until the torrent came to an end. I was experiencing heavy rectal bleeding too. There wasn't a single day of my life that I wasn't in pain.

Visits to GPs left me disheartened. Endometriosis was suspected, but I was told 'it will clear up when you get married' or to 'try getting pregnant'. Eventually I was referred to hospital. The consultant agreed that I had endometriosis and recommended hormone treatment. I declined, as I had heard about the side effects and felt that I was suffering enough without having to deal with further bodily changes.

I started searching the Internet for more information on endometriosis and, one day, I stumbled across Dian's website. My partner ordered her book for me. I started to follow the dietary suggestions; I cut out all wheat products and found to my amazement that the crippling chest and abdominal pains ceased within a couple of days. I was already starting to feel much more in control.

A few months later, I decided to make an appointment to see Dian, as there were still many aspects of my life that were badly affected by endometriosis. I wanted to have regular, healthy pain-free ovulation and menstruation. I longed for uninterrupted sleep and for the day-to-day vaginal, abdominal, joint and muscular pains to end.

At the first consultation, Dian went through the history of my health in great detail, making notes on all of my symptoms. Soon a picture began to emerge of what I would need to eat to improve my health and what food was proving detrimental to it. She recommended quite a lot of supplements to begin with that she felt would benefit me. The prospect of taking seven tablets in the morning and four in the evening did seem a bit daunting, but it was worth a try. The number is reduced as you progress.

For the first few weeks, I didn't notice any change at all, but gradually, I started to realize that the days without pain were turning into weeks and months. The everyday pain that I had grown so used to over the last two years had disappeared. I suddenly realized that ovulation was passing me by unnoticed because I wasn't in pain! My periods started to feel more 'normal'. The blood was no longer rusty brown, but bright red.

Recently, Dian told me I could reduce my intake of supplements to just three in the morning and three in the evening. I have no qualms about taking the supplements for the rest of my life. Later on, I will only need to take a multi-vitamin/mineral, and an evening primrose and fish oil capsule each day. It's well worth it to feel this good!

I find it hard to believe how ill I was and I am baffled as to how I used to struggle through each day. I never thought I would feel so free and full of life again. I really feel as though I've been reborn and it's all thanks to nutrition!

HEALTHY DIETS

Your body is made from the foodstuffs you eat and the water you drink. We are almost 60 per cent water, 23 per cent protein, 14 per cent fats and 3 per cent minerals. The quality of what you put into yourself is clearly a key to the health of the cells and tissues in your body.

What should we be eating to maintain good health? We hear constantly that, if we eat a balanced diet, we will be fine. But what exactly does that mean? For lots of us it would seem to involve confusion and effort: 'Many people regard healthy eating as difficult to achieve and that it requires great psychological effort to maintain a healthy change.'[6] People worry about time spent in food preparation, self-control, and the cost of fresh food, and the fact that 'the experts keep changing their minds' as another fad diet comes into vogue. Sometimes mixed messages are given which can be totally confusing. In the end, most people may feel bamboozled and give up. They continue eating the foods they have grown up with and those they enjoy without thinking.

In the UK, the 'Balance of Good Health' logo used by dietitians and the Health Education Council shows a picture of a plate divided into five segments: fruit and vegetables; bread and other cereals and potatoes; milk and dairy foods; fatty and sugary foods; meat and fish; and alternatives. In the USA, the fourth edition of *Dietary Guidelines for Americans* uses a food pyramid (*see* figure 11.1) to emphasize the number of servings recommended from six food groups to meet the guidelines.[7] For our purposes here in this book, we will use the food pyramid as it comes closer to the desired intake of nutrients. Chapter 12 looks at what foods should be eaten to maintain health, while this chapter concentrates on nutrients and supplements. On looking at the diagram of the food pyramid, it can be seen that we need to keep variety at the forefront of our choice of foods.

The guidelines are as follows:

1   Drink one litre of fresh filtered water each day.
2   Eat three to four helpings of vegetables (two servings of dark-green leafy vegetables, two servings of red or orange vegetables) and two pieces of fresh fruit (no citrus, more berries) every day.
3   Eat two to three servings of wholegrain cereals, such as rice, oats, rye, buckwheat, corn, millet or quinoa, unless you are grain-intolerant – in which case, you can use root vegetables, sago, tapioca or arrowroot, banana or chestnut flours.
4   Eat 30g of fibre foods each day. This comes from fruit, vegetables, wholegrain cereals, or nuts and seeds.
5   Eat some complex carbohydrate foods daily, such as cereals, root vegetables or pulses (legumes) as this supplies slow-releasing sugars into the body to sustain energy levels.
6   Take one tablespoon of fresh cold-pressed cis oils each day (sesame, sunflower, safflower or olive oils) or eat seeds and nuts, or take one tablespoon of ground linseeds with breakfast. Avoid trans fats.
7   Eat 50–75g of protein foods per day, choosing from a variety of sources – pulse vegetables (legumes), grains, nuts and seeds, eggs, dairy foods (cow, goat and ewe), and fresh fish or lean organic meats – so that you take in a wide range of amino acids.

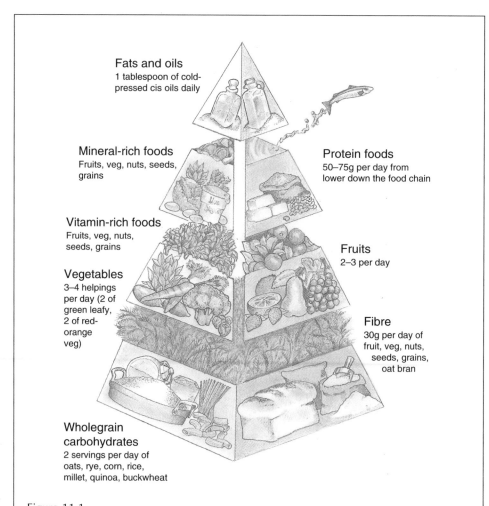

Fats and oils
1 tablespoon of cold-
pressed cis oils daily

Mineral-rich foods
Fruits, veg, nuts, seeds,
grains

Protein foods
50–75g per day from
lower down the food chain

Vitamin-rich foods
Fruits, veg, nuts,
seeds, grains

Fruits
2–3 per day

Vegetables
3–4 helpings
per day (2 of
green leafy,
2 of red-
orange
veg)

Fibre
30g per day of
fruit, veg, nuts,
seeds, grains,
oat bran

**Wholegrain
carbohydrates**
2 servings per day of
oats, rye, corn, rice,
millet, quinoa, buckwheat

Figure 11.1
The Food Pyramid. A guide to the food groups from which you should pick your daily
diet. By choosing the highest quality food you can ensure that the body can reach its
optimum health potential. Remember that your body is entirely composed of the food
you eat and the water you drink. Reproduced with kind permission of P Holford of
ION from Optimum Nutrition Magazine, 9, pp. 3, Autumn 1996

Janet H of Berkshire

*I have found that a combination diet has helped over the last few years, i.e. not mixing
starch and protein foods at the same meal.*

CASE STUDY

The foodstuffs we eat are divided into different groups by their chemical structure and the way in which they act when metabolized by the body. The main divisions are:

1   Macronutrients, composed of the proteins, carbohydrates and fats, and essential oils.
2   Micronutrients, consisting of tiny amounts of vitamins and minerals, essential oils and phytochemicals.

There are also the non-digestible fibres and water that we require to stay healthy. Eating a balanced diet means that we have to choose wisely from all these areas and maintain a variety.

MACRONUTRIENTS

Proteins

In Greek, the word 'protein' means 'I am first'. Proteins are the building blocks of life. Without them, we cannot build new cells, tissues, enzymes, hormones, antibodies, macrophages and neurotransmitters. There are 22 known amino acids and, in different combinations, they build new cells. If you think of the 26 letters of the alphabet and the number of words in a dictionary, you can imagine the many uses of amino acids joined together in chains. The variety is almost endless. The quality of the protein you eat should be the best. Fifteen per cent of our daily food intake should be protein, around 75g (or 3oz), depending on body build. This should come mainly from vegetable sources, with occasional meat, eggs, dairy foods and fish.

Animal protein foods are rich in saturated fats which need to be kept low. Include in the diet small amounts of organic pork, lamb and dairy produced from cows, sheep and goats to reduce your intake of saturated fats. Chicken, turkey, venison, game birds and eggs are good sources of protein and are lower in saturated fats. Fibrous foods bind to cholesterol and oestrogen to remove them from the body, so by balancing these fatty foods with oats and legumes you allow the body to maintain its homeostasis naturally.

Vegetable proteins are found in pulse vegetables (peas, beans and lentils), seed vegetables (broccoli, cauliflower), wholegrain cereals, and nuts and seeds. Nuts and seeds also contain the good quality cis oils which our cells so desperately need. If you are vegetarian or vegan, you need to take in sufficient pulses (legumes), nuts and seeds, and grains to meet your needs as well as make sure that you have adequate vitamin B12 supplements in your diet. Two helpings of vegetable protein each day would be adequate. Dark-green leafy vegetables and apricots help to maintain iron levels.

Carbohydrates

There are three forms of carbohydrate: simple sugars such as glucose, and fructose; double sugars such as sucrose (table sugar), maltose, lactose; and the long-chain carbohydrates such as cereal fibre and vegetables which are broken down slowly and release sugars steadily into the bloodstream. This is the way our bodies evolved to maintain a constant supply of energy production in cells.

Fast-releasing simple sugars dump too much glucose too quickly into the bloodstream for our pancreas and liver enzymes to deal with, and this can lead to illness. In 1907, people ate an average of seven pounds of sugar a year; by 1991, this had risen to 120 pounds per person, and our body's liver and pancreas cells are not designed to deal with such vast amounts.

The eight pints of blood in the body require only two teaspoons of glucose to be circulating at any one moment. Insulin (which requires zinc) and glucose tolerance factor (which requires vitamin B3, chromium and manganese) help to maintain this fine balance. But if you munch on bars of chocolates, cakes and cookies all day, you will use up all the zinc, B3, chromium and manganese, and end up with a stressed pancreas and liver. Eat these foods as occasional treats so that they stay special, rather than as everyday foods. When you are feeling hungry, the body is sending a message that it needs more nutrients. It does not want and cannot use sugars and fats in vast quantities. Eat nuts and seeds or fruits as snacks.

The body burns the carbohydrate glucose in every cell to provide energy, but we do not have to eat sweet foods to provide glucose. Our digestive system makes the enzyme amylase, which breaks down all the complex carbohydrate foods into simple sugars, but this is done at a steady rate so that the bloodstream carries a constant supply of glucose to the cells for energy production. Wholegrain cereals, root and pulse vegetables, and fresh fruits contain these helpful slow-releasing carbohydrates, whereas sweets, cakes, cookies, pastries, honey and most refined foods are laced with sugars which release glucose into the blood too quickly. One Mars bar contains the equivalent of eight teaspoons of sugar, a small pot of yoghurt may have seven, and a glass of alcohol has eight. Sugar excess can lead to problems like diabetes, insulin resistance or low blood sugar (hypoglycaemia), where we suffer from high and low mood swings and dizziness. All refined sugars are unnecessary and should only be eaten occasionally as a treat, as our ancestors ate them when they found a honeycomb.

Complex carbohydrates come neatly packaged with vitamins and minerals combined in bananas, seeds and legumes, whereas refined sugars have been so processed that the essential vitamin and mineral content is depleted. Two-thirds of your daily carbohydrate diet should come from dark-green leafy, legumes (peas, beans and lentils) and root vegetables (potatoes, parsnips, carrots, turnips, swedes), wholegrain cereals and fresh fruits.

Fats and oils

A well-balanced diet is composed of 30 per cent good quality fats and oils. The term 'good quality' means that they should be fresh and not rancid, and should be cold-pressed (the cis form). There are three main groups of fats: saturated fats from animals, and monounsaturated and polyunsaturated vegetable fats. Saturated hard fats from animal sources such as meat, eggs and dairy foods should be eaten in small amounts. An excess can be bad for the heart and the arteries, and can lead to obesity. Too many fat cells equals too much oestrogen and, with endometriosis, this is undesirable. Your body weight should be within health guidelines for your height (*see* the section on body mass index in chapter 5).

The unsaturated oils come from nuts and seeds. Olive oil provides us with monounsaturated fats, and sunflower, safflower and sesame oils give us polyunsaturated fats. The oil which you buy should never be hydrogenated, as this process turns them into undesirable trans fats which act just like saturated fats in the body, plus they lack valuable vitamin E. Only choose oils which say cold-pressed, unhydrogenated or unrefined on the label. As we have seen in chapter 4, the good quality cis oils are responsible for the production of prostaglandins, cell membranes, the all-important steroid hormones, brain cells, and skin cells. A good visual sign of deficiency is a dry skin.

Omega-3 oils, rich in alpha-linolenic acid, come from fish, pumpkin seeds and flax seeds (*see* figure 4.4), while the omega-6 oils, rich in linoleic acid, come from sesame, safflower and sunflower oils (*see* figure 4.3). The body needs fresh supplies of both daily. As heat and light damage these oils, they are best eaten cold in salad dressings, or mixed into yoghurt or soups. They should be stored in the fridge in a can or dark jar. The steroid hormones and prostaglandins are made from the oils you eat.

Two other substances which the body requires are not really 'nutrients' themselves, but they do carry nutrients along with them.

Fibre

On average we should be eating around 30g of fibrous food daily, from fruits, vegetables, wholegrain cereals, nuts and seeds. Fibre is not digested by the body, but in transit through the intestines it absorbs water and binds with toxins as well as with oestrogens and cholesterol, to help remove them from the body. Oat bran fibre is the best. Wheat bran can be too harsh on the villi in the intestine. Fibre prevents constipation, diverticulitis and slow passage of food. Foods which are constipating are wheat, bananas, some cheeses and eggs. Speedy passage of waste prevents harmful toxins being absorbed into the body, where they can lead to a sluggish system and lack of energy. If we become constipated through lack of water and fibre, toxins build up and may lead to bowel cancers. Anyone who has suffered from constipation will know how toxic the body can feel and the feeling of freshness after relief is gained. Food should take 18 to 24 hours to travel through the gut, so test your transit time (see chapter 10 for how to perform the transit-time test).

Water

Water is vital to life. After all, our bodies are two-thirds water. Fruits and vegetables have a high water content and, if we drink plenty of fluid, our body cells can detoxify more easily than if we are dehydrated. Try this test. Sit down and place your hand palm down on your thigh. Gradually you will see that the veins on the back of the hand puff up and stand out. As the veins become full of blood, slowly raise the hand and watch carefully what happens to the veins. If the veins go flat by chest level, the body needs another quart of fluid. If the veins take until chin level to go flat, you are one pint down. If the veins do not stand out when your hand rests on your thigh, you are very low in fluid and need to drink water to replace your electrolytes.

Try to drink about one litre of fresh filtered water each day – this means six to eight full glasses. Coffee, tea and alcohol are diuretics that cause water loss, and also remove minerals that are valuable for the reproductive system. Herb and fruit teas can be useful, especially mint, fennel, ginger, cinnamon (which aids digestion); limeblossom (linden) and chamomile (which are calmatives); and raspberry leaf tea (which relaxes the uterus muscle). One cup of green leaf tea daily is said to enhance the immune system. One cup per day of pau d'arco tea from South America, available in healthfood shops, has an anticandidiasis effect. Always filter all water to remove chemicals. Never drink unfiltered tap water as it is high in chlorine and may contain fluoride, neither of which are helpful if you have endometriosis.

Sarah G of Tyne and Wear

I was diagnosed as having endo when I was 18, I am now 23. For as long as I can remember, I always had the most agonizing period pains, but thought that this was normal. I would spend a good week each month practically overdosing on painkillers which never actually alleviated any of the pain.

Previous to my diagnosis, I started experiencing awful stinging pains in the bottom right of my abdomen. I was told I had a bladder infection and when I suggested endo I was promptly told I was 'far too young' and I specifically remember the comment 'oh, you'd know if you had it'. Know about it? I couldn't sleep because the pain was so bad. I eventually had a laparoscopy privately which revealed that, yes, I had endometriosis. I was unfamiliar with the disease, but was reassured by doctors that drugs could help. Luckily I already knew a nutritionist, who had been treating my brother with nutrition – he has ME. I have avoided taking any of the drugs given for endo. I was advised to change my diet considerably and to start taking a number of supplements. To be honest, at the time, I wasn't really convinced that changing my diet and taking a few supplements would help. It took a while, but finally I went on the diet programme free from yeasts, refined sugars, dairy foods and caffeine. Basically I ate fresh, natural food, nothing processed. I discovered after eliminating wheat from my diet, that I was particularly sensitive to it, to the extent that when I ate it I became tired, bloated and my stomach would hurt.

I also started taking a considerable number of supplements. There was one multivitamin/mineral, a vitamin C, a vitamin B-complex, and acidophilus and four Efamol Marine capsules per day. This may sound like an awful lot to anyone who just takes one regular multi each day. I had also been put onto the contraceptive pill to stop the endo spreading and this leaves you deficient in a number of vitamins. [Author: It puts vitamin A and copper levels up and B vitamins and zinc down.]

Although this regime may seem pretty drastic, especially the diet, it's not, and it really helped me over the past five years. Not only has it helped with the pain, I've had the added bonus of losing a little weight, increased energy and fabulous skin, which everyone still comments on!! For me the most effective supplement was the evening primrose and fish oils, which is great for hair and skin, but most significantly, it acts as an anti-inflammatory, which has subsequently helped control the stomach pains. Since I was diagnosed I have had to have two laparoscopies and extensive laser surgery when my endo spread. However, the inflammation has calmed down, and my surgeon is most surprised.

Nutrition plays such an important part in controlling endo, it seems to me that very few doctors are aware of this fact, and that is why nutritionists can play such an important role in helping to control the symptoms of endo.

Endo is not something that has to rule your life, and from my experience you can at least control the awful pain which is so often associated with the disease. I still stick to the diet and take some supplements, but often I forget why I am taking them in the first place, since I have so few problems today.

MICRONUTRIENTS

Vitamins and minerals

Vitamins are used by the body in minute amounts. If you remember chemistry lessons, you often had to measure infinitesimal quantities of powders and mix them together. Then something amazing would happen and you ended up with a totally different substance – like making a cake!

Vitamins and minerals are catalysts of many reactions in the body, present in tiny amounts but precisely regulating what happens. The body suffers if it becomes vitamin depleted, as processes become unregulated and things can go haywire. They act as keys to our system. Lose the key and you can't open the door. The right key will trigger body processes, making the immune cells, neurotransmitters, enzymes and hormones work effectively. Endometriosis certainly feels like the body has gone haywire.

Vitamins. The vitamin B-complex group and vitamin C are water-soluble, so the body cannot store them. Therefore they should be eaten every day. They are found in plant foods, and the fresher the plant the higher its nutrient content. Vitamins A, D, E and K are fat-soluble (in oily foods) and can be stored in the liver. Vitamins A, C and E are antioxidants which are protective against diseases and pollutants caused by free radical damage. Vitamin D (which is actually a hormone in its own right) ensures that our bones balance their calcium levels. Vitamin E protects our own oil-based cell membrane from going rancid, so it literally keeps us fresh. Vitamin A as retinol from animal foods and as beta-carotene from vegetable foods is vital for skin and tissue health.

Certain vitamins affect the reproductive and endocrine systems. The one everyone knows about is folic acid. Deficiency of folic acid is known to lead to spina bifida in the newborn. Folic acid is required by day 27 after conception and malformation of the fetus may occur if it is low. Many vitamin deficiencies are linked to malformations.

Some vitamins work within the endocrine system and balance its workings. One study of 6,400 adults done in Basle, Switzerland, found that 22.8 per cent of women had low levels of thiamine (vitamin B1).

A deficiency of thiamine in animals begun 11–15 days before they mated caused 83 per cent of the embryos to be absorbed. If the deficiency had begun earlier, still most animals had no implantation and often ovulation was inhibited.[8] Clearly if this applied to mankind the function of the reproductive system would be damaged. A syndrome known as lutenizing unruptured follicle (LUF), where the egg remains trapped within the ovary follicle, has been reported in as many as 79 per cent of women with endometriosis.[9] It has been seen from research to correlate with anxiety. Our adrenal glands help us to cope with stress and anxiety. Vitamin B2 (riboflavin) is essential for adrenal gland function together with vitamin B5 and vitamin C.[10] Endometriosis 'thrives on stress-related immune system weakness, which can control a woman's body and her life'.[11] Riboflavin deficiency also causes hormonal imbalances and is essential for the homeostasis and liver clearance of oestradiol and progesterone. If these hormones accumulate in the liver they inhibit the release of LHRH from the hypothalamus and GnRH secretion from the pituitary which would result in infertility. In animals reproduction fails if enzyme levels of B2 and B5 are low.[12] Vitamin B6 encourages the production of progesterone. Some research indicates that the oestrogen and progesterone levels of women with endometriosis are slightly out of balance (there is not enough progesterone for the amount of oestrogen).[13]

Looking at many other pieces of research we can find thousands of pointers as to how vitamins are needed by the endocrine and reproductive systems. Thiamine is required for ovarian hormone production; a deficiency inhibits ovulation. Riboflavin helps the balance between oestrogen and progesterone. When supplies of B2 are low, production of GnRH in the hypothalamus is inhibited, which slows production of FSH and LH from the pituitary. If vitamin B3 is deficient, it causes a deficiency of folic acid and zinc. Vitamin B6 is essential in the hypothalamus to act as a coenzyme in the production of GnRH. It is also a precursor to progesterone and serotonin (a neurotransmitter in the brain). The macrophages of the immune system cannot do their work clearing endometrial implants if they are B6-deficient. You can see how important just the B vitamins are in keeping you healthy. The pill, HRT and antibiotics all have a harmful effect on the blood levels of B vitamins, so you could take a B vitamin supplement to help normalize levels while taking these preparations. (For more details, see the vitamin section at the end of this chapter, starting on p. 263.)

Minerals. Minerals are also needed in tiny quantities by cells: calcium for strong bones, teeth and the nervous system; magnesium for muscles and nerve cells; zinc for insulin and the brain and immune cells; chromium for blood sugar balance; iron to carry oxygen in the blood and for immune cells; and selenium for protection against free radical damage and disease.

Magnesium deficiency lowers thiamine levels in body cells and it works to produce energy. Research also shows it is very important in relaxing smooth muscle and may be of benefit in relieving menstrual cramps. It is used in the immune system for production of complement which helps to remove invading alien cells. Magnesium also promotes sleep, so insomniacs may find it useful. When thyroid function is low, you feel the cold, and magnesium works with iodine and selenium in the thyroid to help temperature regulation. The function of the ovary is also dependent on the body's supply of magnesium.

Zinc works alongside vitamin B6 in the hypothalamus to aid production of GnRH, which takes the message via the pituitary to tell the ovaries how and when to function. A high intake of wheat may reduce zinc levels, as wheat contains phytic acid which can bind to zinc and block its use by the body. White marks on the fingernails indicate zinc deficiency. Zinc is a component of insulin and may prevent ovarian cysts if balanced with copper, iron and manganese. Both high copper and high oestrogen levels are linked to ovarian cyst formation.

Chromium is essential for balancing the blood sugar levels and has been seen to help reduce cravings for sweet things. It is a part of glucose tolerance factor along with vitamin B3. Chromium deficiency causes excessive sweats, irritability, cravings and drowsiness during the day.

Hair mineral analysis is quite effective at showing if you have low levels of minerals which can then be rebalanced with short-term mineral supplementation. An audit of 150 women with diagnosed endometriosis has shown that they have a common pattern of deficiencies of vitamins C, B1 B3 and B6 and the minerals magnesium, zinc and chromium. Look at the charts at the end of this chapter and ensure that your diet is rich in foods containing these nutrients. If it is, but you are still ill, look to healing your digestive tract which may have been compromised by stress, drugs or surgery. Malabsorption can be having a detrimental effect on your whole body's health. Read chapter 10 again and see what steps you can take to help improve your absorption of nutrients. Some women do not eat nutrient-rich food, but the vast majority try very hard to eat well. We know that endometriosis is systemic, it does not just affect the uterus and ovaries. To help yourself to heal you need to help your whole body. Plenty of fresh fruits, vegetables, nuts and seeds should enhance your intake of vitamins and minerals. At the end of this chapter there is a section to explain the role of each vitamin and mineral in the reproductive system (*see* p. 263).

POOR NUTRIENT INTAKE

Diets are easily unbalanced. Many people cook the same tried-and-tested dishes day after day, year after year and do not eat a varied diet. This reduces the amount of nutrients and phytochemicals eaten, and this, in turn, reduces the strength of the immune army, the production of hormones, enzymes and gastric juices, and neuro-transmitter function. This amounts to a 'domino effect': being low on some nutrients in the diet has a profound effect on the body's production of these vital messengers. Liken it to a large hall in Japan, where for fun they often set out long, swirling lines of dominoes. Someone flicks a switch and the dominoes begin to fall one by one creating amazing patterns, twists and turns. Our body's metabolism flows rather like this. Creation of one enzyme triggers production of a hormone, which causes a gland to produce another hormone – but only if the nutrient is present to help the enzyme key that hormones need. It is as complicated as a road map. But poor nutrient uptake is like removing some of the dominoes in the patterns. For instance, if you remove some of the zinc you could not make the enzymes, therefore the hormone could not be produced, and so the cells cannot work at their optimum level, and they become ill. This is called subclinical deficiency – we function below par. What we need is to reach 'enzyme saturation' level, where every cell has all the vitamins and minerals it needs in order to work efficiently.

Zinc, for instance, is required by over 200 enzymes. Imagine 200 enzyme-dominoes in a row. If you absorb sufficient zinc, all 200 of the dominoes will pass on their energy to a hormone or enzyme. If you absorb insufficient zinc, some of the dominoes may not fall, so the production of a zinc-dependent hormone will fail. Effective production of proteins for hormones, enzymes within body cells will also begin to fail and the body fall ill. Magnesium works over 300 enzymes. If we are deficient in zinc or magnesium, some of the body systems may begin to fail or at least work erratically. This would mean that hormones and immune cells will not be produced at the optimum level to make all the body systems function normally. Vital messages could not be sent or may be garbled, which changes normal cellular functioning.

Vitamins and minerals may be synergistic with one another (they balance one another's reactions), or they may be antagonistic, so that if one is too high, the other will inevitably be too low, if one is deficient, it may trigger deficiency in another, or each may amplify the effect of another. For instance, if vitamin E is deficient, 'this depletes the body of zinc, which in turn raises copper levels. High copper levels have been related to high oestrogen levels and this, in turn, has been connected with ovarian cysts and depression'.[14]

Research shows that 'deficiency in vitamin B6 automatically lowers vitamin B2 levels, which impairs the metabolism of folic acid, B5 and zinc, and affects vitamin C and A uptake. Low vitamin C prevents efficient absorption of iron, allowing excess copper into the system, affecting zinc even more.'[15] Folic acid is not absorbed well without zinc, but excess folic acid reduces all the other B vitamins.

This is like a vicious circle, and it has profound effects on the production of hormones for the reproductive system. As we have seen, vitamin B6 and zinc are vital to the production of GnRH in the hypothalamus, and their levels affect pituitary production of FSH and LH, which trigger the ovarian function. This is why a balanced diet containing all the essential nutrients is vital to health.

ANTINUTRIENTS

Caffeine, alcohol, cigarettes and heavy metals have detrimental effects on our intake of nutrients, as they can act as diuretics and remove nutrients from the body, or they may block nutrient uptake.

Caffeine

Studies have shown that 'women who were heavy coffee drinkers before pregnancy (seven or more cups per day) had, either before or after adjustment, almost a doubled chance of difficulty in becoming pregnant compared with the women who drank little or no coffee (less than one cup)'.[16] Caffeine is also found in colas, tea and chocolate, and some painkillers. Other chemicals associated with caffeine are theophylline and theobromine, both of which are known to be nervous-system stimulants. Caffeine robs the body of thiamine (vitamin B1), inositol, biotin, zinc, calcium and iron. It appears to have an effect on ovarian function.

> Things which matter most must never be at the mercy of things which matter least.
>
> *Goethe*

Alcohol

Research revealed that 'the risk of endometriosis was roughly 50 per cent higher in women with any alcohol intake than in control subjects in research. In the body we know that alcohol is converted into fat for storage and that all fat cells in the body in turn produce oestrogens. Moderate alcohol use may contribute to the risk of specific types of infertility'.[17] Alcohol robs the body of the vitamins A, D, E, K, and all the B-complex group and magnesium. The latest research suggests that women should give up all alcohol if they want to become pregnant. Women who drank less than five units a week were twice as likely to get pregnant as those who consume ten. Dr Tina Kold Jensen, of the National University Hospital in Denmark, reported the research in the *British Medical Journal*. Women had the best chance of conceiving when they did not drink at all. It was felt that alcohol disrupted the ability of the fertilized egg to implant in the womb. So although women conceived, the body would abort a pregnancy.[18] Research from the University of Aarhus in Denmark with 25,000 women shows that drinking five units of alcohol a week may increase the chances of having a baby in the early stages of pregnancy by 3.7 times.[19] Those women with endometriosis who are attempting to become pregnant should note this information.

Smoking

It is common knowledge that smoking causes cancer but less well known that it also affects reproductive health: 'Current and past smokers have reduced gonadotrophin-stimulated ovarian function. Tobacco exposure is associated with decreased oestrogen, and decreased numbers of oocytes. Smoking has an adverse effect on ovarian function.'[20]

Research also suggests that 'women with prenatal exposure to their own mother's cigarette smoking had reduced fecundity; that is they found it less easy to become pregnant themselves'.[21] If you smoke, you may damage your future daughter's ovaries and her chances of achieving a pregnancy. Nicotine robs cells of vitamin C, B1, calcium and the whole B-complex family. For each cigarette smoked the body uses 25mg of vitamin C!

Recent research reported by the American Chemical Society found 'a by-product of cancer-causing chemicals (known as NNK) in the urine of babies born to mothers who smoked. These compounds passed through all of the babies' cells and were present in 22 out of 31 urine samples taken from newborn babies whose mothers smoked, while none were found in the urine of babies whose mothers did not smoke'. As endometriosis cells behave similarly to cancer cells, women with endometriosis may wish to refrain from smoking before and during pregnancy and lactation.[22]

Heavy metals

A diet which is rich in calcium, magnesium, selenium, iron and zinc protects us from the bad effects of 'heavy' metals such as lead, mercury and cadmium. These latter metallic elements are damaging to body cells. Lead is known to be mutagenic, causing abnormalities in the fetus. Contact with these metals should be avoided where possible. Lead is found in paints and petrol and cadmium comes from cigarettes.

Dr Bryan Hellewell, advisor on toxic metals to the Environmental Health Agency in the UK, warns that, 'In the face of mounting evidence of danger and an absence of evidence of safety, it is my duty to advise that the use of mercury dental amalgam tooth fillings in the mouths of women who are pregnant should be discontinued.'

Research shows that 'mercury is seen to cause birth defects and nervous system disorders and it is best to avoid dental fillings while pregnant'[23] and 'copper in excess can also cause problems in the liver and digestive tract'.[24] Eating an excess of chocolate can be a problem for some: 'The total dietary copper intake by males and females was positively associated with the consumption of chocolate foods.'[25] High copper correlates with high oestrogen and women with endometriosis and those attempting pregnancy need to keep oestrogen in balance. High copper is also related to ovarian cyst formation.

Recreational drugs

One in 20 women are reckoned to use cannabis, a study in the British Journal of Obstetrics and Gynaecology suggests. Researchers claim that smoking cannabis at least once a week before and during pregnancy resulted in babies who were, on average, 250g (9oz) lighter and 1cm shorter, and had smaller heads than those born to non-users. It is shown that smoking cannabis at least once a week during pregnancy has the same damaging effects on the baby as smoking 10–15 cigarettes a day. This research shows that we know too little about the long-term effects, and the biological effects on the unborn child and ova/sperm may only be apparent later in life. Drug use may harm ova and blastocyst, so are best avoided.[26]

ASSESSING YOUR NEEDS

Using the food pyramid (*see* figure 11.1 on p. 238), the vitamin and mineral listings at the end of this chapter, and the chart provided, you can analyse the foods you eat over the next two days. With endometriosis, infertility and pain, we are trying to target the nutrients to begin a healing process.

It is therefore very important that you assess your diet in order to work out whether you do take sufficient levels of the B vitamins, magnesium, zinc and essential fats required by the reproductive system. It may take a little time, but as you work through this you will begin to see just which foods you need to add to your diet and which you need to reduce or exclude. Wanting to feel well again can act as the spur.

Make two photocopies of the charts on pp. 250 and 251 and write down absolutely everything you eat over the next four days. *Be honest with yourself* to get the best and most accurate picture of your health. Use the vitamin and mineral charts at the end of this chapter to help you. Try to judge whether or not you are eating a good range of vitamins and minerals. Two examples are given to guide you, one of a good diet and the other of a suboptimal diet.

DAY ONE

Breakfast: ....
....

Lunch: ....
....

Dinner: ....
....

Snacks: ....
....

DAY TWO

Breakfast: ....
....

Lunch: ....
....

Dinner: ....
....

Snacks: ....
....

Self-analysis chart
(fill in the nutrient details to analyse your intake, and highlight wheat in yellow and dairy in blue)

Food group	Breakfast	Lunch	Dinner	Snacks
Protein				
Carbohydrate				
Fats/oils				
Water				
Fibre				
Vitamins				
Minerals				

SUBOPTIMAL DIET

This example is from a woman who was referred by her gynaecologist and was on her third IVF attempt.

Breakfast: Sugar-coated cereal, milk, toast and chocolate spread, two cups of black coffee with sugar.
Lunch: Chips and beefburger with ketchup and fried onions, two cans of fizzy drink and a bar of chocolate.
Dinner: Crisps and chocolate cake, black coffee and two cans of lager.

You can see that the above diet is too high in refined starches, sugars and hydrogenated trans fats. There is no fresh fruit and the only vegetable is the onion. The coffee and alcohol are diuretics and take the few minerals being eaten out of the body. This diet is lacking in vitamin C and B-complex vitamins, and magnesium and zinc. There is no nutrient intake from fresh fruits, vegetables and nuts. The chosen protein source is high in saturated fats. No good quality cis oils are present, only the poor quality trans oils. The high refined starch and sugar content of this diet could lead to low blood sugar and would not sustain energy levels and stamina. This woman was experiencing peaks and troughs in energy levels throughout the day. It took some time to improve her

Food group	Breakfast	Lunch	Dinner
Protein	milk	beef	
Carbohydrate	sugar/cereal chocolate spread sugar in coffee	bread roll chips ketchup onion	crisps/chocolate cake
Fats/oils	chocolate spread cream in milk	beef fat chip fat onion cooked in oil bar of chocolate	crisps fat chocolate cake
Water	in coffee	in canned drink	coffee/lager
Fibre	cereal	potato/onion	crisps
Vitamins	A&D in milk cereal fortified with B vitamins	vitamin C in potato and onion folic acid B6	
Minerals	calcium in milk	potassium calcium	copper in chocolate

health due to the long-term poor nutrient intake. However, she persevered and improved her eating pattern, and had a successful pregnancy.

IDEAL DIET

This example is from a woman with severe endometriosis who had tried many drug treatments, and also had extreme irritable bowel syndrome. Her digestive tract was probably inflamed and she was malabsorbing nutrients, despite her seemingly good diet.

Breakfast: Muesli with nuts, seeds, banana and natural yoghurt, lemon and ginger tea.
Lunch: Mackerel salad with rye crackers, fresh fruit salad, still water with lemon.
Dinner: Stir-fried vegetables with tofu and brown rice, apple, limeblossom tea.

This person was receiving more vitamins and minerals each day than most people. She was eating more good quality cis oils from the olive oil, the fish, and nuts and seeds, as well as vegetable proteins and a good range of fibre foods. All the carbohydrate foods were complex, thus releasing sugars gradually into the bloodstream to keep energy levels even throughout the day. She also ate a wide range of fresh fruits and vegetables. She was sensitive to wheat and, once that was removed and the digestive tract inflammation had been corrected with supplements, this woman's symptoms eased.

Food group	Breakfast	Lunch	Dinner
Protein	nuts, seeds, yoghurt	mackerel	tofu brown rice
Carbohydrate	wheat, oats, rye, millet flakes	Ryvita	brown rice
Fats/oils	in nuts and seeds	mackerel	stir-fry olive oil
Water	herb tea	still water	herb tea
Fibre	muesli banana	salad veg rye fruit	brown rice vegetables apple
Vitamins	A,D, C, B6, E	A, B-complex, E, C	B-complex, A, C, E
Minerals	calcium magnesium zinc	selenium zinc calcium potassium	calcium magnesium zinc potassium

NUTRITIONAL SUPPLEMENTS

Why should we need supplements at all if our diet is balanced? After all, if we eat a balanced diet we should stay healthy. The trouble is that most of us have diets that are unbalanced. If your diet is well balanced and you are healthy, then taking supplements may not be necessary. However, if you are ill and your diet is not the best it can be, then taking supplements for the short term to give the body cells a boost can be beneficial to the healing process. Also digestive problems do affect absorption. Being ill shows that the body is not coping, so short-term supplementation for three to four months to correct imbalances can be tried, while the diet or digestion are being corrected.

Jo R of Slough

•
C
A
S
E

S
T
U
D
Y
•

I am 25 years old and have had painful periods for as far back as I can remember. By the age of 18 the period and preperiod pains worsened and I found myself suffering for two weeks of my cycle, leading up to my period. My preperiod symptoms were stomach cramps, tiredness, water retention and extremely volatile moods, which would last up until my bleeding began. Once my period came, for the first two or three days, the pain in my lower abdominal area would be so excruciating, that at the time I found it difficult to stand up straight. My bleeding would be so heavy that I found it difficult to function at all. Once the first few days had passed, I would have a fairly normal period, which lasted, for approx. three more days and then two fairly pain-free weeks until the cycle began again.

This became increasingly more difficult as it not only affected my work, as I was incapable of working for three days a month, but my social relationships were also affected, as I was so lethargic and irritable.

My doctor's response to my repeated pleas for help were, 'Do you think you're the only woman who has ever had period pains.' Typical.

Out of desperation I changed my doctor and set about the many elimination tests, scans and examinations until finally, following a laparoscopy, I was diagnosed as having a classic case of endo in my pelvis and lower abdominal area.

I was advised that my only form of treatment would be a hysterectomy or hormone treatment. As you can imagine I opted for the latter of the two and began taking Provera three times daily.

After about three weeks of this treatment, my body shook so ferociously that I found it difficult to hold a cup of tea without spilling it. Huge boils appeared on my back and shoulders, and hair began to sprout from my neck, face and lower body. I returned to my consultant who immediately took me off Provera treatment. We discussed the other possibilities but I still kindly refused a hysterectomy! I then tried taking the pill continuously with a break every three months. My mood swings remained and the rest of my body eventually gave up, and I had problem after problem with headaches, haemorrhoids, to greasy hair and acne.

It was at this time that a friend read an article written by Dian. I drove down for a nutrition consultation and found that I gained more answers and satisfaction in the hour I had with her, than the entire time I had been under the various consultants and GPs.

I started a nutrition programme which incorporated diet, exercise and vitamin supplements. I cut out wheat, alcohol and caffeine and supplemented my diet with a multivitamin/mineral, evening primrose oil, vitamin B6, fish oils, acidophilus, vitamin C and magnesium. Within two months, I felt and looked like a new person. My energy returned, my mood swings ceased, my periods regulated themselves and my skin cleared up. Not only did I feel 110 per cent better, but people commented on my appearance!

I will not pretend that this initial step was easy; in fact I found it extremely difficult. But once I came to terms with this fact and changed my way of thinking, it became much easier.

I followed the diet for over a year and now I have reduced my vitamins to evening primrose oil and a multivitamin and magnesium. I now take the pill 2 monthly and my periods remain pain-free.

SUPPLEMENT CHOICE

When you first walk into a healthfood shop or pharmacy, the vast array of nutritional supplements lined up on the shelves can be daunting. You feel overwhelmed in choosing the right one for your needs. The body is a chemical factory and has a need for each nutrient and, although they should be in our food, we have to absorb them efficiently. We have also seen that poor farming with depleted soils have reduced the mineral content of foods (*see* pp. 184–5).

Rest assured that no supplement company is going to produce any tablets containing an unsafe dose. If you stick to the exact recommendations on the label, you can't go wrong. Some people feel that if one tablet is good for you, two must be even better – this is a very dangerous idea. Doses are always very carefully gauged, so you must stick to them. A table of safe doses is given on p. 258, and usually the lower optimum range dose is adequate. For instance, if you are taking a multivitamin/mineral tablet and an antioxidant tablet make sure that you do not overdo the selenium (no more than 150μg per day).

Always check with a nutritionist or nutrition-trained health professional if you need extra guidance. They are trained to find out, through various tests, exactly what your specific nutrient requirements will be. In nutrition consultations, which usually last for an hour, every person is treated as a unique individual and no two people leave with the same 'prescription' of supplements. Very few people absorb the level of nutrients their bodies need to function, and taking the correct ones at the correct dose for your needs can help to get your body biochemistry up and running again at its optimum range. For further information, see www.endometriosis.co.uk.

Keep in mind that the recommended dietary allowances (RDAs) are for healthy people and that they do not allow for those whose needs are affected by illness: 'In the USA alone 100 million people suffer from allergies, arthritis, diabetes, heart disease, etc.'[27] For many people the RDAs are too low.

When endometriosis strikes, it is often a fact that the body's digestive tract is malfunctioning, and that the immune, nervous, endocrine and reproductive systems are undernourished. Short-term supplementation may help your body cells to begin functioning again at an optimum level. Dr Anthony J Verlangieti, Director of the Artherosclerosis Research Laboratories and Professor of Pharmacology and Toxicology at the University of Mississippi School of Pharmacy states that 'it is a myth that we get all the vitamins we need in our daily diets'. He suggests that everyone should take supplementary vitamins. Several economists have estimated that by increasing our intake of vitamins and minerals, we would reduce health-care costs for cardiovascular disease by 25 per cent.

Subclinical deficiencies would 'not normally be discovered in routine physical examinations but subclinical deficiencies affect the body's wellbeing and do show up with hair mineral analysis and blood tests done at specialist clinics'.[28] The health service presently makes no attempt to check the vitamin and mineral levels of sick and dying people in order to treat them and correct their body balance/homeostasis. Instead, drugs are given which mask the symptoms. With good nutrition you begin to heal the tissues the natural way.

Begin to feed your body with the nutrients it needs both from foods and supplements and, in the first three to four months, you may well feel your health begin to improve slowly but surely.

As we have seen from the numerous case histories, supplements alone are not sufficient – you must combine them with a healthy diet. Supplements are only used to kick-start the body, to help cells to reach enzyme saturation levels, where all cells have the nutrients they require to make enzymes work effectively. But the need for good quality food is paramount. Natural, fresh foods contain nutrients if they have been grown in nutrient-rich soil. Processed foods and those grown on overfarmed soils are depleted. It is your choice of nutrient-rich food that counts the most. Try to broaden your horizons and be bold, try different foods to add a wider variety of nutrients to your repertoire. As James I of England (1566–1625) said: 'He was a bold man who first swallowed an oyster.'

To continue to eat low-nutrient high-calorie foods and take supplements alone will not lead to good health. We hope that this book will be a working guide for you to achieve a feeling of total wellbeing again.

Good supplements will tell you the exact form of the minerals (citrates, picolinates, amino acid chelates are best; oxides and carbonates are a waste of time), and they should be wheat-, dairy-, yeast- and sugar-free. *If they are not, do not buy them.* Avoid yeast-based B vitamins, chronium and selenium. If you are intolerant of yeasts, they will make your symptoms worse. Your body is like your car. Would you put cheap inferior oil or petrol into your car and risk it being damaged? Treat your body in the same way; after all, it has to stay healthy for at least 80 or 90 years. 'Picking the right supplements is an art in itself', says Patrick Holford, founder of the Institute for Optimum Nutrition. Choose from the most reputable companies, or ask your local consumer council which companies have the best labelling policies. If in doubt, write directly to the manufacturer. Read up about nutrients from other books. A good healthfood shop should help to guide you in your choice. Some mail order companies produce good quality supplements, and their addresses are at the end of this book (*see* pp. 397–8).

Carl Pfeiffer, MD, PhD, of the Brain Biocenter in New Jersey, USA, says: 'Vitamins and minerals play a crucial role in preserving and maintaining health and restoring it in diseased patients.' Supplements of vitamins, minerals and essential fatty acids taken for three to six months will help to replenish body cells. When the body is ill, it requires the building blocks of life to restore its vitality and renew failing cells. By taking supplements you can support the digestive, immune and reproductive systems and improve the body's healing potential. Remember that the body is striving to be well all the time. The only way the body has to heal itself is through the nutrients we eat. If the diet is depleted in nutrients or the digestive tract is damaged, the body cells will sustain damage. The following is a basic programme for everyone to try. For an individually tailored one, consult a qualified nutritionist and get a full assessment of your needs.

Take each of the following daily, for two to three months, while improving your nutrient intake from foods:

- Multivitamin/mineral (yeast-, sugar-, gluten-, dairy-free)
- Vitamin C with bioflavonoids
- Evening primrose and fish oils (combined)
- Acidophilus (dairy-free)
- Magnesium taurate or malate
- Zinc methionine or citrate
- Digestive enzymes with each meal
- B-complex vitamins (yeast-free) 50mg (optional)
- Selenium and vitamins A, C and E (yeast-free)
  (antioxidants optional).

Table 11.2 is a guide to safe levels of supplements. Always err on the side of caution and take the lower doses in the optimum range to begin with. Higher doses may not be necessary unless you are properly assessed and instructed by a nutritionist to take higher quantities. The maximum figures come from research on the levels at which supplements cause adverse side effects in some individuals. There are a few rules to remember when taking supplements:

1 Always consult a doctor before you try to get pregnant or if you are planning to lose weight. Chosing supplements on these occasions requires trained advice.
2 Ask for various tests, such as thyroid and coeliac checks, to be done. Never undertake a course of supplements if you are already taking orthodox medications unless interactions have been ruled out.
3 Vitamin E should only be taken at 100IU doses if you have high blood pressure. It

Vitamins	Optimum range	Maximum safety level
A	7,500–20,000iu**	33,333iu*
D	400–1,000iu	2,000iu
E	100–1,000iu	1,500iu
C	1,000–4,000mg	6,000mg
B1	25–100mg	140mg
B2	25–100mg	160mg
B3	50–150mg	180mg
B5	50–300mg	400mg
B6	50–100mg	300mg
B12	5–100μ	300μ
Folic acid	50–400μ	2,000μ
Biotin	50–200μ	10,000μ

* For women of childbearing age, the maximum safety level for long-term use is 10,000IU per day.

** When attempting pregnancy or while pregnant, take no more than 2,000IU of vitamin A per day in total.

Minerals

Calcium	400–800mg	3,000mg
Magnesium	300–500mg	1,000mg
Iron	10–25mg	50mg
Zinc	15–30mg	50mg
Copper	1–3mg	5mg
Manganese	5–25mg	100mg
Selenium	50–250μ	500μ
Chromium	50–250μ	500μ

Table 11.2
Vitamins and minerals – how much is safe? Reproduced with kind permission of P Holford of ION, from *Optimum Nutrition*, ION Press, pp. 141, 1994.

should not be taken with magnesium, as they are antagonistic and cancel one another out. (Similarly, never take zinc and iron together.)

4 Always take folic acid with zinc; take a B-vitamin complex with a single B vitamin; otherwise the one taken singly stays high while the others are knocked down low. Vitamin C taken with iron helps its absorption; calcium uptake is improved when evening primrose oil is taken; and boron improves calcium uptake.

5 Evening primrose oil should not be taken by anyone prone to epilepsy.

6   Most supplements are designed to be taken with food.

7   Prebiotics, probiotics and digestive enzymes should be taken with a cold drink.

8   All the supplements you buy should be hypoallergenic, and yeast-, wheat-, gluten-, sugar- and dairy-free.

TAKING ACTION

Think positive. Take control. Consider what you may gain – better health, and improved quality of life. If you have to give up wheat or dairy foods for a time, so what? Providing you use all the alternative foods suggested to maintain the supply of nutrients from other sources, there should be no problem. The benefits far outweigh the disadvantages, as can be seen from the various case studies throughout this book. Once you develop a new set of menus to follow and know which stores to buy from, life all becomes easy again. In fact, easier. Once you start feeling healthier and happier, coping skills improve.

Knowledge is power. If you know that some foods are making you ill and that using supplements occasionally with the right diet makes you well, then you and those around you will benefit if you put this into practice. Try this for one month and see if there is a difference in how you feel. Then we can put your success on our World Wide Web bulletin board (http://www.endometriosis.co.uk) and let other people know how to regain their health. Remember at football games where you watched the 'Mexican wave' go round the arena? Well, we can send this wave round the world via this book and cyberspace. Your story is just as important as those already in this book (e-mail it to dian@endometriosis.co.uk).

Heather Mc of London

At the age of 30, the terrible pain I had been feeling since I was 15 was finally diagnosed as endometriosis. I began taking various courses of drugs, which were of no help, and had surgery on a regular basis. The endometriosis was quite severe and the laser treatment that I was having seemed to accelerate the problem. The various drugs that I took to combat the effect of the endometriosis were also of no help and the side effects were worse than the pain I was getting!

After more laser treatment and LUNA to help relieve the pain, it was suggested that my only hope of beating this disease was to have a total hysterectomy, including removal of the ovaries. By now I was in so much pain that I was collapsing. I couldn't drive and my work was suffering. I reluctantly agreed to the hysterectomy and, a couple of weeks later, I was back in the hospital.

After this, for one year, everything was great – no pain – and I had no problems at all with my HRT (patches). But then, slowly, the pain came back. On one examination, they felt a lump, so I was back at the hospital for yet another op. I found that they were unable to completely remove some of the tissue from one of my ovaries and this has been enough to allow the endometriosis to continue growing. More laser treatment was given and this led to a problem with adhesions from all the scar tissue.

From then on, the endometriosis continued to grow. I couldn't work, drive or play with my children, and had no sexual relationship – the pain was too severe. I was put onto anti-depressants to help me cope.

I came across Dian's website one day while I was off work yet again with severe pains. I had just spent an hour crying to my mother, telling her that if it wasn't for the children, I wouldn't have the strength to carry on anymore. She begged me to look for another alternative and I decided to book an appointment with Dian's clinic that day. I was very sceptical – after all the treatment that I had tried, how could a change of diet help? However, I completed my questionnaire and went along to my appointment. Dian was lovely – for the first time in 20 years, I was talking to someone who understood exactly what I was going through. Her confidence that I may get better filled me with confidence too. I went away determined to give the diet a try.

That was six months ago. My life has changed totally. For the first time in years, I am WELL. I have changed my diet so that I no longer eat wheat, but apart from that, following Dian's diet plan has been easy. I take supplements which, at the beginning, were quite a few, but they are decreasing each month and, eventually, I will take just a couple a day.

However, the benefits are amazing. I can work full time, drive, play football with the kids; I have a good sex life again and I feel great. I came off the anti-depressants three months ago and I haven't looked back! I occasionally get a pain – mainly due to the fact that some wheat has crept into my diet – but these are few and far between, and nothing like the pain I used to feel. I cannot believe how Dian has managed to turn my life around simply by changing my diet. Everyone with endometriosis should be informed about this treatment to stop all the unnecessary surgery and suffering.

PRACTICALITIES

- Give yourself one month from now as a goal to try the programme.
- Assess your diet, exclude whatever food you think is upsetting you for one month, eating the alternatives suggested (see chapter 12).
- Eat the healthiest, freshest foods you can afford.
- Take some basic supplements each day while you are ill.
- Report how you fare onto our webpage (www.endometriosis. co.uk).
- Join in and let us combat this disease.
- Encourage more research into how nutrients affect endometriosis and infertility and pain.

As Mary Lou Ballweg, president of the Endometriosis Association, headquartered in the USA, states: 'Together we make a difference.' The more of you who try this path and achieve good results, the more we can help each other regain health in this way.

The eminent professor of nutrition John Yudkin says, 'The health of the majority of humans depends more on their nutrition than it does on any other single factor. However important and dramatic the advances in hygiene, medicine and surgery have been, proper nutrition has a more important effect on human morbidity and mortality. For this reason, I believe that the ultimate objective of nutritionists must be the nutrition education of the public.'[29] We owe it to the next generation to encourage research in this vital area. We must save the next generation of women from this disease. The Institute for Optimum Nutrition in London has a nutrition homestudy course, consisting of 12 tapes, a study manual and three books. At the end of the 12-week course, there will be a computer-marked assessment, with a certificate awarded to those who are successful in passing the course. For more information, see www.nutrition.us.com.

Some supplement regimes seem to help to deal with the many symptoms which we perceive as being triggered by endometriosis. The following regimes may be useful for those with endometriosis and also for those who also experience premenstrual tension.

ENDOMETRIOSIS

Correction of imbalances of steroid hormones, too much oestrogen in proportion to progesterone, and correction of prostaglandin levels appear to be key factors in improving health, and nutrition is key to controlling hormone levels. The liver requires a constant supply of B vitamins to deal with hormones, as do the immune cells, together with vitamin C, magnesium, zinc and the antioxidants. If periods are extremely heavy, then take iron EAP2 or citrate for one to two months. The recommendations are:

- Evening primrose and fish oils (2,000mg per day)
- Vitamin C with bioflavonoids (1,000mg per day; 500mg if on medication)
- Multivitamin/mineral (yeast-, wheat-, sugar- and dairy-free – one per day)
- Magnesium malate for fatigue/muscles or magnesium taurate for oestrogen breakdown (300mg per day)
- Zinc methionine (15mg per day)
- Probiotics (dairy-free acidophilus, 4–8 billion viable cells daily)
- Digestive enzymes (glandular-free; one with each meal)
- B-complex vitamins (yeast-free and optional)
- Selenium ACE antioxidants (yeast-free and optional).

PREMENSTRUAL SYNDROME

Four distinct types of premenstrual syndrome are recognized. (Often with extreme endometriosis, we seem to have them all!)

- PMS type A: anxiety, nervous tension, mood swings and irritability. Sufferers need vitamin B6 and magnesium-rich diets.

- PMS type B: hydration, weight gain, swollen legs, breast tenderness, abdominal bloating. Sufferers need diets rich in vitamin E, B6 and magnesium.
- PMS type C: cravings, headaches, increased appetite, heart pounding, fatigue. Sufferers need diets rich in B6, magnesium and chromium.
- PMS type D: depression, forgetfulness, crying, confusion, insomnia. Sufferers need diets rich in vitamin B6, magnesium and vitamin C.

The recommendations are:

- Vitamin C with bioflavonoids PMSD
- Vitamin B6 as pyridoxine 5-phosphate
- Magnesium EAP2
- Chromium polynicotinate PMSC
- Evening primrose and fish oils

- Vitamin B-complex (yeast-free)
- Multivitamin/mineral
- Zinc methionine
- Vitamin E (200IU) PMSB

SUMMARY

Eating well can enhance your body's ability to heal and may well aid its recovery from endometriosis, infertility and pain.

1   Eat as well as you can afford.

2   Buy the freshest food you can find and eat while it is still fresh.

3   Cook from fresh wherever possible, and eat some raw vegetables and fruit every day (organic when possible).

4   Eat a wide variety of foods every day, not just usual old favourites. Make it fun to try new dishes and expand your horizons.

5   Use one tablespoon of cold-pressed cis vegetable oils daily and try to avoid trans fats.

6   Follow the food pyramid as your guide to daily choices of foods. Ensure that you eat good quality protein foods every day.

7   Avoid caffeine, refined sugars and alcohol while you are trying to recover from illness.

8   Drink 1.5 litres of fluid daily. Avoid fizzy canned drinks and use diluted fruit juices or fresh water.

9   Include 30g of fibre from fruits, vegetables, nuts, seeds, legumes and cereals in your daily diet in order to keep your intestines healthy.

10   Use only good quality supplements while you are ill. Use them wisely. Stick to the dose on the carton or bottle. They will only help you if your eating pattern is healthy and once you have corrected your digestive problem.

> It is only with the heart that one can see rightly; what is essential is invisible to the eye.
>
> *The Little Prince*

VITAMINS AND MINERALS

> Our first line of defence against endometriosis may come from our food.
>
> *Dian Shepperson Mills*

DEFINITIONS

Good sources Foods with the highest nutrient levels per calorie are listed in descending order. So the first foods are the best. All foods listed are excellent sources of these vitamins.

Deficiency. When the body lacks optimal levels of vitamins it cannot work efficiently. Early warning signs, such as joint pains, headaches, rashes and bloating, suggest that your nutrient intake from diet and supplements may need increasing.

RDA. These recommended dietary allowances are based on the European Union figures or, in cases where there are none, McCance and Widdowson. These are the levels designed to prevent serious vitamin deficiency. They are not necessarily optimal intakes.

Optimum intake. These are optimal nutrient allowances derived from research testing the level of vitamins needed for optimal health taken from the book *What is Optimum?* by Dr Cheraskin. (You should only ever take a B-complex supplement, never just one B vitamin on its own, as they tend to compete with each other. If you need more of one in particular, say B6, you should take a B-complex plus an extra amount of B6.)

Helpful. Vitamins and minerals need each other in order to work. Eat a healthy, wholefood diet as priority and, if you are ill, supplement a good multivitamin and mineral, before adding extra nutrients.

Harmful. Our diet and environment expose us to 'antinutrients'. The more of these you are exposed to, the higher will be your need for supplements.

VITAMIN C (ASCORBIC ACID)

RDA. Adults: 60mg
Optimum intake. Adults: 500mg

Effects. Antioxidant, antiviral, antibacterial, antihistamine. Used for immune system. Fights infection. Needed for collagen for skin, muscles, joints. Detoxifies pollutants. Protects against cancer. Necessary for energy and stress resistance. Supports adrenal function. For white blood cell function. Used in cells for energy production. Used for sperm production. Thins blood. Potentiates Clomid. Increases absorption of nutrients in the gut. Softens stools. Removes heavy metals from the body. Enhances phagocytosis. Needed for antibody production. Reduces pain. Analgesic.

Deficiency. Frequent colds and infections, lack of energy, bleeding gums, easy bruising, nosebleeds, slow wound healing. Causes poor uptake of iron.

Helpful. Bioflavonoids. Works with B vitamins, Co Q10 and iron to produce energy within cells. Vitamin E. Take with food. Iron is more effectively absorbed when vitamin C is present.

Harmful. Smoking (every cigarette burns up 25mg of vitamin C), alcohol, pollution, stress, fried food.

Good sources. Blackcurrants, berries, peppers, lemons, watercress, strawberries, oranges, grapefruit, new and sweet potatoes, cauliflower, broccoli, melon, spinach, tomatoes, savoy cabbage, green leafy vegetables, jacket potatoes, kale, cantaloupe and honeydew melons, turnip, peas, apples.

VITAMIN B1 (THIAMINE)

RDA. Adults: 1.4mg
Optimum intake. Adults: 7.1mg

Effects. Energy production in cells. Brain function. Used in digestion by protein. Strengthens heart muscle alongside magnesium. Reproductive system, enriches womb lining, needed for ovarian hormones. Works liver enzymes which degrade oestrogen. Suppresses pain. Analgesic.

Deficiency. Tender and weak muscles, eye pains, irritability, poor concentration, 'prickly' legs, poor memory, stomach pains, constipation, tingling hands, rapid heartbeat. Reduces fertility. Depression, insomnia. Reduces endorphin production. Inhibits ovulation. Increases pain.

Helpful. B5, B-complex vitamins, magnesium, manganese.

Harmful. Antibiotics, tea, coffee, stress, birth control pills, alcohol, alkaline agents, e.g. baking powder, sulphur dioxide (preservative), destroyed by cooking/food processing.

Good sources. Peas, red kidney beans, milk, lamb, brown rice, oatmeal, peanuts, pork, lamb, chicken, legumes (peas, beans, lentils), potatoes, watercress, mushrooms, most vegetables, lettuce, cauliflower, tomatoes, Brussels sprouts, spring cabbage.

VITAMIN B2 (RIBOFLAVIN)

RDA. Adults:1.6mg
Optimum intake. Adults: 2.0mg

Effects. Turns fat, sugar, protein into energy. Repairs skin. Regulates body acidity. Hair, nails and eyes. Works liver enzymes which degrade oestrogen. Needed for ovarian hormones.

Deficiency. Hormonal imbalances of oestrogen and progesterone, inhibits GnRH production for FSH and LH, burning/gritty eyes, sensitivity to bright lights, sore tongue, cataracts, dull/oily hair, eczema or dermatitis, split nails, cracked lips.

Helpful. B5, B vitamins and selenium. Take as B-complex with food.

Harmful. Alcohol, contraceptive pill, tea, coffee, alkaline agents (baking powder, sulphur dioxide [preservative]), food processing.

Good sources. Mackerel, mushrooms, potatoes, broccoli, muesli, natural yoghurt, skimmed milk, whole milk, green leafy vegetables, watercress, wholemeal bread, spring cabbage, blackcurrants, beans, eggs, fish, tomatoes.

VITAMIN B3 (NIACIN)

RDA. Adults: 18mg
Optimum intake. Adults: 25mg

Effects. Energy production. Brain function. Skin. Balances blood sugar. Adjusts cholesterol levels.

Deficiency. Lack of energy, diarrhoea, insomnia, headaches or migraines, poor memory, anxiety, depression, irritability, bleeding gums, acne, eczema/dermatitis. Causes deficiency of folic acid and zinc.

Helpful. Works with B-complex vitamins and chromium. Best taken with food.

Harmful. Antibiotics, tea, coffee, contraceptive pill and alcohol, refined sugars.

Good sources. Canned tuna, smoked mackerel, roast turkey, roast chicken, steamed salmon, lamb chops, wholemeal bread, cornmeal, potatoes, broccoli, mushrooms, tomatoes, carrots, fish, eggs, peanuts, avocado, prunes, cauliflower, cod, new boiled potatoes, cabbage.

VITAMIN B5 (PANTOTHENIC ACID)

RDA. Adults: 6mg
Optimum intake. Adults: 25mg

Effects. Energy production. Fat metabolism. Improves function of brain and nerves and anti-stress hormones. Skin and hair. Anti-allergy vitamin. Supports adrenal function. Needed for ovarian hormones.

Deficiency. Muscle tremors/cramps, apathy, poor concentration, burning feet/tender heels, nausea, lack of energy, exhaustion after light exercise, anxiety, teeth grinding, nervousness.

Helpful. Other B-complex vitamins. Biotin and folic acid. Best taken with food. Magnesium.

Harmful. Stress, alcohol, tea, coffee. Destroyed by heat, food processing.

Good sources. Boiled eggs, mushrooms, grilled pork chops, lean meat, green leafy vegetables, nuts, chicken, sea fish, wholemeal bread, celery, strawberries, tomatoes, boiled potatoes, baked cod, cabbage, beans, peas, watercress.

VITAMIN B6 (PYRIDOXINE)

RDA. Adults: 2mg
Optimum intake. Adults: 10mg

Effects. Protein digestion. Brain function. Sex hormone production GnRH in hypothalamus. Reduces symptoms of PMS, menopause. Anti-depressant and diuretic. Precursor to progesterone and seretonin. Needed for macrophage function. Works enzymes in liver which degrade oestrogen. Natural diuretic. Needed for ovarian hormones. Improves immune function. Healthy blood and blood vessels. With zinc works in metabolism of EFAs. Analgesic.

Deficiency. Infrequent dream recall, water retention, tingling hands, depression due to low serotonin levels, irritability, muscle cramps, lack of energy. Causes deficiency of B3 and B2. Anaemia. Poor immune system response. Causes cracks around the mouth and dermatitis on the face. Macrophages cannot remove cell debris in the abdomen.

Helpful. Works with B-complex vitamins, plus zinc and magnesium. Take with food and zinc.

Harmful. Alcohol, smoking, birth control pill, high protein intake, processed foods, penicillin, stress.

Good sources. Bananas, turkey, oat bran, egg yolk, leeks, cod, trout, salmon, sardines, herrings, mackerel, tuna, kale, red kidney beans, broccoli, Brussels sprouts, lamb chops, watercress, cauliflower, spring cabbage, carrots, beans, chicken, peas, potatoes, spinach, cantaloupe melons, onions, almonds.

VITAMIN B12 (CYANOCOBALAMIN)

RDA. Adults: 1mcg
Optimum intake. Adults: 2mcg

Effects. Use of protein. Helps blood carry oxygen. Essential for energy/nerves. Synthesis of DNA. Detoxifies tobacco smoke. Improves sperm count and motility. Analegsic action on pain.

Deficiency. Poor hair condition, eczema or dermatitis, mouth oversensitive, sterility.

Helpful. Works with folic acid. Best taken within B-complex, with food. PABA.

Harmful. Alcohol, smoking, lack of stomach acid.

Good sources. Lamb's liver, sardines, tuna, plaice, Edam cheese, shrimp, eggs, lamb chops, whole milk, cheese, pork, miso paste, herrings, mackerel, cod, chicken legs. Vegetarians may need to take a supplement.

VITAMIN B-COMPLEX – (FOLIC ACID)

RDA. Adults: 200mcg
Optimum intake. Adults: 800mcg

Effects. Early development of brain and nerves, by 27th day of fetal development. Energy production. Reduces inflammation. Oestrogenic action. Improves immune function. Promotes cells to divide.

Deficiency. Eczema, cracked lips, prematurely greying hair, anxiety or tension, poor memory, lack of energy, poor appetite, stomach pains, depression.

Helpful. Works with other B-complex vitamins, especially B12. Best supplemented as part of B-complex with food. Zinc and folic acid levels must be balanced.

Harmful. High temperature, light, food processing, contraceptive pill.

Good sources. Peanuts, spinach, green leafy vegetables, carrots, egg yolk, apricots, melons, beans, pumpkin, hazelnuts, broccoli, walnuts, cauliflower, wholemeal bread, tuna, avocado, dark rye flour, corn tortilla.

VITAMIN B-COMPLEX – (BIOTIN)

RDA. Adults: 150mcg
Optimum intake. Adults: 200mcg

Effects. Important in childhood. Essential fats use, healthy skin, hair and nerves. Made by bifido bacteria to support immunoglobulins.

Deficiency. Dry skin, poor hair condition, premature greying hair, sore muscles, poor appetite/nausea, eczema.

Helpful. Works with other B vitamins, magnesium and manganese. Best supplemented as part of a B-complex with food.

Harmful. Raw egg white, fried food.

Good sources. Almonds, oatmeal, eggs, herring, smoked mackerel, whole milk, lamb, chicken, cheese, rice, tomatoes, boiled cauliflower, grapefruit, lettuce, peas, cherries, apples, white cabbage.

VITAMIN A (RETINOL AND BETA-CAROTENE)

RDA. Adults: Retinol 800mcg, beta-carotene 2,000mcg
Optimum intake. Adults: Retinol 800mcg, beta-carotene 5,000mcg

Effects. Healthy skin and cell membranes. Protects against infections. Antioxidant. Immune system. Protects against cancers. Essential for night vision. Reduces menstrual cramps.

Deficiency. Mouth ulcers, poor night vision, acne, frequent colds/infections, dry flaky skin, dandruff, thrush or cystitis, diarrhoea, menstrual cramps. Used inefficiently if thyroxine is low. Abnormality of sperm.

Helpful. Works with zinc. Vitamin C and E help protect it. Best taken within a multivitamin with food.

Harmful. Heat, light, alcohol, coffee and smoking. Low fat diet.

Good sources. *Retinol*: butter, single cream, hard cheeses, boiled eggs, whole milk, fish liver oils. *Beta-carotene*: carrots, watercress, green and yellow vegetables, cantaloupe melons, tomatoes, broccoli, dried apricots, white cabbage, tangerines.

VITAMIN D (ERGOCALCIFEROL)

RDA. Adults: 5mg
Optimum intake. Adults: 10mg

Effects. Strong and healthy bones by retaining calcium. Precursor to cholesterol (which is the precursor to progesterone).

Deficiency. Joint pain or stiffness, backache, tooth decay, muscle cramps, hair loss.

Helpful. Exposure to sunlight (vitamin D is made in the skin). Under these conditions dietary vitamin D may not be necessary. Vitamins A, C and E protect D.

Harmful. Lack of sunlight, fried foods. Low fat diet.

Good sources. Herrings, salmon, smoked mackerel, boiled eggs, salmon, tuna, butter, hard cheeses.

VITAMIN E (D-ALPHA-TOCOPHEROL)

RDA. Adults: 10mg
Optimum intake. Adults:100mg

Effects. Antioxidant, protecting cells from damage, including cancer. Helps to oxygenate red blood cells, preventing blood clots. Improves wound healing and fertility. Promotes healthy skin. Reduces hot flushes. Improves breast tenderness. Aids sperm. Thins blood. Anti-inflammatory action. Needed for antibody production. Aids egg implantation.

Deficiency. Lack of sex drive, exhaustion after light exercise, easy bruising, slow wound healing, varicose veins, loss of muscle tone, infertility. Low testosterone.

Helpful. Vitamin C and selenium.

Harmful. High temperature cooking, especially frying. Air pollution, contraceptive pill, excessive intake of refined or processed fats and oils. Low fat diet.

Good sources. Sunflower seeds, soya beans, cold-pressed olive oil, safflower and sunflower oils, broccoli, sprouts, green leafy vegetables, spinach, wholegrain cereals, rye, hazelnuts, almonds, peanuts, avocados, salmon, eggs, asparagus, tuna, bananas, brown rice, oatmeal, carrots, peas, pilchards, runner beans.

VITAMIN K (PHYLLOQUINONE)

RDA. Adults: 1mcg/kg/day (sufficient amounts made by beneficial bacteria in the gut)
Optimum intake. Adults:10mcg

Effects. Controls blood clotting. Anti-inflammatory effect. Strong bones.

Deficiency. Haemorrhage (easy bleeding), osteoporosis.

Helpful. Healthy intestinal bifidobacteria, then no need for dietary source.

Harmful. Antibiotics, hormone treatments. For infants, lack of breastfeeding. Low-fat diet.

Good sources. Cauliflower, Brussels sprouts, lettuce, beans, peas, broccoli, cabbage, potatoes, watercress, corn oil, tomatoes, milk.

MINERALS

CALCIUM

RDA. Adults: 800mg
Optimum intake. Adults: 1,000mg

Effects. Health of the heart, nerves, muscles, skin, bones and teeth. Relieves aching muscles, bones, menstrual cramps. Classic complement pathway. Needed for ovarian hormones. Speeds up macrophages' ability to fight infections when the body runs a fever.

Deficiency. Muscle cramps, insomnia or nervousness, joint pain, arthritis, tooth decay, high blood pressure. Menstrual cramps.

Helpful. Works with magnesium and vitamin D, boron. Phosphorus must be in ratio to calcium.

Harmful. Caffeine depletes the body of calcium. Stress causes excretion. Hormone imbalances, alcohol. Phytic acid in wheat. Phosphates in fizzy drinks.

Good sources. Kelp, Gouda cheese, hard cheese, sardines, almonds, whole milk, sunflower seeds, green beans, wholegrain bread and cereals, boiled cabbage, natural yoghurt, carob flour, rhubarb, corn, prunes.

MAGNESIUM

RDA. Adults: 300mg
Optimum intake. Adults: 300mg

Effects. Strong bones and teeth. Regulates and relaxes smooth muscles, uterine muscle, heart muscle. Central nervous system calmative. Energy production. Carbohydrate metabolism. Alternative complement pathway. Strengthens cell membranes. Used by 300 enzymes (30 enzymes for cell growth). Promotes sleep. Regulator of temperature in thyroid function. For red blood cells. Natural diuretic. For ovary function. For myelin sheath. Softens stools. Needed for antibody production and a strong cell membrane. The anti-allergy nutrient.

Deficiency. Muscle spasms, insomnia, nervousness, high blood pressure, irregular heartbeat, constipation, fits/convulsions, hyperactivity, depression, miscarriage, mutagenic changes in sperm, infertility, mitral valve prolapse. Weak integrity of cell membrane.

Helpful. Vitamins B1, B5 and B6, and zinc.

Harmful. Large amounts of calcium, vitamin D, proteins and fats decrease magnesium absorption. Fizzy drinks. Alcohol. Phytic acid.

Good sources. Kelp, sunflower seeds, wheat germ, buckwheat, millet, green beans, barley, crab, bananas, yams, blackberries, broccoli, cauliflower, carrots, sweetcorn, dried figs, aubergines, chicken, onions, apples, celery, lettuce, fresh peas, almonds, Brazil nuts, peanuts, oatmeal, wholemeal bread, soya beans, brown rice, garlic, raisins, peas, baked potatoes in skin, crab, tuna.

IRON

RDA. Adults: 14mg
Optimum intake. Adults: 15mg

Effects. Iron helps transport oxygen to all cells for energy production. Red blood cells. Precursor for IL-1 production. Needed by macrophages to work, for ovarian hormones and for antibody production.

Deficiency. Pale skin, sore tongue, fatigue or listlessness, loss of appetite or nausea, heavy periods or blood loss, infections, impairs cell-mediated immunity, natural killer cells stop recognizing tumour formation.

Helpful. Vitamin C increases iron absorption, and vitamin E, also calcium if balanced but not in excess. (Iron EAP2 is well absorbed and does not cause constipation.)

Harmful. Oxalic acid in spinach, tea, antacids, soya protein, wheat bran, high zinc intake, phosphates in soft fizzy drinks, food additives.

Good sources. Sunflower seeds, almonds, dried prunes and apricots, raisins, Brazil nuts, walnuts, oat bran, pumpkin seeds, millet, parsley, almonds, cashews, dried dates, pecans, eggs, lentils, tofu, peas, brown rice, pork, lamb chops, red kidney beans, sesame seeds, wholemeal bread, cottage cheese, apples.

ZINC

RDA. Adults: 15mg
Optimum intake. Adults: 25mg

Effects. Works over 200 enzymes in the body (20 in the brain). Protein synthesis. Carbohydrate metabolism. DNA synthesis. Healing – skin health. Strong antibodies. Insulin production. Healthy sperm and ova. Alcohol metabolism. Sex hormone production (GnRH in hypothalamus, testosterone in testes). For ovarian function. Stomach acid production. Helps with dyslexia and anorexia. For cell-mediated immunity. Helps convert EFAs to prostaglandins. Natural diuretic. Anti-inflammatory. Healthy sperm. Allows egg to implant in womb.

Deficiency. Poor sense of taste or smell, white marks on fingernails, frequent infections, stretch marks, acne/greasy skin, low fertility, pale skin, tendency for depression, loss of appetite. Infertility.

Helpful. Vitamin B6 and magnesium, vitamins A and C.

Harmful. Phytic acid in wheat prevents uptake, high calcium intake, low protein intake, alcohol, white sugar prevents uptake, stress. Lead, cadmium, aluminium, iron, manganese. High copper. High oestrogen. Fizzy drinks. High meat and dairy food intake.

Good sources. Fresh oysters, ginger root, lamb chops, pecan nuts, haddock, green peas, shrimps, turnip, parsley, potatoes, Brazil nuts, boiled eggs, wholemeal bread, rye crispbread, oatmeal, peanuts, almonds, walnuts, sardines, chicken, buckwheat, hazelnuts, tuna, garlic, carrots, corn, grape juice, olive oil, cauliflower, spinach, cabbage, lentils, butter, lettuce, cucumber, spices, chicken legs.

CHROMIUM

RDA. Adults: 25mcg
Optimum intake. Adults: 100mcg

Effects. Strengthens heart. Balances blood sugar. Improves life span. Balances cholesterol. Turns glucose into energy. Makes insulin work effectively. Aids building of new proteins. Improves weight loss when on a diet.

Deficiency. Excessive/cold sweats, irritability after six hours without food, need for frequent meals, cold hands, drowsiness during the day, excessive thirst, 'addicted' to sweet foods, problems with cell renewal.

Helpful. Vitamin B3, improved diet and exercise.

Harmful. Refined sugars and flours, additives and pesticides, petroleum products, processed foods.

Good sources. Wholemeal bread, rye bread, oysters, potatoes, wheat germ, green peppers, eggs, chicken, apples, butter, parsnips, cornmeal, lamb chops, Swiss cheese, bananas, spinach, pork, carrots, shrimps, lettuce, oranges, green beans, cabbage, mushrooms, strawberries.

SELENIUM

RDA. Adults: 60mcg
Optimum intake. Adults: 100mcg

Effects. Protects against cancer. Disarms FoRs, Boosts the immune system. Needed by thyroid gland. Potentiates iodine. Anti-inflammatory effects. Antioxidant. Needed for prostaglandin production. Sperm production. Ovarian function. Antibody production. Protects the liver. Detoxifies pollutants.

Deficiency. Family history of cancer, signs of premature ageing, cataracts, high blood pressure, frequent infections, infertility, low sperm count, low thyroid function (hypothyroid).

Helpful. Vitamins A, C and E, iodine.

Harmful. Mercury, cadmium, lead.

Good sources. Butter, herrings, wheat germ, Brazil nuts, cider vinegar, scallops, barley, wholemeal bread, lobster, shrimps, kippers, tuna, shrimps, oats, crab, whole milk, oysters, broccoli, cod, brown rice, lamb, turnips, garlic, orange juice, egg yolks, chicken, Swiss cheeses, cottage cheese, radishes, pecans, almonds, hazelnuts, green beans, onions, carrots, cabbage.

IODINE

RDA. Adults: 150mcg
Optimum intake. Adults: 500mcg

Effects. Essential for thyroid glands (controls the body's metabolism), vitality, stable weight, sex organ development, ovarian function, strong teeth, good circulation, temperature regulation, ovarian function.

Deficiency. Breast cancer, lack of energy, hypothyroidism, weight gain, bulging eyes, brittle nails, low resistance to infection, fuzzy brain, obesity, persistent cough and sore throat, constipation, hair loss. Relieves fibrocystic breast with selenium and vitamin E.

Helpful. Selenium, magnesium, copper, manganese.

Harmful. Low fish diet, low vegetable intake, imbalance of calcium and phosphorus, low selenium intake.

Good sources. Shrimps, scampi, haddock, halibut, oysters, cod, salmon, sardines, pineapples, strawberries, tuna, boiled eggs, peanuts, natural yoghurt, hard cheeses, pork chops, lettuce, spinach, green peppers, butter, cream, cottage cheese, lamb, raisins, fried onions.

MANGANESE

RDA. Adults: 2.5mg
Optimum intake. Adults: 15mg

Effects. Used in energy production, bone formation, protein metabolism, metabolism of fats and cholesterol production. SOD (superoxide dismutase) needs manganese to fight FoR damage and protects the cell membrane. Formation of thyroxine. Protects mitochondria. Required by liver. Helps fertility.

Deficiency. Reduced fertility due to defective ovulation, rheumatoid arthritis, cancer, leads to calcium deposition in arteries and soft tissue, abnormal bone and cartilage, backaches, sore knees, glucose intolerance, birth defects, growth retardation, inner ear balance, convulsions, epilepsy, irregular heartbeat, weight loss, dermatitis, loss of hair colour, reduced levels of dopamine, high copper levels, testicular degeneration, inhibits synthesis of cholesterol.

Helpful. Lecithin, choline, increase liver uptake.

Harmful. Excess calcium, phosphorus, iron, cobalt, zinc and copper, pesticides and insecticides, milling process for grains, soya protein.

Good sources. Pecans, Brazil nuts, almonds, barley, rye, buckwheat, split peas, wholewheat, walnuts, fresh spinach, peanuts, oats, raisins, Swiss cheese, corn, cabbage, peaches, butter, tangerines, peas, eggs, beets, coconut, apples, oranges, pears.

BORON

RDA. Adults: none given
Optimum intake. Adults: 3mg

Effects. Boron works very much like oestrogen to prevent the loss of minerals from bone. It is useful combined with vitamin D, calcium and magnesium to help improve bones in menopause to prevent osteoporosis.

Deficiency. None have been identified.

Helpful. Vitamin D, calcium, magnesium, zinc.

Harmful. Caffeine, alcohol.

Good sources. Fresh fruits and vegetables.

12 Food – the best choice for health

Nothing becomes real until it is experienced.

John Keats

WHAT TO EAT?

This is easy. You just have to eat the freshest food available. If you are vegetarian, buy fresh fruits, vegetables, beans, peas, lentils, nuts and seeds and organic dairy foods. If you are carnivorous, choose organic meat which is hormone- and antibiotic-free and find the most unpolluted source of fish (deep-sea fish is probably the best). Then you cook from fresh as often as possible. Try to avoid foods with additives and flavour enhancers and preservatives unless they are natural ones like vinegar or vitamin C. The healthier your food, the healthier you will become.

In *Gulliver's Travels,* Jonathan Swift writes, 'He had been eight years upon a project for extracting sunbeams out of cucumbers.' Indeed this is what our food really is – trapped rays of light and energy from the sun. Plants grow by using the energy of the sun directly to convert nutrients from the soil and elements from the air into plant tissues. The secret to this miracle is the chlorophyll molecule found in plants. Chlorophyll is magnesium-based and it captures the energy of the sun and uses it to synthesize new carbohydrates, proteins and fats in the plants. The plants are eaten by herbivores and we consume plants and/or herbivores. So we are all dependent upon the sun as our major source of energy. Vital energy allows our cells to work at their best.

The Soil Association (*see* p. 395) can provide a list of suppliers in your area who deliver organic vegetables weekly. If you buy foods which have been sprayed with pesticides, herbicides and fungicides, peel them; scrubbing will not be effective. You need to reduce the load of oestrogenic (xeno-oestrogens) chemicals which you take in.

We should not be anxious about food, but by being aware we can make more informed choices about what we choose to buy and eat. Health is such a precious commodity. We do not realize until we lose it, how much it should be treasured and valued. However, food is not a commodity, although great profits are made by food manufacturers and retailers. Your food should be seen as something which can bestow good health.

Think of our ancestors. What did they eat? When times were hard and it was survival of the fittest, you grew what you ate or bartered food, which had to be eaten fresh as storage was a problem. Crops were rotated and fields were allowed to lie fallow to renew the soil. You ate what was in season. Obviously we cannot go back to this, but we should eat from fresh whenever possible. We all have manic days when we arrive home shattered from work and need to take short cuts, but we should try to eat fresh food as often as possible. Meals do not have to take a long time to prepare. Some recipes are given later on in this chapter to help you.

Avril G of Sussex

When I have managed to stick to a natural diet of fresh fruits and vegetables I do definitely feel less sluggish and ill. As soon as I eat something 'unnatural', such as chocolate or sweets, I almost immediately feel ill again. I feel like the substance is poisoning me, which being totally unnatural to the human body, it probably is. I am now expecting a baby in June! Thanks for all your help.

CASE
STUDY

SHOPPING STRATEGIES

Many people shop once a week at the local supermarket. They push trolleys laden with food. But stop and think. Those vegetables and that fruit – how many days ago were they picked? We take them home and they sit at the bottom of the fridge for how many more days? This is not good. Most of the vitamins oxidize as they sit around. We need to eat fresh foods. Our grandparents grew their own or bought fresh local produce so it was still vibrant and full of nutrients. They did not have fridges so could not store food as we do. We should shop for fruits and vegetables every two days to ensure they are still full of vitamins.

Boring diets can also lead to poor intake of nutrients; we need to be more adventurous when cooking. Dishes which are quick to prepare do not have to be the convenience foods we throw in the microwave after an exhausting day. Salads and soups take very little time to prepare. Once you have sorted out your digestive system and begun to absorb nutrients efficiently, you need to keep your body supplied with a wide variety of nutrients, which means a wide variety of foods. Use the weekends to experiment with new recipes – there are some in this book for you to try. Some are wheat- and dairy-free for those who wish to try sensible exclusion diets. The word 'diet' is misleading; this is not a diet, it is eating for health.

Stock your store cupboard up with useful items. You will need some balanced mineral salt, black pepper, spices and herbs for lots of lovely flavours. When you try a wheat-free or dairy-free diet, you need to stock all the alternatives for the moments when you are hungry. Tins of tuna, salmon, beans, vegetable soups and tomatoes for occasional use on exhausted nights are handy. Frozen vegetables and fruits are also useful, as are sugar-free jams. A tour around your local healthfood store will yield a lot of foodstuffs – a yeast-free vegetable stock powder, organic rice and corn crisps. Keep organic fruit and nut bars, dried apricots, fresh coconut and carob bars to snack on should you crave anything sweet. Keep nuts and seeds in your desk drawer at work or sesame sticks. Experiment with other grains, such as quinoa and millet, and look for wheat-free muesli. There are many alternatives to try so you need never feel as though you are hungry. Just look around the shelves of your local healthfood store for other alternatives. You won't starve.

Feeling healthy will come if there is a problem with your present diet. Maybe you are eating a food which doesn't suit you or taking in too many processed foods and not enough fresh ones.

It is crucial to read product labels carefully when buying foods, as modern manufacturing processes add many ingredients to foods which you may not expect to be there. They can be used as fillers and thickenings, so be careful in choosing your products to avoid a reaction if you are sensitive.

Sugar-free eating: Some people find that they react to sugar by becoming lethargic and bloated. If you are sugar-sensitive, then watch out for:

corn syrup, dextrose, fructose, fruit sugar, glucose, glucose syrup, golden syrup, honey, invert sugar, malt syrup, maple syrup, molasses, sucrose, treacle.

Egg-free eating: Very few people are intolerant of eggs, but it may be the additives you react to, so the organic variety may be the most suitable. If any food makes you ill, however, it is best avoided. If eggs affect you, then watch out for labels stating:

albumen, conalbumen, egg white, egg yolk, ovalbumen, ovomucoid, ocoglobulin, vitellin, vitellenin.

Yeast-free eating: If you suspect *Candida albicans* overgrowth in the gut, then the following foods should be avoided for three months (see Appendix B). If you are yeast-sensitive, then avoid:

breads, wines, dried fruits, marmite, B vitamins and selenium obtained from yeasts, vinegars, pickled and fermented foods.

Wheat-free eating: Wheat-free or gluten-free, or both – that is the question. Around 80 per cent of women with endometriosis are finding that, by cutting wheat out of their diet, their abdominal pain is reduced or vanquished. In researching this phenomenon, it has been discovered that wheat, having been genetically modified in the early 1970s, has had two hormones added into its genetic sequence. Further research in this area is about to begin at the Endometriosis and Fertility Clinic.

In the spring of this year, eight women with endometriosis gathered together for a television recording. They ate a pleasant lunch, which consisted of gluten-free bread, rice pasta, gram-flour pastries and salad. Yet, overnight, seven out of eight were very ill with abdominal pain – which was so severe in two cases that they passed out. All had been on wheat-free diets and all had remained pain-free for several months beforehand. It was discovered that only the gluten-free bread canapés had contained wheat flour in the form of coeliac flour (wheat with the gluten washed out). This clearly indicates that it was not the gluten that was causing the problem, as all the other foods were wheat- and gluten-free, but strongly implies that it is some other substance in the wheat that may be triggering the endometriotic implants to become more inflammatory. This substance could be phytic acid, phytoestrogen, xeno-oestrogens from pesticides (wheat is sprayed between 9 to 12 times as it grows), excess bran or the two hormones in the plant's genes which were not present naturally.

Eating a wheat-free exclusion diet for one month will show whether or not boycotting wheat will be of any help to you. If you suffer from constipation, headaches, brain-fag or fatigue and have fertility problems, then it may prove helpful.

Any of the following could indicate the presence of wheat or a derivative:

modified starch, dextrins, maltodextrins, wheat flour, thickening, bran, wheatgerm, wheatgerm oil, farina, cereal filler, couscous, semolina, rusk, soy sauce, lagers and beers.

If you are gluten-sensitive, then you should avoid:

wheat, barley, oats, rye, spelt, amaranth, triticale, bran, malt.

Alternatives to wheat-based foods include:

rye crispbread, 100 per cent rye bread, rye pasta, oatcakes, porridge oats, oat muesli, corn tortillas and tacos, corn pasta, polenta, corn crispbread, rice pasta, lentil pasta, poppadoms, onion bhajis, Bombay mix, buckwheat pancakes, ricecakes, brown rice, rice noodles (angelhair), millet, millet flakes, pastry made from brown rice flour, ground almonds and margarine in equal proportions, potato-based pizza made from creamed potato and rye flour, Breton pancakes made from cornmeal and buckwheat flour.

Various companies now produce wheat-free bread and pizza bases; see the address section (p. 398) for mail order details, although many supermarkets now stock these items.

Have on hand a selection of nuts and seeds to snack on. Un-flavoured crisps, tacos and poppadoms are also fine in moderation.

Dairy-free eating: People with a family history of atopic conditions usually find that excluding bovine dairy foods from the diet can benefit their general health. If any members of your family suffer from asthma, eczema, hayfever or arthritis, then this may be of help to you. Signs of dairy intolerance include diarrhoea, indigestion, sinus and catarrh problems, and subfertility. A one-month exclusion diet may show if you have problems when diary is reintroduced. Any of the following could indicate the presence of milk:

lactose, casein, whey, caseinates, ghee, hydrolized casein, whey powder, milk solids, non-milk fat solids, skimmed-milk powder, whey proteins and sugars, yoghurt.

Choose to eat dairy foods which are not from bovine (cows) sources, such as goats, ewes, buffalo, soya, rice, oats and almonds. If you are trying a dairy-free regime, stock up with various alternatives to cow dairy foods such as:

ewe's (sheep's) milk and yoghurt, cheeses such as Feta, Ossau, Manchego, Spenwood, Shepherd's Purse, Roquefort, Pecorino Romano (Parmesan); goat's milk and yoghurt, and cheeses such as Halloumi and Village Green; buffalo Mozzarella cheese (delicious in salads and on pizzas); non-dairy alternatives like hummus, vegetable pâtés (carrot, mushroom, chestnut), nut butters, poor-man's caviar or black olive spread, avocado and egg pâté, or tuna, mackerel or crab pâté; even Tofutti ice cream and Plamil's dairy-free chocolate for special occasions.

RULES FOR A HEALTHY DIET

1 **Eat two fresh fruits and four fresh vegetables daily.** Whenever possible, eat fruit and vegetables raw, as they are rich in vitamins and minerals needed by the body. Cooking destroys many of the vitamins, and breaks down the fibre in the food making it less effective in the intestines. Green leafy vegetables are rich in the B vitamins and magnesium which are needed by the reproductive system daily. Red-orange vegetables and fruits are rich in vitamin A. Dried apricots are a good source of iron.

2 **Eat wholegrain cereals and unrefined foods**. Include a variety of cereals in your diet, not just wheat. Use oats, rye, spelt, barley, millet, rice, corn, quinoa or buckwheat. If you have a problem with gluten use the last five cereals only. Nuts and seeds are rich in vitamins and minerals, as well as important cis vegetable oils. As far as possible use only fresh, unprocessed foods as a basis for your meals, such as lean meat, poultry, fish and game. Oily fish like herrings, tuna, mackerel, sardines, salmon, pilchards and trout contain essential fatty acids which your body needs to build healthy tissues, so eat them twice a week.

3 **Drink at least a litre of fresh water daily.** Try diluting unsweetened fruit juices, or various herb teas. Chamomile helps sleep, lime- or lindenblossom aids relaxation, mint, ginger and fennel aid digestion. Dandelion tea is a diuretic. Carrot juice also helps digestion. V8 vegetable juice helps to cleanse the liver.

4 **Use only cold-pressed vegetable oils.** Our bodies require essential cis oils to strengthen cell walls, vegetable oils to build the anti-inflammatory series 1 prostaglandins and fish oils for omega-3 fats. It is very important to use unprocessed vegetable oils which have not been chemically or heat treated. The

container should say unrefined, unhydrogenated or cold-pressed for sunflower, safflower, corn and olive oils. Evening primrose oil is a good source, but expensive. Edible food-grade linseed oil from a healthfood shop is also useful. Try grinding one tablespoon of linseeds each day and mix into muesli or salad dressings. Butter can be used in moderation (organic butter can be found) or choose un-hydrogenated margarine from your healthfood store.

5 **Half your diet should consist of alkaline-forming foods**, such as vegetables, fruits, sprouted seeds, live yoghurt, almonds, Brazil nuts and buckwheat. The other half should be acid-forming foods, such as grains, pulses, nuts, seeds, eggs, cheese, fish and poultry. This helps to balance your digestive enzymes.

6 **Reduce your intake of sugary foods.** Try to avoid needless refined sugar consumption as it can cause fluid retention and may prevent other vital nutrients from being absorbed. Sugar also thickens the blood and stops immune cells from working efficiently for four hours after intake. Avoid chocolate, sweets, biscuits, cakes, puddings, ice cream, sugary fizzy drinks, sweet tea or coffee, jams and honey. Find other treats to give yourself instead. Chocolate can be saved as a special treat for birthdays, anniversaries, Christmas and Easter. Try Green & Black's organic chocolate. Carob bars or fruit and nut bars are far more nutritious snacks.

7 **Avoid excess salt intake.** Too much salt causes fluid retention and PMS symptoms. Reduce the amount of salt added to cooked foods and avoid eating salty crisps, nuts, bacon and kippers. Use herbs, spices, lemon juice or root ginger to impart flavour instead. You require only 3g salt per day (0.1oz) and most diets allow up to 10g (0.3oz). If you suffer from low blood pressure, then a little salt is fine, but there is danger with high blood pressure.

8 **Cut down your intake of tea, coffee, alcohol and tobacco.** Caffeine and excess alcohol are thought to impair ovarian and testes function, and so affect fertility. Tobacco and alcohol can aggravate some PMS symptoms. Try herb teas or coffee substitutes. Caffeine and alcohol are diuretics and literally throw out of the body some of the precious minerals needed by our reproductive system.

9 **Avoid excess fatty foods,** like beef, lamb and pork. Red meat supplies the proinflammatory series 2 prostaglandins, so should be eaten in moderation. Game is often less fatty meat. Use white meat and fish. Avoid fried foods, and grill or bake instead. If you must fry, use a little cold-pressed olive oil and butter, and gently cook on a low heat. Steam vegetables whenever possible. Eat a sensible amount of dairy foods. If eaten to excess, the calcium in them can prevent absorption of magnesium, which helps muscles to relax. Balance dairy foods with lots of fresh, green leafy vegetables. If you are a vegetarian, use more legumes (pulses).

10 **Exercise regularly.** Gentle exercise and exposure to fresh air and sunshine are vital in maintaining health. Take walks, go swimming or cycling if you are able. Gentle exercise helps the body produce endorphins (natural painkillers) and stimulates the digestive tract.

11 **Eat a high-fibre diet.** We need to include more fibre in our diet to ensure the stools are well-formed and that waste can pass through us at an even rate, avoiding the build-up of harmful toxins in the intestines. Fibre of the type provided by fructo-oligosaccharides (FOS) also helps to maintain the good bifido gut flora which produce the B vitamins needed by the liver enzymes. The fibre in the diet also stimulates peristalsis, and binds to cholesterol and oestrogens to escort them from the body. Fibre can be from wholegrain cereals (especially oats), nuts, seeds or from fruits and vegetables. Only 30g (1oz) of fibre is needed each day, and a diet rich in plant fibre easily supplies this.

12 *Candida albicans.* If you think you have an overgrowth, or an allergy or sensitivity to the yeast *Candida albicans* in your digestive tract and suffer abdominal bloating after meals, then remove the foods which 'feed' the yeast for two or three months – refined sugars, yeasts, wheat, fermented foods, dried fruits and dairy foods. The following foods have anti-yeast properties and should be used frequently – garlic, onions, cabbage, broccoli, Brussels sprouts, kale, watercress, mustard cress, cauliflower, turnips, cinnamon, olive oil, aloe vera juice and pau d'arco tea (see Appendix B for dietary guidelines).

SUGGESTIONS FOR WEEKLY MENU PLANS

(Recipes are given for those in boldface type)

The following suggested weekly menus can serve as a starter for your HELP – healthy-eating lifestyle plan. They can also act as a guide for food exclusion diets (*see also* p. 326).

> When we are flat on our backs, there is no way to look but up.
> *Roger W Babson*

Wheat-free diet – Week 1

	BREAKFAST	LUNCH	TEA/DINNER
1	Prune juice Ricecakes & hummus Mint tea	**Potato & leek soup** Oatcakes & apple Figs	Turkey breast Rice, broccoli, carrots
2	Sheep's yoghurt with ground almonds, oat bran & banana Prune juice Fennel tea	Mackerel Mixed salad Baked potato Dates	Chestnut pate Pumpernickel rye bread Tomato & celery Apple
3	**Breton pancakes** Blueberries Mint tea	**Chicken with lemon & olives** Boiled rice Broccoli, carrots Figs	**Carrot & almond soup** Corn tacos Apple
4	**Rye bread** & poached egg Carrot juice & herb tea	Grilled chicken Green beans, swede Jacket potato Dates	Vegetable & lentil soup Rye crackers Pineapple
5	Potato cakes Sugar-free baked beans Mint tea	Stuffed aubergine (eggplant) Grilled tomato & green salad Pear	Turkey breast Boiled potato Brussels sprouts, beetroot
6	Greek sheep's yoghurt with banana, oat bran & almonds Herb tea	**Bean & rice casserole** Green salad Soya yoghurt with mint & cucumber	Salmon pâté & ricecakes Tomato, celery Apple
7	Oatcakes & hummus Prune juice Fennel tea	**Vegetable cobbler** Cabbage, carrots Potato	Green leafy salad **Tuna pâté** & cornbread Pear & figs

Menu suggestions – Week 2

	BREAKFAST	LUNCH	TEA/DINNER
1	Scrambled eggs Ricecakes Herb tea	**Cream of watercress soup** Apple Beverage	**Chickpea & spinach curry** Rice Oat crumble
2	Soya yoghurt with dates, ground almonds & banana Tea	Chicken Spinach salad Jacket potato Figs	**Avocado pâté** & ricecakes Salad
3	Rye bread & spreads Herb tea	**Nut loaf** Boiled new potatoes Broccoli, carrots Banana	Courgette (zucchini) & spinach soup Oatcakes Apple
4	Rye crackers & poached egg Herb tea	Poached salmon Green beans, sweetcorn Jacket potato Melon	**Lentil & apricot soup** Rye crackers Dates
5	Potato cakes Scrambled egg Tea	**Potato-based pizza** Watercress salad Grilled tomato, peas Pear	Grilled pork chops Boiled potato Green beans & red cabbage Kiwi
6	Soya yoghurt with banana Herb tea	**Aubergine loaf (eggplant)** Green salad & jacket potato Soya yoghurt with mint & cucumber	Tuna pâté & rye crackers Tomato, celery Apple
7	Oat crackers & nut butter Herb tea	**Tuna & sweetcorn flan** Broccoli, carrots Melon	**North African salad Tomato salad** Pear

Snacks between meals

Nuts
Sunflower seeds
Date & fig bars
Raisins & sultanas
Savoury popcorn
Hazelnut butter on crispbreads
Replace cow's milk with soya milk in recipes

These are merely suggestions to give you an idea of how several days' meals can be wheat- and dairy-free should you want to try an exclusion-style diet. There are so many alternatives and you need not feel hungry. In fact, the meals are very tasty. Experiment with some of the following recipes at weekends and get a feel for what you like. Wander round the local healthfood shop and see what they have to offer as alternatives to crisps and bars of chocolate. Try some of their corn pastas and rice couscous. The following recipes should give everyone something to try. Many are quick and easy to prepare, and we hope that you enjoy eating them. (All recipes are for four people.)

> Happiness: a good bank account, a good cook, and a good digestion.
>
> *Jean-Jacques Rousseau, Philosopher*

SOUPS

Lentil and apricot soup

50g/2oz red lentils, washed
50g/2oz dried apricots, washed
1 large potato
1.2 litres/2 pt vegetable stock

juice of half a lemon
1 tsp ground cumin
3 tbsp chopped parsley
seasoning

1 Put lentils and apricots in large saucepan.
2 Chop potato and add to pan with remaining ingredients.
3 Bring to the boil, cover and simmer for 30 minutes.
4 Leave to cool.
5 Place in a blender and liquidize until smooth.
6 Reheat, adding seasoning to taste.

Carrot and almond soup

400g/1lb carrots
1 potato
1 large onion
celery leaves
1 large cooking apple
2 tsp wholegrain mustard

1 tbsp chopped parsley
1 tsp vegetable stockpowder
juice of half a lemon
1 tsp mixed herbs
50g/2oz ground almonds

1   Dice all the vegetables.
2   Cook in 1.2 litres/2 pt of water, simmering gently. Add the apple last of all.
3   After 25–30 minutes, remove from the heat. Cool for 5 minutes.
4   Add the mustard, vegetable stock powder, lemon juice and herbs.
5   Blend or liquidize until smooth.
6   Add the ground almonds and reheat.
7   Garnish with flaked almonds and parsley to serve.

Potato and leek soup

1kg/2lb potatoes
400g/1lb leeks
0.7 litres/1 pt milk (soya)

½oz butter
Seasoning
Parsley to garnish

1   Peel and boil the potatoes until soft.
2   Clean the leeks, finely chop and fry gently until soft.
3   Mash the potatoes with some of the milk and butter.
4   Mix in the leeks and rest of milk. This may be liquidized.
5   Bring to the boil and serve garnished with parsley.

Cream of watercress soup

1 medium onion
1 small potato
25g/1oz butter
1 bunch of watercress

0.35 litres/½ pt milk (soya)
0.35 litres/½ pt vegetable stock
salt and pepper
4 tbsp single cream (optional)

1   Chop the onion and potato.
2   Melt the butter in a saucepan and sauté the onion until transparent.
3   Add potato, watercress, milk and stock. Bring to boil, cover and simmer for
    20 minutes.
4   Allow to cool slightly, then blend until smooth.
5   Return to pan, season to taste, stir in cream and reheat to serving temperature.

Avocado soup/dip

1 ripe avocado
6 spring onions (scallions)
175g/7oz sheep's milk or soya yoghurt

2 tbsp cream
salt and pepper (optional)

1   Peel and stone the avocado.
2   Slice into a tall jug.
3   Add the chopped onions, milk or yoghurt, cream and seasoning.
4   Liquidize or blend to make a dip.
5   Add 0.35 litres/½ pt water to make a cold soup.

MAIN MEALS

Chicken with lemon and olives

2 tbsp olive oil
3kg/6.5lb chicken, cut into 8 pieces
100g/4oz chopped onions
1½ tsp paprika
1 tsp ground ginger
1¼ tsp turmeric

½ tsp salt
black pepper
2 fresh lemons, quartered
0.3 litres/⅜ pt water
24 small green olives

1   Warm the olive oil and brown the chicken pieces. Place in a dish with the stock
    they make.
2   Pour off the remaining oil from the pan and fry the onions gently until soft
    and brown.
3   Stir in the paprika, ginger, turmeric, salt and pepper.
4   Add the fresh lemon, chicken pieces and the stock.
5   Add the water and bring to the boil, then reduce the heat and cover, and simmer
    for 30 minutes until the chicken is tender.
6   Add the olives, and cover and simmer for 5 minutes. Taste for seasoning.
7   Serve with rice and green salad or steamed vegetables.

Bean and rice casserole

225g/8oz black beans, soaked overnight
   and drained (or use tinned kidney
   beans)
1 green pepper, cored, seeded and sliced
1 clove garlic, peeled and crushed
1 red chilli, finely chopped (optional)
300ml/½ pt chicken stock

2 tbsp cold-pressed sunflower oil
1 medium onion, peeled and chopped
4 large tomatoes, skinned and sliced
1 red pepper, cored, seeded and sliced
1 tsp coriander
salt and pepper
225g/8oz long-grain brown rice

Garnish
Fresh coriander leaves, avocado slices, lemon juice

1 Cook the beans in fast-boiling, unsalted water for 15 minutes. Reduce heat and
   simmer for 45 minutes until tender. Drain.
2 Heat oil, fry onion over moderate heat for 3 minutes. Add garlic, peppers and
   chilli (if used). Stir well, cook for 2 minutes.
3 Add tomatoes, salt, pepper, coriander and cook for 1 minute. Add rice, stock,
   beans. Bring to a boil.
4 Cover pan. Simmer for 45 minutes until rice is cooked and stock is absorbed.
5 Garnish.

Potato-based pizza

225g/8oz boiled potatoes
50g/2oz butter
100g/4oz rye flour/buckwheat/cornmeal

salt
freshly ground black pepper

Topping
2 tbsp olive oil
225g/8oz onions (thinly sliced)
1 red pepper (thinly sliced)
1 clove garlic (crushed)
2 tbsp tomato purée
50g/2oz frozen sweetcorn

½ level tbsp oregano
2 tsp lemon juice
salt
freshly ground black pepper
175g/6oz Feta or buffalo milk
Mozzarella cheese

1   Boil the potatoes until they are soft, then mash them to a pulp with the butter.
2   Sift in the flour and a little salt and pepper. Now mix to a dough.
3   Transfer to a floured surface and knead lightly until the mixture becomes soft and elastic.
4   Roll out to a 10in (25cm) round. Place on oiled baking sheet.
5   Heat the olive oil in a large frying pan and fry the onions, red pepper and garlic for 5 minutes.
6   Stir in the sweetcorn, oregano and lemon juice, and season with salt and pepper.
7   Spread the tomato purée on the pizza base and then top with the onion mixture.
8   Place the cheese on top and bake on a high shelf at gas mark 6 or 400°F or 200°C for 40 minutes.

Parmesan polenta-based pizza

Base
1 litre/1¾ pt water
125g/4oz butter
salt and pepper

375g/13oz instant polenta
150g/6oz grated Pecorino Romano
 (Parmesan) cheese

Coating
80g/3oz instant polenta
2 beaten eggs
olive oil for frying

50g/2oz grated Pecorino Romano
 (Parmesan) cheese

Topping
250g/8oz Manchego, Mozzarella,
 Spenwood or Village Green cheese,
 sliced

4 chopped tomatoes
Black olives anchovies (optional)

1 Boil water in a large saucepan and pour in the instant polenta, cook for 2 minutes until thickened.
2 Remove from the heat and beat in the butter, cheese and seasoning. Cook for 15 minutes.
3 Place the polenta into a length of cling film and roll into a long sausage shape 10in long (20cm). Chill for 2 hours in the fridge.
4 Mix the dry polenta and finely ground cheese in one dish and have the beaten egg in another.
5 Slice the chilled polenta 'sausage' into 10 pieces. Dip each piece into the egg and then roll in the dry mixture, like making fish cakes.
6 Shallow fry each circle until golden brown and crispy.
7 Top with a slice of cheese and tomato, and garnish with olives and anchovies. Grill for a few minutes until the cheese has melted.
8 Serve with a crisp green salad. Freeze leftovers for another day.

Tomato and courgette tian

1 medium aubergine	2 courgettes
1 onion	1 beef tomato
125g/4oz Feta cheese	225g/8oz basmati rice
4 tbsp fresh chopped parsley	4 tbsp olive oil

1 Slice the aubergine and cover in salt. Leave for 20 minutes, then wash and pat dry on kitchen towel.
2 Boil the basmati rice for 15 minutes in salted water.
3 Fry the onions for 3 minutes. Add the aubergine slices, fry until softened. Add the courgettes and cook until soft.
4 Beat the eggs, then add the cheese and half the parsley.
5 Add the cooked rice to the vegetable mixture.
6 Stir in the egg mixture.
7 Place half the mixture into a buttered ovenproof dish. Place the sliced tomatoes down the centre. Place the rest of the mixture on top.
8 Bake for 25 minutes in the oven at gas mark 5 or 380°F/190°C.
9 Sprinkle with the rest of the parsley to serve.

This can be served with a fish dish or with crisp green salad.

Potato cakes

3 large potatoes	1 onion, finely grated
3 medium eggs	Mixed herbs, salt, pepper
1 tablespoon cornflour	

1 Boil the potatoes and cream until smooth, adding the sieved cornflour a little at a time.
2 Add the grated onion and seasoning.
3 When cooled, add the beaten eggs.
4 Shape into potato cakes and lightly fry in olive oil or freeze between sheets of greaseproof paper.

Tuna and sweetcorn flan

100g/4oz ground almonds
50g/2oz brown rice flour
50g/2oz oat bran

100g/4oz tub margarine (Vitaseig or
  Vitaquell)
salt and pepper

Filling

2 eggs
150ml/¼ pt soya milk or small carton
  of sheep's or goat's yoghurt

175g/7oz tin tuna
175g/7oz tin sweetcorn
1 tbsp fresh parsley (chopped)

1   Mix the ground almonds, brown rice flour and oat bran with a little salt and pepper.
2   Mash together with margarine to form a soft dough.
3   Grease a pie/flan dish. Press the mixture to form a solid base and walls.
4   Beat the eggs and yoghurt together.
5   Place the tuna, then the sweetcorn evenly in the dish. Season.
6   Sprinkle over the chopped parsley. Pour over the egg mixture.
7   Bake until pale gold. Oven gas mark 5 or 375°F or 190°C for 30 minutes.

Shortcrust pastry may be used for the base (150g/6oz flour and 75g/3oz of margarine using the rubbing-in method).

Aubergine loaf (eggplant)

1 large or 2 medium aubergines
100g/4oz cooked millet or rice
2 tbsp parsley
1 clove garlic
a few drops Worcestershire sauce
salt and pepper

3 eggs
75g/3oz grated cheese (Feta or
  Mozzarella)
150ml/¼ pt olive oil
2 tbsp tomato purée
75g/3oz flaked almonds or pine nuts

1   Wash aubergines. Cut in half lengthways. Sprinkle with salt, leave for ½ hour to sweat.
2   Place all the other ingredients, except the nuts, into blender and liquidize until smooth.
3   Rinse the aubergine and chop roughly.
4   Place the aubergine and nuts into the mixture and stir.
5   Grease a 1kg/2lb loaf tin with oil. Pour in the mixture.
6   Cook for 20 minutes at gas mark 6 or 400°F or 200°C. Reduce heat to gas mark 4 or 350°F or 180°C and cook for a further 20 minutes.
7   Test with a skewer. Leave for 10 minutes to cool, then loosen gently and turn out.
8   Serve with rice or jacket potato and a crisp salad. Garnish with apple slices. Lovely cold too!

Nut loaf

1 onion
75g/3oz butter
4 tbsp medium oatmeal
350ml/½ pt milk (soya)
2 beaten eggs (or 1 egg + 2 yolks)

100g/4oz sweetcorn
8oz/225g nuts (peanuts/cashew) or
   dried, soaked chestnuts/almond
1 tbsp oat bran or sesame seeds

1   Peel and chop onion finely.
2   Melt the butter in a pan. Add the onions. Fry for 5 minutes.
3   Add the oatmeal, stir well.
4   Add the milk, stir until thickened. Allow to cool.
5   Stir in the beaten eggs and the sweetcorn.
6   Add the ground nuts and mix well. Season.
7   Oil tin. Line with oat bran or sesame seeds.
8   Place mixture in tin, bake for 1 hour in oven gas mark 4 or 350°F or 180°C.

Chickpea and spinach curry

2 onions
1 tsp chopped root ginger
1 clove garlic chopped
1 tsp mild curry powder or
¼ tsp each of salt and pepper, cumin,
   coriander, ginger, cinnamon
0.25 litres/10oz natural yoghurt
2 tbsp tomato purée

15oz can of tomatoes
1 tsp creamed coconut
450g/1lb chickpeas (soak overnight,
   boil 10 minutes, simmer 2 hours, or use
   a tin)
450g/1lb fresh spinach (250g/8oz
   frozen)

1   Chop the onions finely and fry until soft in 2 tbsp olive oil with ginger and garlic.
2   Add curry powder and fry 2–3 minutes. Lower heat.
3   Add most of the yoghurt a little at a time. Cook gently until the oil separates out.
4   Add the tomatoes and paste. Cook gently 30 minutes until a rich curry sauce
    is produced.
5   Add the chickpeas and spinach. Simmer gently for 20 minutes (add a little water if
    the sauce becomes too dry).

Any meat, fish, vegetables or beans may be used in the curry sauce, or it may be used
to stuff aubergines and sweet peppers (capsicum).

   Serve with mango chutney, banana slices, brown rice or millet, yoghurt and mint,
lime pickle and tomato slices.

   To cook the millet, add 1 cup of millet to 4 cups water. Simmer 15 minutes. Millet
can also be used with stir-fried vegetables. This is the most nutrient-rich grain of all
and the only one which is alkaline.

Vegetable cobbler

Base

3 medium carrots
½ small cauliflower
50g/2oz butter
3 leeks

50g/2oz sweetcorn
1 tbsp cornflour
150ml/¼ pt chicken stock
2 tbsp fresh parsley

Topping

40g/1.5oz margarine
175g/6oz rye flour
½ tsp baking powder
75g/3oz oat bran

50g/2oz Feta cheese
1 egg
2 tbsp natural soya yoghurt

1 Cook carrots and cauliflower in boiling water for 5 minutes.
2 Drain. Place into a casserole dish.
3 Melt 25g/1oz butter. Fry leeks and sweetcorn 4 minutes. Stir.
4 Melt 25g/1oz butter. Stir in cornflour to form a roux paste.
5 Remove from heat. Slowly blend in the stock. Season.
6 Boil. Simmer 3 minutes. Add chopped parsley. Stir continuously.
7 Place all vegetables in the casserole dish. Pour sauce over top. Put in oven for 40 minutes at gas mark 4 or 350°F or 180°C.
8 Scones (rubbing-in method): Rub the margarine into the sieved flour and baking powder. Add the bran and ¾ of the grated cheese.
9 Add the beaten egg and yoghurt to form a firm dough.
10 Roll out. Cut 15 scones. Arrange over the vegetables.
11 Sprinkle with rest of cheese. Bake for 15 minutes at gas mark 6 or 400°F or 200°C, till golden.

SNACKS

Tuna pâté

1 tbsp (level) live soya yoghurt
½ tbsp (level) mayonnaise

¼ tbsp tomato purée
1 small tin tuna

1 Mix the yoghurt, mayonnaise and tomato purée together.
2 Add the tuna and mix in.

Avocado pâté

1 hard-boiled egg	½ lemon
1 avocado	salt, pepper, paprika

1 Chop the hard-boiled egg finely into a bowl. Add salt and pepper.
2 Cut the avocado flesh into the bowl.
3 Chop together. Add the lemon juice.
4 Place in a small dish. Garnish with paprika.

Tomato salad

4 tomatoes (peeled and thinly sliced)	Salt
2 tbsp olive oil	Freshly ground black pepper
2 tsp lemon juice	1 tbsp chopped fresh chives

1 Place the tomatoes in a shallow salad dish.
2 Mix together the oil, lemon juice and salt and pepper to taste.
3 Pour over the tomatoes. Sprinkle with the chives. Chill for at least 1 hour
   before serving.

North African salad

175g/6oz long grain rice	4 tbsp olive oil
1 small cucumber (sliced)	4 tsp lemon juice
2 medium bananas (peeled and sliced)	large pinch ground coriander
1 avocado (peeled and diced)*	large pinch ground cumin
1 tbsp pinenuts or almonds	salt and pepper

1 Cook the rice in boiling salted water for 15 minutes or until it is tender. Drain and
   allow to cool.
2 Put the rice, cucumber, bananas, avocado and pinenuts in a salad bowl and
   stir well.
3 Mix together the oil, lemon juice, coriander, cumin, salt and pepper in a bowl and
   beat well.
4 Pour dressing over the rice mixture and mix well. Serve with tuna pâté.

*2 tbsp raisins can be used in place of the avocado.

Celery, apple and walnut salad

½ medium head of celery (finely
   chopped)
2 red eating apples (cored and diced)
2 tbsp live yoghurt

juice of half a lemon
1 tbsp mayonnaise
25g/1oz shelled walnuts or pecans
   (chopped)

1   Mix together the celery, apples, yoghurt, lemon juice and mayonnaise in a
    salad bowl.
2   Chill for 30 minutes.
3   Just before serving, stir in the walnuts or pecans.

Salad niçoise

½ small lettuce (separated into leaves)
2 tbsp olive oil
juice of half a lemon
150g/6oz French beans (cooked)
3 tomatoes (peeled and quartered)

75g/3.5oz can tuna (drained and
   flaked)
black olives (stoned)
3 medium potatoes (cooked and diced)

1   Arrange lettuce leaves on a shallow serving dish.
2   Mix the oil and lemon juice together to form a dressing.
3   Cut the beans into 1in (2.5cm) lengths and mix together with the potatoes,
    tomatoes, dressing and tuna.
4   Toss gently to combine. Spoon the mixture over the lettuce leaves and garnish
    with the black olives.

Green tossed salad

Lettuce
Celery
Watercress

Chopped spring onions (scallions)
Baby spinach leaves

Choose a selection of the above and toss together with a mixture of olive oil and
lemon juice. For flavourings, add honey, mustard or tahini (sesame seed spread) or
black olive pâté.

BREADS

Shaker corn bread

1 cup cornmeal (polenta)
$1/3$ cup soya flour
$1/4$ cup fine oatmeal
3 tsp baking powder

$1/2$ tsp salt
1 egg
$1–1 1/4$ cups soya milk

1　Heat the oven to 190°C.
2　Grease a 20cm x 10cm loaf tin.
3　Mix the dry ingredients in a bowl.
4　Beat the egg and milk together.
5　Whisk the egg milk mixture into the dry ingredients and pour into the tin.
6　Bake until golden (30 minutes approx).
7　Eat hot or cold or toasted.
8　For a lighter texture, add 2 whisked egg whites after the milk and egg, or 4 tbsp grated cheese.

Flat rye bread

2 cups rye flour
2 tsp baking powder
$1/2$ tsp salt

2 tbsp melted butter
1 tbsp honey
1 cup milk

1　Heat the oven to gas mark 6 or 400°F or 200°C.
2　Mix the dry ingredients together.
3　Melt the butter and honey and add to the milk.
4　Beat the liquid ingredients into the flours until a smooth dough forms.
5　Oil a round pizza baking sheet and spread the dough.
6　Prick with a fork.
7　Bake until golden (approx 20 minutes).

Breton pancakes

1 cup buckwheat flour   1 cup cornmeal
1 beaten egg   1¾ cups soya milk

1 Mix the dry ingredients together.
2 Beat the egg and milk together.
3 Add the egg and milk mixture to dry ingredients and beat well.
4 Heat a knob of butter on a hot griddle or frying pan.
5 Pour in ⅓ cup mixture and fry one side until brown and then the other.
6 Keep warm under a low grill (makes 6–8 crisp-edged pancakes).
7 Serve with maple syrup and stewed blueberries for breakfast or dessert.

Serve with tuna or salmon in parsley sauce or with chicken in mushroom sauce for a savoury meal.

Flapjacks

75g/3oz butter   50g/2oz soft brown sugar
2 level tbsp golden syrup   175g/6oz rolled oats

1 Grease a 7in (17.5cm) cake tin.
2 Melt the butter, sugar and golden syrup over low heat.
3 Mix in the oats, then press into the tin.
4 Bake in an oven for 20 minutes at gas mark 4 or 135°F or 180°C until golden.
  Cool in tin and mark into six slices.
5 When firm, cut the slices and remove from the tin.

Lemon and almond cake

2 lemons
225g/8oz castor sugar
1 heaped tsp baking powder

6 large eggs
225g/8oz ground almonds

Syrup
Juice of 3 lemons
crème fraîche

100g/3oz castor sugar

1   Boil the lemons for 1½ hours, keeping an eye on the water level. Cool.
2   Remove the lemon pips and cores and liquidize/blend.
3   Add the eggs, 6oz of sugar and the ground almonds. Beat in the baking powder.
4   Pour into the baking tin. Bake until golden brown.
5   Place the juice of 3 lemons into a sieve. Add the sugar and boil. Simmer to reduce to half.
6   Bake in an oven for 50 minutes at gas mark 5 or 380°F or 190°C.
7   When the cake is done, pierce it with a skewer and pour the syrup over the surface. Leave to cool.
8   Serve the cake with crème fraîche.

Caribbean bananas

25g/1oz butter
1 tsp allspice berries
2 tbsp brandy
Greek ewe's yoghurt and berries to serve

8 bananas, peel and slice
3 tbsp soft brown sugar
2 oranges, rind and juiced

1   Melt the butter in a frying pan. Add the banana slices, sugar and spice.
2   Fry gently until the bananas are soft.
3   Pour over the brandy. Transfer the bananas into a serving dish. Stir in the orange juice. Serve with yoghurt or ice cream.

Cheese sables

175g/6oz cheddar cheese
75g/3oz ground almonds
50g/2oz butter

75g/3oz ground rice
salt and pepper

1 Mix the cheese, ground rice and ground almonds together.
2 Rub the butter into this mixture.
3 Add 5–6 tbsp water and mix to a firm dough.
4 Roll out on a floured surface (rice flour). Cut into small rounds.
5 Place onto a greased baking tray and bake in an oven for 10–15 minutes at gas mark 4 or 350°F or 180°C until golden brown.
6 Store in an airtight container when cool. Keep for one week.

Savoury cheese flapjacks

50g/2oz finely chopped onion
150g/5oz porridge oats
¼ tsp mustard
salt

175g/6oz grated cheddar cheese
1 beaten egg
pinch of rosemary
pepper

1 Gently fry the finely chopped onion in butter for 5 minutes.
2 Add the cheese and oats. Stir well.
3 Beat in the egg and seasoning.
4 Press into the greased tin and bake in the oven for 40 minutes at gas mark 4 or 350°F or 180°C until golden brown.
5 Cut into 8 slices and serve warm or cold.

Thai rice pudding cake

250g/9oz Thai jasmine rice
125g/4oz castor sugar
1 stem lemon grass
6 large eggs, separated

1 litre soya milk
4 cardamom pods
300ml/10 fl oz double cream (goat's)

Topping:
500g tub crème fraîche and berries

1 Bring to the boil the milk, rice, sugar, lemon grass and cardamom seeds, and stir.
2 Reduce the heat and simmer very gently for 25 minutes until the mixture thickens.
3 Remove the lemon grass and cardamom seeds and cool.
4 Stir in the cream and egg yolks.
5 Whisk the egg whites to form stiff peaks.
6 Fold gently into the mixture. Place into a deep 9in (22.5cm) lined cake tin.
7 Bake in the oven at gas mark 3 or 340°F or 170°C until golden brown, and cool before turning out.
8 Serve with the crème fraîche and berries.

Sephardic cake

2 whole large oranges
225g/8oz ground almonds

6 eggs, separated
150g/6oz castor sugar

1 Boil the oranges for one hour until soft. Drain and remove the stones. Liquidize/blend until smooth. Cool.
2 Grease a 10in (25cm) round, loose-bottomed baking tin.
3 Whisk the castor sugar and egg yolks until thick and creamy.
4 Fold the ground almonds and orange pulp very gently into the egg mixture.
5 Pour into the greased tin and bake in the oven for 1½ hours at gas mark 7 or 425°F or 200°C until firm to the touch.
6 Cool and melt chocolate to run down the sides.

Almond and polenta cake

225g/8oz castor sugar
225g/8oz quick-cook polenta

225g/8oz ground almonds
225g/8oz butter, softened

1 Grease a 7in (18cm) loose-based fluted tin with butter.
2 Mix the castor sugar, ground almonds and polenta together in a bowl.
3 Stir in the softened butter until the mixture forms a ball of dough.
4 Press the mixture into the greased tin.
5 Bake in the oven at gas mark 5 or 380°F or 190°C until golden brown and firm to touch.
6 Cool, then turn out onto a plate. Cut into triangular slices and serve. Keeps for three days.

Chocolate fudge cake

250g/9oz plain chocolate
125g/7oz ground almonds
5 tbsp apricot jelly/jam

175g/6oz butter/margarine
4 eggs, separated

1 Preheat the oven. Line an 8½in cake tin with greaseproof paper and brush with melted butter.
2 Break 6oz of chocolate into pieces and place in an ovenproof bowl over hot water to melt. Stir until soft.
3 Cream 4oz of butter with the sugar until pale and fluffy.
4 Stir in the ground almonds, 4 egg yolks and melted chocolate.
5 Whisk the egg whites in a clean bowl until they stand in peaks. (This is the only air you will have in the cake to make it rise.)
6 Fold the egg whites very gently into the chocolate mixture, saving as much of the bubbles as possible.
7 Pour into the tin and bake in the oven for 50 minutes at gas mark 4 or 350°F or 180°C until firm to the touch.
8 Leave to cool for a few minutes, then carefully tip onto a plate.
9 Spread the apricot jam on top.
10 Melt 3oz of chocolate and spread over the top, allowing it to run down the sides – yummy!

This is for those special occasions or for that happy birthday.

There are many good wheat-free, dairy-free and *Candida* recipe books around. Make or buy sodabreads or sour-dough breads. Explore different foods in your diet and, if the changes you make help you, then stick with them for three months. As it can take up to four days to react to a food, leave at least that much time between introducing different foodstuffs. You may wish to try a rotation diet of rye on the first day, potato on the second day, oats on the third day, rice on the fourth day and corn on the fifth day.

This is a quest in which you are trying to determine whether a particular food is upsetting your digestion or immune system. Allergy Care and Lifestyle (*see* Useful addresses, p. 398) have mail-order catalogues which may help you find alternative foods if you live far from a good healthfood shop.

SUMMARY

1   Eat organic fruits and vegetables if you can. If not, peel everything.

2   Eat more foods from lower down the food chain, such as fruits, vegetables, nuts, seeds and cereals. Avoid an excess of meat and dairy foods, so less pesticides will be absorbed from animal fat.

3   Stock your cupboard with interesting foods, especially when undergoing an exclusion diet. Make sure that you have corn tacos, oatcakes, rye crispbreads or ricecakes on hand. Add exciting dishes to your repertoire and try some of the recipes included here.

4   Look around healthfood shops for all the alternative foods and healthy cis cold-pressed oils and organic grains, nuts and seeds. Find out about organic food delivery services from the Soil Association.

5   Try to cook most of your meals from fresh food, so you have control over their content.

6   Make changes and give your new 'diet' three months to help your body renew itself, and stimulate the cells to work efficiently at producing hormones, enzymes and prostaglandins.

7   If you suspect one or two foods are upsetting you – such as wheat or dairy – exclude them one at a time for one month. If it makes a difference to the way you feel, you are halfway there and the second half of the journey will get much easier. Once you begin to taste that feeling of wellness, there is no going back.

8   Variety is the spice of life! Be bold – experiment!

13 Furthering research: let's find the cure

There is no medicine like hope, no incentive so great, and no
tonic so powerful as expectation of something better tomorrow.
Orison Swett Marden

Endometriosis has the dubious distinction of being one of the major enigmas of
modern gynaecology. It rightly deserves this honour of being classified as an enigma
for the simple reason that science has yet definitively to determine the cause of the
disease and, more importantly, has yet to develop a permanent cure. It is especially
enigmatic since it is not a newly discovered disease. Sampson gave an elegant
description of endometriosis in the early 1920s and we have not made much
progress in medically understanding this disease for the 50 years following his
landmark observations. However, since the 1980s, things are beginning to happen at
a rapid pace. Over the past 10 years, more and more scientists have taken on the
challenge of uncovering the nature of these rogue implants and hopefully in our
lifetime we may see the development of a cure for endometriosis.

The reason for the absence of a cure for one of the most prevalent gynaecologic
disorders of our society can be summed up in one statement: 'nobody dies from
endometriosis'. Although women may at times feel like they could die from the pain,
there have been rare reports of serious complications. Endometriosis is a benign
disease. Because of this, most governments are not willing to give much financial
backing for scientific investigations of endometriosis. Just 15 years ago you could count
on your fingers the number of scientists around the world who were actively engaged
in research on endometriosis. But the good news is that this attitude has abruptly
changed over the past 10 years, primarily through the 'grassroots' efforts of afflicted
women. Working through organizations like the International Endometriosis
Association, headquartered in the USA, who aid associations in countries all over the
world, and the separate National British Endometriosis Society, the Endometriosis
Association of Australia, the New Zealand Endometriosis Foundation, and the Nordic
and European groups (and fertility self-help groups like the American Resolve and
British Issue groups), more money has recently become available to scientists through
the lobbying of governments to release more money for this specialized research.
Often women are too ill to raise money on their own behalf to give to drug companies
for research. This new research has begun to shed light on the cause and development
of endometriosis, and will hopefully lead to an understanding of the disease that will
eventually evolve into a medical cure. It would be so wondrous to have at our disposal

a one-application cure that would rid womankind of the pain and infertility of endometriosis, though healthy eating relieves symptoms.

The authors would like to share with you some of the promising areas of scientific investigation that may lead to the cure that women so desperately crave. Current scientific research seems to be centred on investigations of the cause of endometriosis, the biochemistry of the endometriotic implant and therapies, and the design of new drugs to suppress the disease or new surgical techniques to cut out damaged organs. More thought needs to be applied to finding the cause in order to elicit the cure. Only by actually knowing what is triggering this disease can we hope to develop a real cure, instead of just suppressing symptoms. Nutrition is a key player in this discovery as it rules all body biochemical processes.

THE CAUSES OF ENDOMETRIOSIS

In chapter 2 we discussed the current theories of what causes endometriosis. The theory with the most support is that proposed by Sampson in the early 1920s. He noted that endometriosis may be a result of endometrial tissue falling into the abdominal cavity, instead of flowing out of the uterus at the time of the menstrual period. This endometrium attaches to the walls of the abdomen and grows under the influence of the ovarian steroids. However, there is a problem with this theory. It seems that nearly all women have free-floating endometrium in their abdomen at the time of the menstrual period, yet many women do not develop endometriosis. The obvious question thus arises – 'Why do some women appear to be "immune" to endometriosis while other women readily develop the disease?' To answer this question scientists have been actively examining what mechanisms are involved in the attachment of endometrial tissue to the abdominal wall.

ATTACHMENT OF CELLS

The most exciting research has been on molecules that allow two cells to attach or become integrated into each other. The three major types of substances involved in the attachment and growth of endometriotic implants are growth factors, remodelling enzymes and integrins.

The growth factors are hormone-like substances that stimulate cellular growth. They are required for normal cells to divide to form new cells and therefore they allow for tissue growth.

The remodelling enzymes are compounds that enzymatically digest away the connections between cells. These are the enzymes that some cells secrete to digest away the cement that allows cells to be attached to each other. They must be secreted in order for cells, like endometrial cells, to invade or wiggle their way in between the cells of the abdominal cavity.

The physical attachment of cells to each other involves the third type of molecules, the integrins. Integrins are molecules on the surface of cells that allow cells to attach to each other. They are like the glue that allows the endometriotic implant to become permanently attached within the abdominal cavity.

Growth factors

Many cells of the body produce a class of stimulatory molecules that have been called growth factors and cytokines. These factors are very diverse and have been given names which would seem unusual to most people. Since these names can be confusing we will use their initials as we describe them. In women with endometriosis, growth factors and cytokines are secreted primarily by the endometrium itself and also by immune cells (*see* chapter 9). These factors are dumped into the fluids of the abdominal cavity and stimulate the cells of the endometriotic implant to grow. Growth factors are involved in wound healing and cell division, and send signals over short distances, cell to cell.

The five major growth factors and cytokines found in the fluids of the abdominal cavity are IGF (insulin-like growth factor), EGF (epithelial growth factor), VEGF (vascular epithelial growth factor), IL-1 (interleukin-1) and TNF (tumour necrosis factor).[1] Laboratory experiments have shown that abdominal fluid and some of these compounds stimulate the growth of the endometrium. Furthermore, the abdominal fluid of women with endometriosis contains more VEGF, IL-1 and TNF than that of women who do not have the disease. We have not yet investigated all of the growth factors/cytokines, but by understanding these substances better we may come up with a means of preventing growth of endometriotic implants.

Remodelling enzymes

As the endometrial tissue attaches to the abdominal wall, the cells of the abdominal wall must be separated to allow the endometrial cells to wedge themselves in between the cells of the abdominal wall. This remodelling of the cells of the abdominal wall is controlled by two groups of proteins, the MMPs (metalloproteinases) and TIMPs (tissue inhibitors of MMPs). MMPs (which are based upon the minerals zinc and magnesium) digest the connections between cells, and TIMPs inhibit this action. As the endometrium attaches to the wall of the abdomen MMPs are secreted, and the endometrium worms its way into the abdominal wall. TIMP molecules are secreted at the same time to prevent the digestion of the abdominal tissue next to the endometrium. For endometrial tissue, the production of the remodelling enzymes is controlled by the ovarian steroid hormone progesterone.[2] This may be why the endometriosis reattaches and gets worse with each menstrual cycle. The oestrogen and progesterone produced in each menstrual period is conducive to endometrial implantation into the abdominal wall. Another exciting bit of laboratory research has been the discovery that suppression of MMPs prevents the attachment of endometrium to abdominal cells.[3] This has not been tested in humans, but if a form of treatment could be developed that did not have bad side effects, the potential therapeutic benefits would be great. Remember that magnesium, vitamins A, E and C and cis fatty acids give cell membranes their integrity so harmful drugs are unnecessary.

Integrins

Each cell has to be able to 'stick' to another and the surrounding tissue to form our body structure. This adhesion material is collectively known as 'integrins'. In addition to maintaining the structure of our body, integrins are important in the healing of wounds and for the development of the embryo. Once again the 'stickiness' has to be just right. The mesh formed by integrins is made of gel-like chains of sugars and proteins, as well as collagen. It is rather like the cell having Velcro made of proteins on the outside. This Velcro surface sticks to the protein scaffold on the next cell wall, which makes up the connective tissue known as collagen (using vitamins A, C and zinc).

Over 20 different types of integrins have been found so far and the number of integrins discovered in the human endometrium and in endometriosis continues to grow.[4] Additionally, the integrins of the endometriotic implant are different from those of the endometrium of the uterus.[5] The role of these differences is still under investigation. When and how the first regurgitated endometrial fragment comes into contact with the peritoneal lining, and how it apposes, attaches and subsequently invades remains enigmatic.

The integrins can have a very powerful effect on cells. If these contacts are lost, dividing cells stop proliferating and die. The messages passed via integrins from outside and inside all cells depends upon the quality of integrins. If we could selectively inhibit the integrins of the endometriotic implant, it would cause the death of the endometriosis. There is some evidence that the function of integrins is modulated by lipids, so again the type of cis oils in the diet may play a role.

By studying the molecules involved in the growth and development of the endometriotic implants, scientists may be able to better understand why some women get endometriosis and others do not. It is hoped that we can mimic the effects seen in the abdomens of the women without endometriosis as a cure for women who develop endometriosis.

THE IMMUNE SYSTEM

One of the more promising areas of research has been the role of the immune system in the development and maintenance of endometriosis. As we discussed in chapter 9, the immune system of the endometriosis patient appears to be altered, and this alteration may be one of the main reasons why some women develop endometriosis while others do not. The first indication that the immune system may have gone awry was the observation in the early 1980s that the macrophages of the abdominal cavity were different in patients with endometriosis to those in disease-free patients.[6, 7] We now know that these macrophages make some of the growth factors/cytokines mentioned above and that they stimulate endometrial growth and therefore the endometriotic implant.[8] 'Neutrophils and macrophages produce FORs, including superoxide anion and hydrogen peroxide. Studies have shown that hydrogen peroxide at a low dose can stimulate progesterone secretion from midcycle luteal cells (of the ovary). However, higher doses inhibited progesterone secretion.'[9] More recently, laboratory experiments were presented by Nothnick and Vernon at the international endometriosis meetings in Yokohama, Japan, that suggest that implant growth will not progress in the absence of macrophages.[10] The administration of a compound that inhibits the activation of macrophages (pentoxifylline) prevented the invasion and development of endometriotic implants. Research by Nothnick and colleagues has suggested that pentoxifylline reduces endometrial implant size independent of steroid levels (no effect on cyclicity, or ovarian or uterine macrophages).[11] These studies have not been tested in long-term human studies, but the initial results are encouraging, although a loss of macrophages and weakening of the immune system could lead to major health problems and death.

THE ENDOMETRIOTIC IMPLANT

One of the reasons why very little progress has been made in endometriosis research is related to the fact that most research over the past 30 years has dealt exclusively with treatment. Very little work has been directed towards the study of the pathology and physiology of the disease. Money can only be made by drug companies in developing drugs so the crucial basic cellular science work is neglected.

However, there has been a recent interest in studying how the endometriotic implant functions. In particular, the implants have been examined for their capacity to secrete substances that may be of physiological importance. We have already seen from the above discussion that many scientists have examined the implants' ability to produce a variety of substances (such as growth hormones, cytokines and integrins). There has also been an interest in examining the proteins produced by implants. Drs Sharpe and Vernon have shown that endometriotic implants are prolific in manufacturing proteins and that they produce hundreds of different proteins.[12] However, when they compared the implant with the endometrium, they noted that two unique proteins were produced by the implant, and not by the endometrium of the uterus. These two proteins were called endo 1 and endo 2 (endometriotic implant proteins 1 and 2). Dr Sharpe has purified, isolated and determined that these proteins are TIMP (see pp. 79, 306) and a large protein called haptoglobin.

These are exciting discoveries since these proteins may serve as markers of the disease. It may be possible some day to collect a blood or abdominal fluid sample to determine if a person has endometriosis and perhaps even be able to tell how severe the disease is. This would be much better than performing a laparoscopic examination under general anaesthesia.

PRION PROTEINS

Strange prion proteins, responsible for 'mad cow disease', have been cast as 'social deviants' because their only known function was to wreak havoc. But new research is beginning to show that prion proteins may have an important role to play in health. A geneticist at the National Institute of Health in Washington DC has discovered prions in yeasts. Some researchers believe that prion proteins may help the fertilized egg to become a multicellular organism. At some point in this transformation the embryo cells decide whether to become liver, muscle or other tissue. Once they have made that decision, all their progeny have to stick with it. Yet all cells carry the same genetic code, so it is unclear just how these cells pass on this vital information. Prions could be responsible. Cells in different tissues manufacture different types of protein, some of which keep the correct genes for that tissue turned on. If these regulatory proteins had the ability to spread their influence as prions do, then dividing cells within a tissue would automatically know which genes to turn on. Some of these phenomena could be to do with prions.[13]

When a group of cells in the developing animal begin to change into a different type of tissue, large amounts of regulatory proteins appear in a cascade which later subsides. Researchers have identified these prion proteins which allow yeasts to change between the two types, though it is too early in the research to see specifics. This new area of research may show why normal endometrium tissue within the uterus turns into endometriotic implants outside the uterus, producing its own oestrogens and proteins. We have to wait and see …

BEHAVIOUR OF ENDOMETRIUM

'The early phases in the pathogenesis of endometriosis are still poorly understood. When and how the first regurgitated endometrial fragment comes into contact with the peritoneal lining, how it apposes and attaches, and subsequently invades remains enigmatic. These fragments in a direct or indirect way cause damage to the peritoneal, mesolthelial lining, thus exposing the extracellular matrix and creating adhesion sites for the endometrial implants. Mesothelium has Teflon characteristics rather than Velcro, and forms the first line of defence against penetration by endometrial fragments.'[14] This research is trying to deduce the way in which the cell membranes are being breeched by the endometrial fragments. By looking at how the cell membrane functions, it may be possible to work out how to prevent these fragments from invading the tissue. It is working out how to stop the adherence which will provide the cure.[14]

Tracking the growth patterns

Other research is looking at the monthly shedding of the endometrium and how it grows and disintegrates cyclically. 'The critical part of the process of endometrial growth and regression is the growth and regression of blood vessels that supply the endometrium.'[15] This study is looking at how protein and messenger RNA (mRNA) determine gene expression and, thus, the protein levels in the endometrium. They are trying to track and understand biological functions such as the growth and the development of endometrial cells to see how they degenerate into endometrial implants growing outside the uterus cavity and how they develop their own blood supply.[15]

The Genome Project report

Familial endometriosis is well recognized from several studies that have described smaller clusters and sister-pairs with a five- to nine-fold higher risk in first-degree relatives. The relative risk is not only raised among sisters, but also cousins. The disease can be inherited through the paternal as well as maternal side. Studies of families suggest two phenotypes in relation to close family members – one with an early onset of disease characterized by severe dysmenorrhoea and more subfertility, the other with a later onset and shorter prodroma (time between onset of first symptoms and development of the disease) before diagnosis, and less effect on fertility. This research in Iceland is linked closely with the Genome Project at Oxford with Stephen Kennedy. Iceland is a useful research area as the community is very tightly knit, and clear records have been kept for hundreds of years, such that endometriosis on the islands has been traced down to just seven families. You can log on and add your own family's history of endometriosis at www.medicine.ox.ac.uk/ndog/oxegene.htm.[16]

Environmental and genetic factors

There is one review of all studies investigating the association between endometriosis and various genetic and environmental risk factors. Prevention of endometriosis may only be possible if we understand more about the ways in which we can modify the environmental and genetic factors that influence the development of this disease. 'Greater exposure to retrograde menstruation (heavy, frequent and long duration of bleeding) and oestrogen (unopposed ovulation, high body mass index) are likely to increase endometriosis risk. Smoking and exercise may decrease the risk through the reduction of oestrogen levels. Dioxins appear to increase the risk in primate studies. It is important in all studies to have consistent disease definition and good design in order to replicate the findings.'[17]

Endometriosis Association data

Since 1980, the Endometriosis Association in the USA has grown to include members and support groups in 66 countries. Data on the symptomatology of endometriosis from the EA research registry encompasses the medical and family histories of over 4,000 women, with particular focus on pain, onset of symptoms and how the disease affects overall quality of life. Pain is the most common symptom – and menstrual pain is a particular problem in 98 per cent of those whose symptoms started before the age of 20. An important trend observed in comparison to data collected in the 1980s shows that endometriosis appears to now be starting at a younger age, and that severe pain is significantly more common in those whose first pelvic symptoms began before the age of 15. In fact, 60 per cent had their first symptoms before the age of 20 (38 per cent before the age of 15). Attention needs to be paid to early diagnosis in teenagers, and preventative treatment needs to be found in order to devise the best long-term treatment plan to manage this chronic disease.[18]

Emerging research

Some examples of the progress in research on endometriosis were reported, at the April 2001 National Institutes of Health Symposium, by Kevin Osteen for the Endometriosis Association's Research programme:

- A focus on what's happening at the very beginning of implantation of endometrial tissue – presumably the very early stages of the pelvic disease – has also highlighted the extremely important role of progesterone in endometriosis. It is felt that, in endometriosis, one of two progesterone receptors is not working.
- A return of interest in prostaglandins, overlooked since the early and mid-1980s, bodes well for increased attention to the inflammatory aspects of endometriosis and a deepened understanding of the immune system's role in creating the disease and symptoms. This, in turn, should lead to more immunological treatments in the future.
- Work supported by the EA shows that certain immune reactions originally noted in cancer further the understanding of endometriosis as a potential autoimmune disease and offer promise for a non-invasive diagnostic technique, as well as helping gain acceptance for immunotherapy treatment.
- Sherry Rier, PhD and holder of the Tracy H. Dickinson Research Chair of the Endometriosis Association, presented her just-published research showing that certain PCBs previously unsuspected in endometriosis appear to play key roles. (PCBs are a type of dioxin.)
- A representative of the Environmental Health Science Bureau of Health in Canada presented work in which exposure to dioxin resulted in a significantly higher survival of endometrial implants in monkeys and significantly larger implants compared with the control group. The conclusion was that dioxin made it easier for endometrial implants to thrive. Analysis of the fluid around the ovaries in women going to fertility clinics reveals a broad range of chemicals, including PCBs and pesticides.
- The Endometriosis Association has an open research fund to aid clinical research and looks forward to receiving more clinical research proposals.[19]

Designer oestrogens

A variety of oestrogen-like molecules are being developed to reduce or avoid the 'bad' effects of the hormone and/or mimic 'good' effects. Such molecules are popularly called 'designer oestrogens'. Pertinent examples are tamoxifen and raloxifene. Other drugs are targeted just to one aspect of oestrogen function – for example, the bisphosphonates, such as alendronate, which act specifically on bone metabolism.[20] This ongoing research is trying to find ways in which oestrogen dominance may be rebalanced within the body. Because the growth of endometriotic implants is dependent upon oestrogen, women with endometriosis feel that they must find a way to balance the oestrogen to stop it causing harm to healthy tissue. However, oestrogen does many good things in the body (*see* p. 223 on how to make oestrogens safer using indoles and phytonutrition).

Endometriosis and cancer: similar yet different

The EA has been struck by the similarities between endometriosis and cancer. The cancer data from the North American survey brought home how prevalent cancer is in women with endometriosis and their families. Endometriosis has long been considered as 'benign cancer' by some experts. This is not to say that it will develop into cancer, as it never happens in the vast majority of women. But there may be some mechanism involving lifestyle choices or diet, or a weak genetic link that may be a trigger factor in susceptible people. By trying to improve health, it may be possible to counteract the risk. Dioxins have long been considered one of the most powerful cancer-causing agents known to man. It is therefore logical to assume that if some women with endometriosis have been exposed to dioxins, this may also make them susceptible to cancer. There is some research looking at all the links and parallels between these two diseases.[21] Women who believe they may be at risk with a strong family history of cancers should ensure that their doctors are kept informed. All women are advised to eat a low-fat diet rich in the good cis fatty acids, and avoid excess saturated and trans fats in their diet. Also, the avoidance of talcum powder is suggested. As Mary-Lou Ballweg states, 'No one knows better than a woman living with endometriosis that good health is not "given". No-one has a greater stake in our good health than we do.'

NUTRITION RESEARCH

There has been a lack of well-controlled experiments involving sufficient numbers of women with the specific condition of endometriosis. However, there have been other trials which have looked at the role of nutrients in relation to symptoms of pain, fatigue, heavy periods and fertilization. There have been numerous studies on nutrition and its effects on reproduction and the uterus, but to our knowledge there has only been one endometriosis study that has looked at women's health and symptomatology with regard to the use of supplements and diet. Research into the nutritional status of the endometriosis patient looked at 20 women diagnosed with endometriosis and 10 women with no history of female complaints (acting as controls), for a three-month period. The women were matched in pairs according to deficiency symptoms; each pair was then randomly split into two groups – A and B. A placebo or nutrition supplement containing thiamine (100mg), riboflavin (100mg), pyridoxine (100mg), magnesium amino acid chelate (300mg) and zinc orotate (20mg) was taken for three months. During the three months the women with endometriosis in the placebo group showed no statistically significant change in their symptoms, whereas the women with endometriosis on the supplement showed a statistically significant (98 per cent) improvement of their symptoms. The study suggests that nutritional supplementation and/or an improvement in the diet may offer significant alleviation of some of the symptoms which we perceive to be linked to endometriosis.[22] Much of this information is included in this book and it is hoped that this information will stimulate an increase in awareness of the importance of doing nutritional research on endometriosis.

Further detailed research assessing the vitamin and mineral status of women with endometriosis may well show up certain anomalies in body biochemistry that we may be able to use to our advantage in treating the symptoms of endometriosis. Whether these anomalies are due to a poor diet, malabsorption or a genetic enzyme failure may hold a clue to the elusive cure for endometriosis. By assessing B vitamin levels, red cell, magnesium, white cell, zinc, liver enzyme status, hair mineral analysis, thyroid profile, thyroid auto-antibodies, allergy screen, gluten sensitivity evaluation, gut fermentation study, liver profile, *Chlamydia* species specific antibody screen, and hormone profiles, we may find a commonality to help research follow the right path. Research has shown ways in which nutrients and changes in diet may be used to alleviate pain, inflammation, fatigue and PMS symptoms. We can harness that information to help improve our health. Orthodox treatments currently fall short of curing the disease; correcting the basic body biochemistry of each individual may be a start. We are at a crossroads when a combination of research in different fields may combine to provide the cure.

Research beginning in 2002 is looking at the effect of wheat on endometriotic implants to ascertain whether it impacts on the inflammatory status. This research will also assess whether or not the hormones in the wheat genome have an effect on oestrogens.

THE ELUSIVE CURE

The bottom line for endometriosis research is to develop a cure. It should be evident from the above discussion that there is much hope for a cure. What we should learn from the study of endometriosis is that the body is not a set of disparate organs. We can no longer compartmentalize the organs into the separate digestive, immune and endocrine systems as they all work together. Gynaecologists need to become immunologists and gastroenterologists, and vice versa, or work very closely together. Nutrition helps the body as a whole; it is true holistic and preventive medicine for the future. Orthodox medicine has not yet reached this point of knowledge but it must if we are to find a cure. Nutritional assessment should be a major part of the cure.

The main driving force behind the development of a cure is the procurement of the funds required by nutritionists to continue their research. Through the efforts of many 'grassroots' groups, funding has increased for endometriosis research, but we must guard against slowing down our efforts when we are so near having a potential cure. We must unite to encourage increases in the government funding of endometriosis research. Our daughters must not have the threat of this illness hanging over them like the sword of Damocles; it is currently estimated that 'one in 20 sufferers will be teenagers'.[23] How could we ever want any of our daughters to suffer what we are going through? Present statistics demand action: 'With the present world population of six billion, not less than 200 million women should therefore have endometriosis. By the year 2025 the world population could reach 10 billion with the potential of half a billion women suffering from this disease.'[24] Women need to push forward the research effort on endometriosis.

Let us all hope that a second edition of this book will not be needed because of the development of a cure. What a pleasant thought!

> There is nothing so far removed from us to be beyond our reach, or so hidden as to be that we cannot discover it.
>
> *René Descartes, French philosopher*

SUMMARY

1 Encourage government funding of basic research to find a cure.

2 A cure will only come when we know why endometriosis occurs. Suppression by drugs is not a cure. When the drugs are stopped the endometriosis comes back, often within 18 months.

3 Encourage research which shows how cells function.

4 Support your local endometriosis charity, even if you do not attend the meetings. Stay in contact with the group leader to encourage and support research. Local companies may be willing to give to the charities. Persuade family members to leave a legacy in their wills. (Look up www.endometriosis.co.uk.)

5 Watch little girls at play. Do you really want them to grow up and experience what women with endometriosis have to go through? The answer is always NO. No one should have to endure this pain. Make yourself heard either through your local group or at a national level.

6 The interest in medical research has increased greatly over the past 10 years. However, relative to other areas of science, very few governmental resources have been applied to endometriosis research.

7 Some promising areas of research include those which look at growth factors, the immune system, integrins and specific proteins which are excreted, as well as looking at basic body biochemistry and cell behaviour.

8 Although nutrition can have an amazing impact on endometriosis there has been a lack of well-controlled research. By looking at a large group of women and comparing their basic body chemistry, we may be able to find exactly what imbalances exist in body cells which could be common to us all. This could point to a cure and treatment for the source of the problem. Healthy eating often alleviates the symptoms.

9 Nutrition affects all body systems, the reproductive, immune, digestive and nervous systems, which are all interlinked. We have to move away from the idea that just the womb and ovaries are involved in endometriosis. As we have seen in this book, this disease is systemic. It affects the whole body.

10 Become informed of research and the choices open to you. You can only make a true choice for your own treatment if you have been given an informed choice. If access to some orthodox and holistic treatments are being hidden or even denied you, then be suspicious. Ask questions until you are happy with the answers. Ulterior motives abound, usually to do with profit, not your health.

> Whatever you can do, or dream you can, begin it. Boldness has genius, power and magic in it.
>
> *Johann Wolfgang von Goethe, 1749–1832*

14 Colour the body healthy: key steps to recovery

> Tell me and I forget, teach me and I learn, involve me and I remember.
>
> *Benjamin Franklin*

The key to healing endometriosis lies in healing the whole body. This ability is in your hands should you choose to use it. As we have seen time and time again, all body systems are linked to one another by receptor cells which respond to hormones and enzymes. The whole body behaves as one entity for a good reason – it is!

Nutritional medicine is not magic – it merely helps you to improve the workings of each system and so that you can correct all the imbalances. These happen due to stress, environmental pollution, poor digestion or contaminated foods, or long-term use of antibiotics, steroids or non-steroidal anti-inflammatory drugs (NSAIDs). Stress and trauma can also upset the apple cart, so that normal homeostasis in the body gets flung sideways. It happens to us when we least expect it, often after illness when the body is run down or after a very stressful episode in one's life. Family and friends who love you will support you through the bad times.

THE INDIVIDUAL APPROACH

Individually orientated nutritional medicine is a unique approach in which the consultant tries to discover everything that can possibly be done to bring that particular person back to optimum health. Conventional medicine uses protocols for each disease state, and the attitude is that whatever is found to be wrong rises above individuality and forms a pattern of treatment that can be applied to everyone else with that condition. Doctors develop 'protocols' for each illness and everyone with that illness is treated according to the prescribed protocol regardless of whether or not it suits them. Thus, treatments are the same for everyone with a given disease, with no consideration for individuality in body biochemistry.

In contrast, nutritional therapy tries to harmonize each person's unique body biochemistry. The body is constantly synthesizing, manufacturing, creating and rebuilding. A key feature of this chemical factory is the communication system used between cells. If that goes wrong, then the whole body can no longer function. Each cell produces prostanoid hormones that are involved in this long-distance message-carrying which are dependent upon the oils and proteins we choose to eat. There are $100,000,000,000,000$ or 10^{13} cells that have to communicate each second. The cell membrane is as fine as the gossamer wings of a fairy, and requires oils and magnesium to maintain its integrity. The whole working of our body is passed between these vital cell membranes, and its size is vast, the equivalent of 10 football fields, so a lot of good oils are required.[1]

Your body has developed an array of features to test whether or not foods suit you as an individual. Smell and taste are the obvious ones. If something is not right for you, you avoid it. If you do eat something wrong, you may develop bad indigestion, or even be sick or have terrible diarrhoea as the body rejects it. The liver is fairly efficient at expelling anything foul if it cannot detoxify the substance. We all have to work within these senses. If we sense that a particular food makes us feel queasy, or causes heartburn or makes us bloated or constipated, then we should have the sense to avoid it. Listen more to what your body is telling you. Once foods are metabolized, they become a part of you. Everything that you have eaten in the past seven years is now firmly embedded within your structure. This is how anthropologists can work out the past lives and diets from the bodies found in ancient burial grounds and in mummies.

A good nutritionist will listen very carefully to what you tell them about all your health problems. Nothing is irrelevant, and alongside the information taken from a questionnaire are all the little niggly details adding up to the big picture of how the body is malfunctioning. The most important facts of each patient's story may often seem to be the irrelevant details of past illnesses and exposures to pollutants. The question, 'Could the sticky brown blood at period time be causing worse pain symptoms?' or 'I eat paper every day – could this be making me ill?' is pertinent to the problem. Some people can easily be made ill by a food that nourishes and sustains another, and the nutritionist is like a detective who listens and learns from you in order to solve the mystery. Modern medicine often only sees a truth in medical textbooks after peer-reviewed papers have been selected. What we need most is a dialogue between clinicians who have direct experience with patients who show convincing positive reactions to a diet and academics who are more focused on drug trials.

DECISIONS, DECISIONS, DECISIONS

You need to make a decision as to how to proceed. Having read through this book, it is essential to sort out the stages that are necessary for you to follow for your particular situation. Because we are all so different and because endometriosis can manifest itself in so many different guises in the body, it is crucial that you assess each body system and decide what needs sorting out first. Work with your diary and plan a time when it will be best for you to start. Plan meals and sort out recipes. Write out a weekly shopping list so that it becomes easier to follow. Spend some time looking at the different healthfood shops in your area – the small independent ones are usually the best for variety. Try out some of the alternative foods at weekends and try out some different dishes. If you like what you make, perhaps on another weekend you could batch-bake and put portions into the freezer. This will be helpful once you are in the swing of things. Planning will help you to stay on track. When eating out at cafés and restaurants, begin by sussing out the menu to find what you are able to eat once you are on the programme. Start looking at food for its health-giving properties and the ways in which you are going to use it to regain your life.

By contacting a well-qualified nutritionist and following the HELP system, a healthy eating life programme (for this is what a diet truly is), you can aid the body in working at its most optimum levels. What is required for health is for all the enzyme and hormone systems and neurotransmitters to be working at peak form as a result of absorbing nutrients. The digestive system disassembles nutrients and sends them into body cells, where they are reassembled into the forms that the body needs to rebuild and heal itself.

The questions we need to ask of ourselves are:

1   What kind of foods and nutrients does this person need to get in order to thrive?
2   What kinds of foods and environmental pollutants should this person avoid in order to thrive?

Remember these facts:

* The bone marrow makes 2.5 million red blood cells every second
* The human stomach produces a new layer of mucus every two days to prevent it from digesting itself
* The lining of the digestive tract is replaced every four days
* All the amino acids you eat are made into 50,000 different proteins and 20,000 enzymes that the body requires daily
* White blood cells are replaced every 10 days
* New skin is replaced every 24 days

If the body can work at this pace and be so efficient, then we owe it some effort to work with it so that it will at least have a chance of making us well again.

> When you are in the company of angels and starshine, things are looking up.
>
> *Douglas Pagels*

FOOD FOR HEALTH

Modern medicine does not consider food to have health-giving qualities. Instead, food is seen as a commodity to be bought and sold for profit. The connection between body biochemistry and vitamins and minerals as cofactors and coenzymes in body cells is not taught in medical schools. We need to move back to this form of medicine, where both drug therapy and food are used side by side as preventative medicine. They go hand in hand. Indeed, a healthy diet may be thought of as preventative medicine, as healing the gut membrane and replenishing the vital gut flora are the first goals of treatment when someone is ill.

In 1971 the World Health Organization set up a repository of information on healing plants at the University of Illinois' pharmacy department. They studied 50,000 scientific references concerning the healing substances found in foods. When they compared 140 com-pounds in 90 plants, they found that 74 per cent correlated with the purified active chemical and the condition they were used to cure in folk medicine. Looking back at Ayurvedic scripts and Chinese scrolls from 1500 BC, the same knowledge existed even then, yet is still undergoing rigorous trials in modern medical laboratories. Research which has been carried out by nutrition departments in world-renown universities is not believed by the medical Establishment. Excellent research is not accepted by medical journals, so it is only published in nutrition journals. But unless these papers are peer-reviewed for publication in, for example, *The Lancet, British Medical Journal* or *JAMA*, this nutrition research goes unheard of and unseen by the medical profession who do not take the time to read nutrition journals. Good nutrition research therefore never gets published in mainstream medical journals unless it is repeated by a medical team – a very sad state of affairs.

Nutrition is no longer taught adequately in schools as 'home economics' became too expensive to fund. The government expects the public to buy the food in shops and supermarkets which all looks very healthy and is brightly packaged. We know from research by Professor Tim Lange at South Thames University that 44 per cent of the population buy convenience foods only and rarely cook. Food is just something to be bought and sold, and it is this attitude that needs to be changed. After the 'mad-cow disease' crisis, the genetic modification that threatens natural foods and the horrors of the foot-and-mouth epidemic, we can all understand the need for us to have pure and healthy food to eat, untainted by chemicals and manipulation by humans.

How are we to change the attitudes of people who think of food as a commodity to thinking of food as something to use to maintain health and support us into a healthy old age? Only by teaching good nutrition and by understanding the very nature of food itself. The Nordic countries have a nutrition policy in which they state that they do not want their elderly population to be ill. Therefore, they are advising the younger members of their countries on how to eat healthily and maintain health into old age.

RAINBOW-COLOURED MEALS

The most important thing you can do is choose the foods you eat wisely. Food costs may increase as you try to plan what is best for you to buy. But if you are eating less expensive meat, dairy foods and chocolates, and more legumes and fish, then it should balance out. Changing from bread- and wheat-based foods to rye- , oat- , corn- and rice-based foods may cost a little more now. But in the long term, these changes will be beneficial, and the difference in your health will be worth the small sacrifices along the way. Try to avoid all processed foods as much as possible and use only those that are full to the brim with nutrients. This means buying the freshest foods you can find and going back to a basic 'Stone Age'-type diet, consisting of fresh fruits, vegetables, cold-pressed oils, lean meat, fish, pulses/legumes, and nuts and seeds. It is not difficult to do once you get into the swing.

The colours of foods are a key to the ways in which they may benefit the body. The colour usually equates to the phytochemicals found in the food – flavonoids and indoles are contained in green vegetables, carotenoids in red/yellow/orange fruits and vegetables, proanthocyanidins in blue/red berries. Using a wide variety of foods with different colour schemes on your lunch and dinner plates can help to ensure that a range of these helpful phytochemicals are taken into the bloodstream to aid the body in its healing process.

Eating rainbow-coloured meals ensures that you obtain the variety of nutrients your body needs. When eating out, choose the options that provide the largest amount of fresh vegetables and fruits. By eating the more natural option, we increase our ability to stay healthy.

> The more we depart from the state of nature, the more we lose our natural tastes.
>
> *Jean-Jacques Rousseau, French philosopher*

When choosing foods to eat, we need to consider the quality:

First quality:	fresh and raw
Second quality:	fresh and lightly cooked
Third quality:	frozen
Fourth quality:	tinned.

The top two levels of quality should be our first choices; frozen is reasonable – as the food is rapidly processed and packaged after picking, the nutrients are still fairly well preserved. Tinned foods should be at the bottom of the list as emergency foods for when you are in a hurry or pressed for time.

When choosing ready-made meals, we need to be discerning. A lot of packaged foods contain various food additives, pesticide residues and added synthetic growth hormones. Small amounts of prepared foods are fine, but they should not be consumed as an everyday meal. Besides, manufactured dishes cost far more to buy than when they are made from fresh. At weekends, you could do a batch-bake and make one dish for that day and freeze three or four others for those busy evenings when you are too tired to cook.

FOOD CHOICE QUIZ

What is the quality of your choices of foods at present? Look at the following and choose one food from each group that is closest to what you are currently eating at this time.

1 Typical breakfast
   a Bowl of wholegrain cereal with nuts and berries
   b Fresh fruit salad with a fruit & nut bar
   c White toast with marmalade
   d Iced Danish pastry

2 Typical midmorning snack
   a Piece of fresh fruit
   b Handful of nuts and seeds
   c Few sweet biscuits
   d Chocolate bar

3 Typical sandwich lunch
   a Salad platter with turkey
   b Wholegrain bread with salad and tuna or salmon filling
   c Egg mayonnaise and bacon with lettuce
   d Fast-food beefburger and chips

4 Typical afternoon tea snack
   a Hummus and crudités
   b Fresh fruit
   c Tea and wholemeal biscuits
   d Chocolate bar and coffee

5 Typical evening meal
   a Steamed fish and fresh vegetables
   b Pasta in tomato and basil sauce with tuna
   c Roast beef with roast potatoes and parsnips
   d Sausage and mash with baked beans

6 Typical main meal vegetables
   a Steamed broccoli and carrots
   b Frozen peas and sweetcorn
   c Sweetcorn and tomato on a pizza or in pasta sauce
   d Chips and beans

7 Typical supper dish
   a Fruit and mineral water
   b Herb tea and oatcakes
   c Milky drink and biscuits
   d Crisps and drinking chocolate

8 Typical restaurant meal
   a Salad and white meat or steamed fish and vegetables
   b Vegetable curry and boiled rice
   c Roast pork and vegetables
   d Pizza and chips

9 Typical dessert
   a Fruits and cheese board
   b Yoghurt and berry fruits
   d Cheesecake and cream
   c Death by chocolate

10 Typical drinks throughout the day
    a Mineral water and herb teas
    b Fruit juices and tea
    c Coffee and squash
    d Tinned fizzy drinks containing aspartame.

If most of your answers are a and b, then you are choosing the best-quality and freshest food choices. If you are choosing c most often, then you are missing a lot of nutrients from the fresher foods. If your main answers are d, then you are probably taking in very low levels of vitamins and minerals, and need to reassess your food choices and try to include more fresh food into your diet.

Look at a typical office worker who rises early, struggles into work via a long train journey, has no time to eat well at lunchtime so snatches and grabs a meals at the desk, then rushes home. Once at home, he or she is so tired that they prepare a fast-food meal and flop.

Often, food in modern diets is high in refined carbohydrates (starches and sugars), which should be replaced by complex carbohydrates to provide more fibre to soak up the excess oestrogen and cholesterol. These high levels of sugars will cause sugar to be dumped into the bloodstream, which creates an insulin response. The body then converts the sugar into fats. This is an easy way to put on excess weight and, in the long term, there is the risk of diabetes developing as the pancreas is overstimulated. Fibre from complex carbohydrates, on the other hand, will cleanse the bowels and absorb more waste toxins, thus protecting the intestinal membranes.

The present foods are low in vital nutrients whereas the new food choices contain far more vitamins, minerals and essential fatty acids of the cis variety. The old diet was high in trans fatty acids, which we know behave more like saturated animal fats in the body. The fresh fruits and vegetables in the new diet will also provide soluble fibres and phytochemicals that benefit the body through their protective antioxidant effects.

Eating meals should be a relaxed affair. Modern life, with its snatched meals, does not allow for the release of digestive enzymes whereas leisurely mealtimes do. We have also removed the vast amounts of caffeine from the diet and added more drinks which

Meal	Food now	New food choice
Breakfast	Danish pastry Coffee	Fruit & nut bar Herb tea
Midmorning snack	Chocolate bar Coffee	Nuts and seeds Mineral water
Lunch	Cheese & pickle sandwich Biscuit and coffee	Salmon salad sandwich Fruit Tea with lemon
Midday snack	Crisps Coffee	Fruit & nut bar Mineral water
Dinner	Pasta in tomato sauce Coffee and Ice cream	Trout in lemon sauce Broccoli Grilled tomato New potatoes Herb tea Fruit
Snacks	Sweets, biscuits, coffee and chocolate	Fresh fruits, nuts & seeds

aid the function of body cells and the kidneys. More fish is eaten – this should be deep-sea fish wherever possible to reduce the pesticide load. Also, less processed and packaged foods and more fresh foods are eaten.

Office workers tend to drink an excess amount of coffee as it is easy to get from machines. Caffeine is a diuretic and locks up minerals such as calcium, magnesium and zinc, preventing their uptake. In the long term, this could lead to osteoporosis.

Fizzy drinks contain phosphorus, which reduces absorption of calcium, so these should also be kept to a minimum to protect the bones. Weight may be lost dramatically once a healthy diet is eaten. Many people often remark that they are eating more on a healthy diet and yet have lost weight. Try it for one month and see if your energy and vitality improve. Avoiding empty-calorie foods and replacing them with foods rich in nutrients will have a dramatic effect on health in most people.

MENU SUGGESTIONS

Breakfast

Muesli with berries, nuts & seeds
Porridge with berry fruits & honey
Egg-fried rice with vegetables
Potato cakes and eggs or beans
Smoked salmon and scrambled eggs
Kippers or haddock
Rice cakes and nut butters
Corn crispbreads and hummus
Poached egg and toast
Omelettes
Beans/egg/tomatoes/mushrooms on toast

Hors d'ouevres

Crudités and dips
Avocado soup
Green salad
Fruit sorbet/salad
Tuna and avocado

Soups

Vegetable soup
Avocado soup
Watercress soup
Vichyssoise soup
Courgette and spinach soup
Carrot and almond soup

Main meals

Salads with meat or fish, eggs or beans
White fish with steamed vegetables (red and green)
Oily fish with salad and jacket potato
Corn tortilla and salad, avocado dip, beans and cheese
Nut loaf with jacket potato and green vegetables
Stuffed aubergine or pepper and salad with rice
Lentil bake with mixed vegetables
Omelette and salad or Spanish style
Lamb with lemon and olives with rice and green salad
Poultry dish with vegetables

Desserts

Fruit salads
Poached pears with cinnamon and apple juice
Stuffed peaches with ground almonds and apricots, and orange juice
Baked egg custard
Baked apple with berry yoghurt
Grilled banana and honey
Brown rice pudding
Bread and butter pudding with stewed apples

Snacks

Fruits and nut bars
Nuts & seeds
Poppadoms
Corn crispbreads and dips
Plain crisps
Corn tacos

Drinks

Filtered or mineral water
Herbal teas
Barleycup, Caro or Yannah coffee substitutes
Diluted fruit juices
Elderflower cordial
Earl Grey, darjeeling, lapsang souchong teas with lemon

Gabi of London

This is a typical week of what I eat. It's quite varied and illustrates that there is life without wheat, citrus, chocolate, coffee and processed foods. After a week, I found I really looked forward to some foods – fruits and yoghurt or fish. Not all the foods are organic, but the fact that they are fresh makes them much more enjoyable and good for me.

Before I changed my diet, my mouth often felt 'claggy', which must have been due to all the additives I was consuming. In the old days, I'd rather have had a bar of chocolate than an apple, but now a chocolate bar would be too sweet and leaves a taste in my mouth for hours. Although I must admit I do indulge in fish and chips (I remove the batter) from the chippie very occasionally, it's a real treat, and I tell myself the fish is good for me. I really don't miss bread; it made me feel so ill.

This is why my change of diet has been so easy to stick to. If I don't eat properly, I feel ill – it's as simple as that.

CASE STUDY

GABI'S MENU SUGGESTIONS FOR A WEEK

SUNDAY

Breakfast: Dried fruit, nuts and seeds
Midmorning snack: Apple
Lunch: Ricecakes, hummus, yellow and green pepper, cherries, mango juice
Midafternoon snack: Dried fruit salad
Dinner: Omelette with potatoes, peas, onions, peppers; salad: tomato, kiwi, olives, rocket, French dressing
Drinks: Three glasses of water, one tea, one herbal tea, one juice

MONDAY

Breakfast: Dried fruit, nuts and live yoghurt, cranberry juice
Midmorning snack: Dried fruit, nuts and seeds, pear
Lunch: Greek salad: Feta cheese, olives, cucumber, tomatoes, rocket, oil dressing; tropical smoothie, water
Midafternoon snack: Apple
Dinner: Risotto: celery, bacon, borlotto beans, onion, chargrilled asparagus, sardines, peppers, tomatoes and parsley
Drinks: Four glasses of water, two teas, two juices

TUESDAY

Breakfast: Sesame Ryvita, liver pâté, mango juice
Midmorning snack: Dried fruit, nuts and seeds
Lunch: Salade Niçoise: tuna, potato, olives, red onion, green beans, egg, water
Midafternoon snack: Two kiwis, banana
Dinner: Grilled chicken in honey, spring onions, garlic; peas and roast potatoes
Drinks: Three glasses of water, two teas, one juice, one lager

WEDNESDAY

Breakfast: Sesame Ryvita, liver pâté, apple juice
Midmorning snack: None (optional)
Lunch: Pesto salad with rocket and tomato, water
Midafternoon snack: Banana and yoghurt
Dinner: Grilled chicken with spring onions, garlic; herb salad with avocado and olives
Drinks: Five glasses of water, three teas, one juice

THURSDAY

Breakfast: Apricots, nuts and yoghurt, mango juice
Midmorning snack: Dried fruit, nuts and seeds
Lunch: Prawns, rocket, celery, tomato, banana, cranberry juice
Midafternoon snack: Pear, a very small piece of birthday cake (!)
Dinner: Grilled aubergine, feta cheese, apple, herb salad with olives, water
Drinks: Five glasses of water, one tea, one herbal tea, two juices, two lagers

FRIDAY

Breakfast: Rice cakes, cream cheese, apple juice
Midmorning snack: Dried fruit, nuts and seeds
Lunch: Greek salad: Feta cheese, cucumber, onions, tomatoes, water
Midafternoon snack: Apple, nuts and seeds
Dinner: Grilled salmon steak, asparagus, new potatoes, banana and live yoghurt, water
Drinks: Four glasses of water, three teas, one juice

SATURDAY

Breakfast: Strawberries, raspberries, banana live yoghurt
Midmorning snack: Fruit flapjack
Lunch: Ryvita, tuna pâté, carrot, cucumber, tomato
Midafternoon snack: Apple
Dinner: Chilli, basmati rice, rocket salad, tomato, cucumber, coriander; strawberries, raspberries and cream, water
Drinks: Four glasses of water, two teas, two juices

HEALTH AND VITALITY RESTORED

Many women comment that their feelings of wellbeing and vitality make it easy to follow the diet as, once they feel their energy returning and the pain lessening, they never want to return to the bad days of exhaustion and pain. Getting through the first month may be the most arduous time. But unless you try this wholeheartedly, you will never know. It may be that you need to try two modalities together, such as herbs and nutrition or homeopathy and nutrition. We are all unique individuals and so have different needs.

Whatever you do, you need to plan your attack on endometriosis and then carry it through. Sometimes, you may go through a patch of feeling worse before you can get better. This is why throwing yourself into a *Candida*-style diet first may be too harsh, and you need to move forward and feel much stronger before trying a full-blown candidiasis diet. Also, the symptoms of 'die-off' can be very debilitating as the bloodstream fills up with toxins and you feel ill all over. Some nutritionists advocate this as the first step – a complete detox. With endometriosis, it is vitally important to get the feel-better factor back first. Endometriosis symptoms are bad enough so it is better to take it one step at a time, and reduce pain and improve energy for two months before embarking on a detox or candidiasis diet. Always be aware that as you detox, dioxins may be released from fat cells. This must therefore be done slowly as it could make the endometriosis pains worse.

So what to do and in which order? Women question how they should tackle the illness through diet and supplement use. It usually takes at least three to four months to feel fully well. For some, it happens in two months whereas for others, like one of the authors (DSM), it took one year. Remember too that, having been ill for a long period of time, it may take several months to get back to your old self. Perseverance is the key. As already mentioned, nutrition does not work like drugs – it takes time, and can follow along the lines of a game of shutes/snakes and ladders. However, changing your diet is trying to correct body biochemistry, and not masking symptoms as many drugs do. The case histories scattered throughout this book should be helpful to you. Everyone has their own story to tell and their own joy in their healing pathway. It is a change for life and should help your long-term health.

A FIVE-STEP PLAN

Take control and begin with a plan to follow for a few months. Help your body rebalance its biochemistry and bring everything back to an even keel. Photocopy the diet pages in chapter 11 and keep a chart on how you feel for the next two months (*see* Appendix C). Keep your thoughts honed on what you are trying to achieve. The things that you may have to give up are not as important as your health.

Knowledge is power and the authors hope that they have provided you with sufficient information to seek your own path back to good health. Remember always that the body wants only to be well. An ill body is crying out for key nutrients and providing them for all your cells will allow them to work their magic. Whether you are trying to rid yourself of pain or attempting a pregnancy, the use of good food and nutritional supplements can only be beneficial. It allows your body to fight back!

Ask your GP to do a few tests, and be assertive. If you have been working and pay health insurance, then this is one of your rights. It is important to know your iron count, thyroid and liver function, and gluten sensitivity (both IgE and IgG), even lactose intolerance tests.

> Don't be afraid to take a big step if one is indicated. You can't jump a chasm in two small steps.
>
> *David Lloyd George*

FIVE-BIG STEPS TO TAKE

Step one: digestion

Take a one- or two-month course of slippery elm, acidophilus and a digestive enzyme alongside a multivitamin/mineral and an essential fatty acid (fish and evening primrose oils or flaxseed oil). They must all be wheat-, sugar-, dairy- and yeast-free in order to work.

Step two: pain reduction

Stop taking the slippery elm once digestion has improved and add a magnesium supplement. The best one is in malate form (as malic acid works in Kreb's cycle to aid energy production), but if this cannot be obtained, try magnesium citrate or amino acid chelate. Magnesium relaxes tense and taut muscles that are in spasm, while essential fatty acids reduce internal inflammation. Therefore, the use of magnesium should continue until the pain begins to abate. Marine fish oils from the Efamol range have been proven by research to be among the best formulations available, and are lowest in dioxins and PCBs. Vitamin C can also relieve pain due to its antihistamine properties. D,L-Phenylalanine (DLPA) can be used for a month if the pain is daily and severe to see if it works for you. Once it has reduced the pain, you can reduce the dose (*see* chapter 4 for details).

Step three: energy levels

Iron is essential for energy, along with vitamins C, B1, B2, B3 and B5, magnesium and coenzyme Q10. If your periods are very heavy with clots, add an iron supplement for one to two months. The best form is iron EAP2 or citrate, as they do not cause constipation or turn the stools black, as do those available on prescription. Vitamin C taken alongside iron can also be beneficial in its gentler form of magnesium ascorbate (rather than the acidic ascorbic acid). Many vegetarians find they require iron, but meat-eaters may also find themselves iron-deficient if they are bleeding internally from endometriotic implants and have heavy periods. Coenzyme Q10 can be beneficial for some people by aiding energy production at a cellular level. Iodine-containing kelp may aid energy levels by its action on speeding up thyroid function. If you are truly drained and can barely move, then take one 500mg L-tyrosine tablet for one day. It should provide that extra boost to flagging energy. Use this sparingly on odd occasions, not as a daily supplement (*see* p. 147).

Step four: reproductive system support

To aid fertility or even simply to support the endocrine system, it is crucial that the diet be supportive. Modern Western food intake appears to fall short of the nutrients necessary for the endocrine glands to work in harmony. A multivitamin/mineral (with a limit of 2000 in vitamin A), essential fatty acids, acidophilus and digestive enzymes, plus an antioxidant and magnesium may help to ensure that all the endocrine glands are restored to an improved condition. In some cases, the use of kelp may aid thyroid function if you have a borderline low thyroid function reading. It usually takes more than four months on a good nutrition programme before women can become pregnant, so persevere. Many women with endometriosis – be it mild, moderate or severe – can achieve a pregnancy; very few do not succeed. A healthy body stands a much better chance of producing a healthy baby. It is crucial that you eat a balanced diet with a little protein at each meal and take in good cold-pressed oils. Remember that your partner should strive for a healthy diet for three months too, to optimize sperm health.

Step five: immune support

The use of an antioxidant can be beneficial in the long term to prevent cellular damage from free oxidizing radicals (FORs). We know that some of the damage to the cell membranes that allows the endometriosis to attach may be in part due to FOR damage. Avoidance may therefore help to prevent further damage to DNA and cell membranes. A supplement of vitamins A, C and E and yeast-free selenium may be helpful. An efficient immune system may help to keep the endometriosis at bay.

PLANNING THE SHOPPING

Everyone has to shop for food. To buy food to maintain health, we need a basic shopping list which we can work around.

BASIC WEEKLY SHOPPING LIST

> Green leafy vegetables
> Red vegetables
> Salad vegetables
> Fruits (no citrus, but more berries)
> Nuts and seeds
> Oily fish (deep-sea)
> Lean meat (preferably organic)
> Eggs, organic, free range
> Peas, beans, lentils
> Goat or ewe's dairy foods: cheeses, yoghurt or fromage frais
> Breakfast cereals, porridge, oat muesli
> Rye breads, oatcakes and corn crispbreads
> Fruit juices, such as apple, pineapple, cranberry
> Bottled water.

It might be worth making a three-week plan of the meals you wish to have. Everyone has favourite dishes that are quick and easy to prepare, but then we get stuck in a rut. We eat the same meals week in and week out. Perhaps we need to be more adventurous at weekends and try out one new dish as a possible addition to our repertoire. If you are vegetarian, then make sure that you do not rely solely on dairy foods for protein. Try some peas, beans, lentils, nuts and seeds in your meals. We have included a few recipes for you to try. If you are buying packet foods, then choose the healthy option. Some labels may be misleading, so read carefully. Some products contain cheap fillers like saturated fats or rusk to bulk them up or flavour enhancers like sugar, salt or monosodium glutamate.

The fresher your food, the healthier you will be, as fresh food is higher in vitamins and minerals. Older fruit and vegetables contain much less as many of the vitamins are oxidized during storage. In fact, we should all try to buy our fresh produce every other day.

HOW TO BE ECONOMICAL WHEN SHOPPING

- Use chicken and turkey for low-fat meat.
- Trim fat from red meat and reduce intake to once a week.
- Have a vegetarian dish once a week, as it costs less to make a vegetable curry (like chickpeas and spinach, or parsnip, butter bean and banana curry).
- Have an omelette and salad one day.
- Try a vegetable and bean casserole another day.
- Try to be more adventurous because, that way, you take in different nutrients.
- Buy foods when they are in season as then they are cheaper.
- Buy food on special offer only if you are going to use them.
- Avoid buying from open sacks as the food may be spoilt.

The sayings 'eat in moderation' and 'variety is the spice of life' may be the most important to adhere to when it comes to staying healthy.

> An idea for leftover turkey is to wrap it in aluminium foil, and throw it out.
>
> *Anon*

CANDIDA REDUCTION

Not every woman with endometriosis has *Candida*. *Candida albicans* is a potent immune agent, exhibiting many immunomodulatory effects.[2] The International Endometriosis Association, headquartered in the USA, has shown that many women with endometriosis often test positive for allergy to *C. albicans*, luteinizing hormone (LH), oestrogen, chemicals and foods, but any combination of sensitivities is possible, including sensitivity to moulds, pollens and progesterone.[3]

A large number of women show no overt signs of *C. albicans* overgrowth, but symptoms may increase if yeast-based foods and supplements are used. A number of supportive doctors are using immunotherapy to treat their patients alongside conventional medical treatments, but very few doctors in the UK follow this line of approach. Antifungal treatments are the main line of attack (*see* chapter 10 for details). The use of caprylic acid, Mycopryl, grapefruit seed extract and pau d'arco tea can all aid the fight against yeast overgrowth. Taken alongside a course of acidophilus, these will help you regain control of the gut flora and redress the balance. (Appendix B on p. 343 shows a two-month programme you can follow.)

GUIDELINES FOR A HEALTHY APPETITE

- Enjoy your food; savour the tastes and textures.
- Eat a wide variety of different foods.
- Eat only when you are hungry and stop eating once you are full.
- Eat complex carbohydrates to maintain a balanced blood sugar.
- Eat plenty of fresh fruits and vegetables.
- Eat fresh fish, nuts, seeds and legumes for extra protein.
- Use only the cold-pressed oils.
- Avoid refined sugars and starches.
- Avoid caffeine most of the time.
- Avoid food with additives.
- Reduce alcohol to five glasses per week.
- Reduce red meat and use more poultry and game.
- Exclude wheat for one month to see if there is any effect.
- Exclude bovine dairy on a different month to see if that has any effect.

This style of eating should benefit you 10-fold:

1 Increase energy
2 Maintain a healthy weight
3 Protect cells from premature ageing
4 Improve memory and concentration
5 Protect the skeleton
6 Protect against heart disease
7 Support the reproductive system
8 Support the immune system
9 Maintain a sense of wellbeing
10 Support pain-control mechanisms in the body.

Does this all seem too arduous? When we are functioning below par, it takes extra energy to do the smallest thing. If this seems a big step, then take heed of what Henry David Thoreau said – 'Even a journey of 10,000 miles starts with a single step. Take the small steps and the big changes will then take care of themselves. If you have built castles in the air, your work need not be lost; that is where they should be. Now put foundations under them.' The Chinese had another way of stirring us into action – 'Be not afraid of going slowly, only of standing still.' American Ralph Waldo Emerson said that we should 'Always do what you are afraid to do'. My headmaster joined them in this philosophical mindset, always chiding the class that 'there is no failure except in ceasing to try'. We all have to work through this quest for health alone. There are guides around but, ultimately, we are alone in this body and only we can sense what feels right and what feels wrong. It is important that we seek out the right course of action for us individually.

> My right hand is being held by someone who knows more than I,
> and I am learning.
> My left hand is being held by someone who knows less than I, and I
> am teaching.
> Both my hands need thus to be held for me – to be.
>
> *Natasha Josefowitz*

Guiding one another is what this is all about. We all have to work with women and young girls around the world to help one another to learn how the body works, what a miracle it is, and how to maintain health through our use of foods and nutrients. This is knowledge that has been lost before, so we need to teach it again to everyone. Health throughout life is the greatest gift. Growing old and remaining healthy are very important. In our reproductive years, we should be full of the joys of life, not languishing in agony in a corner, weeping inside because of all the pain. The body knows instinctively how to heal itself. Your support for that process is what this book is about.

> Take control, be healthy, be happy and spread the word.[4]
>
> *Richard Helfrich*

15 The keys to wellness are in your hands

There's no elevator to success. You have to take the stairs.

Live and Learn and Pass it On,
quote from the Central Baptist Hospital 1997 calendar

Endometriosis is a serious, debilitating disease which can manifest itself in so many ways. This is the crux of the problem. Every woman's endometriosis pain is different. The whole condition remains a mystery to the medical profession and lay people alike. Women need a cure. This is the cry of distressed women the world over. Drugs and surgery can allay some symptoms, but often bring others. Getting to the root of the problem and working with the body are all-important. After all, we are what we eat. To help the body heal requires good food rich in nutrients. The body is trying to heal itself all the time. Look at the speed with which it can work, given the right building blocks:

- Blood circulates through the body every 20 seconds. In one minute, it has travelled through the liver three times!
- You produce 100 billion red blood cells every day.
- Over 2,000 immune cells per second are produced by the body.
- Touch something and you send a message to your brain at 124 mph.
- You make one litre of saliva every day.
- Every four days the whole lining of the gastrointestinal tract is renewed.
- When you smile, you exercise 30 different muscles.

Seek happiness in the present, and you'll find it in the future.

Kazuo Suzuki, Karate Master

We need to work with the body, not against it. The environment contains harmful substances, as do some foodstuffs. We have to try to avoid these to give our immune and reproductive systems a fighting chance. Health can be regained, as you have read in this book.

We are all unique and we can only do our best. Eating well gives your body the ability to heal itself. Remember, the main nutritional premises of this book are:

1 Eat as well as you can afford.
2 Buy the freshest food you can find.

3 Cook from fresh whenever possible, or eat fresh, raw food in salads daily.
4 Eat as wide a variety of foodstuffs as possible, remembering that 'variety is the spice of life'.

Nutrition is not an easy option, as some of the women have stated in the case studies. It requires some determination and perseverance. You can but try. Women can all help one another through this healing process. The support network can be found on the Internet. Log on to: www.endometriosis.co.uk and www.makingbabies.com. These websites offer a holistic approach, including both orthodox and complementary options, information on medical ethics, and contacts around the world who may be able to answer your questions and allow you to make an informed choice.

Being positive in the face of an illness for which no medical cure is offered requires a lot of faith and hope and the will to be well. Helping yourself along the path to recovery is a start. Let this book be a guide; we want to take you on a journey back to wellness.

This book should help to lead you into discovering the power of good nutrition. Use it well and pass the message on. When women meet at endometriosis symposia all over the globe, we try to metaphorically hold hands around the world, because we are all a part of a whole. Never feel alone with endometriosis – women are all guides for one another. There are many roads back to wellness, and when you have the strength you will find the right combination for you. Have faith in the body's ability to heal.

> We only grow when we push ourselves beyond what we already know. Every great achievement was once considered impossible.
> *Live and Learn and Pass it On,*
> *quote from the Central Baptist Hospital 1997 calendar*

WHAT YOU CAN DO

To help to guide you down the right path to health, we have some suggestions for supplements which you may wish to use while you adjust your eating pattern. No one woman will require the same supplements as another because of your unique 'biochemical individuality'. Just as our endometriosis manifests itself in a different way in each of us, the pattern of nutrients needed by each of us will be subtly different. As a nutritionist assesses your specific needs, they will be different from the next person. The consultation may take an hour or more and various tests may be suggested. These tests will show the vitamin and mineral status of your tissues, gut fermentation and food intolerances. From this, any deficiencies can be seen and adjusted. This is why no clients who come for nutrition consultations ever leave with the same dietary advice or 'prescription' for supplements.

It is important to understand that the nutritional regimes found at the end of each chapter are not like orthodox or complementary medicine. Both of these approaches require you to take a 'medicine' – be it a pharmaceutical drug, a herb or homeopathic tablet – until you are well. Nutrition works when you assess your present lifestyle and nutrient intake. The changes you make will hopefully improve the integrity of the digestive tract and thus the absorption of the vital nutrients the body requires to heal. You may need to take supplements for a short time to speed this healing process up. Many of the changes you make will stay with you for a long time, once you are eating foods which supply the nutrients your reproductive system needs. Knowing how good it can feel when you are well again often keeps you focused on the goal of maintaining that sense of wellness, and continuing with healthy eating habits.

Often, the author (DSM) has been asked to formulate a little 'green' tablet for everyone to take. This is impossible. Endometriosis is multifactorial and women have symptoms which are too varied. Also, not all symptoms may be due to the endometriosis – some may be vitamin and mineral deficiencies, enzyme failures or genetic weak links. Everyone has to be treated according to their individual needs. That way, the treatment is individually tailored and that uniqueness is followed-up at each visit.

No one person ever has exactly the same regime as another as your needs may be entirely different. Then, over two to six months, the diet can be adjusted to improve nutrient absorption, and supplements taken until the body biochemistry has been corrected. After this the healthy eating pattern should be maintained, and supplements may be used on and off as necessary. The body should be able to correct itself and maintain this balance while good quality food is eaten, with supplements only taken if ill health strikes again. Some people like to take a maintenance dose at weekends only.

The role of nutrition should be to correct imbalances. Once health has been obtained, the body should – given a good quality nutrient-rich balanced diet and an efficient digestive system – maintain that health without the constant need for supplements. Supplements alone will not suffice – what you eat is all important. The two need to be combined at first for the body to recover its equilibrium, its balance. Just taking supplements alone and continuing to eat an overprocessed high-sugar, high-fat, low-fibre diet will not improve health.

One should always take a low-dose multivitamin/mineral supplement as a background upon which to build up those that need replenishing. Remember that if a specific, single B vitamin is required, then a B-complex should be taken either alone or as part of a multi-vitamin/mineral supplement. Then the single B vitamin can be added on top. All the supplements you buy should be hypoallergenic, and yeast-, wheat-, gluten-, sugar- and dairy-free. Many can be obtained by mail order if a good supplier is not available locally. The quality is very important, as cheaper supplements may have less absorbable forms of minerals or contain yeast-based vitamins. Never begin a treatment until you have consulted a qualified nutritionist.

All substances are poisonous if taken in excess – even water. Manufacturers always put safe doses in their pots. The danger comes when people think they know better and that, if one is good, then two must be even better. It is NOT! Follow the instructions and check with the chart in chapter 11 as to safe levels. Never exceed these. It is best if you seek out a nutritionist in your area to work with you.

The following are symptoms which many women report alongside their endometriosis.

FATIGUE

Low energy reserves are common with endometriosis, when you are constantly fighting pain and anxiety from wondering what is going to happen next. The emotional toll from stress wears out the nerves.

Coenzyme Q10 (ubiquinone)
B-vitamin complex
Iron EAP2 or citrate
Vitamin C with bioflavonoids
Evening primrose and fish oils

Magnesium malate
Pantothenic acid (B5)
Zinc citrate
Chromium polynicotinate

DEPRESSION

Deficiencies of various vitamins and minerals – such as calcium, magnesium, potassium, iron, vitamin C, biotin, folic acid, pyridoxine, thiaminr and B12 – plus an excess intake of copper or magnesium are associated with depression. Balance is all important with all nutrition. Certain food allergies can be problematic, especially sugar and wheat in susceptible people. Some foods become addictive and, often, it is the food which you crave that is doing you the most harm.

B-complex vitamins
Folic acid
Magnesium EAP2
Vitamin C
D,L-Phenylalanine OR L-tyrosine
Evening primrose and fish oils

Biotin
Calcium citrate
Iron EAP2
Chromium polynicotinate
Multivitamins/minerals

MITRAL VALVE PROLAPSE

This has been found to be fairly common in women with endometriosis. The heart requires vitamin B1 (thiamine) and magnesium to help the muscle relax. Avoid all foods containing aspartame, caffeine and phosphorus fizzy drinks. Potassium levels should be checked, so eat plenty of fresh fruits and vegetables.

Magnesium EAP2
Coenzyme Q10

Vitamin B1 (thiamine)
Multivitamins/minerals

OSTEOPOROSIS

As oestrogen levels decline, we may be liable to osteoporosis; some hormone treatments may also provoke this condition if they simulate menopause. Maintaining a healthy diet containing all the nutrients required by bone can be a start. Bone is living tissue with nutrients constantly flowing into and out of it. It needs magnesium, phosphorus, boron, manganese, silicon, strontium, zinc, copper, sodium, vitamins K, D and B6, folic acid and protein, not just calcium. Again the balance is all-important. Three brisk 20-minute walks each week help to put calcium into bone.

Boron 3mg/day	Calcium gluconate
Magnesium malate	Multivitamins/minerals
Vitamin D	Efamarine

HOT FLASHES

Research has shown vitamin E to be very effective in reducing the frequency of hot flashes and painful breasts. If you are wheat-intolerant, look for vitamin E that is not from wheatgerm oil.

Vitamin E	Multivitamins/minerals
Vitamin C with bioflavonoids	Evening primrose oil

INSOMNIA

Foods high in the amino acid L-tryptophan may be helpful. This amino acid is the precursor to serotonin, a neurotransmitter that is important in inducing sleep. Evening meals containing turkey, milk, soya, cottage cheese, peanuts or lentils may be helpful. Never take B vitamins at night as they keep you awake!

Magnesium malate	Vitamin B3 (niacinamide)
Chamomile or limeblossom tea	

We wish you well in your quest for health. Just be sensible and eat as well as you are able, taking supplements only when necessary. Two to three months should be adequate if you have milder symptoms but, for some, you may need to follow a sensible eating pattern for six months to a year. It all depends on how ill you are to begin with.

Listen to what your body is telling you about foods and supplements. There is life after endometriosis and you can retrieve good health by making your body as strong as possible. Take heed of the comments of other women found throughout this book. They have trodden this path before you. Let them lead the way. A thank-you to all of them for their trust and perseverance. Good luck with your quest. May good health be yours – it is the most precious thing you own.

Eat well, sleep well – deeply. For tomorrow comes and it's all yours.

Ancient Proverb

SUMMARY

1 Your body is trying to heal itself. Have faith in your body's ability to heal.

2 You can give your body the building blocks it needs. Changing your eating pattern will help. Taking supplements will enhance the healing process, but just taking supplements without improving digestion and nutrient intake will have no effect.

3 Heal your digestive tract first.

4 You are unique and thus need individual treatment. What works for one person will not work in the same way for another.

5 You need to muster some determination and perseverance in your quest for good health. It takes some time to heal a body which has been ill for some time. Use this book's nutritional suggestions as a guideline.

6 Never feel alone with endometriosis. Know that all over the world women are sharing your pain and working to overcome it.

7 Assess your present lifestyle and nutrient intake carefully and honestly.

8 Eat healthy food and avoid greasy, fatty, sugary, starchy processed junk – it will make you ill. Cook from fresh often.

9 Be sensible about nutritional supplements. They are a support while you improve your eating pattern and/or correct your digestion.

10 Let the women who have trodden this path before you lead the way. Health is a pleasure we should grasp in both hands.

Never doubt that a small group of thoughtful, committed people can change the world. Indeed, it is the only thing that ever has.

Margaret Mead, anthropologist

Join us at www.endometriosis.co.uk and www.makingbabies.com .

Appendix A

American Society for Reproductive Medicine Revised Classification of Endometriosis

Patient's Name _____ Date_____

Stage I (Minimal) - 1-5
Stage II (Mild) - 6-15
Stage III (Moderate) - 16-40
Stage IV (Severe) - >40
Total_____

Laparoscopy_____ Laparotomy_____ Photography_____
Recommended Treatment_____

Prognosis_____

PERITONEUM	**ENDOMETRIOSIS**	<1cm	1-3cm	>3cm
	Superficial	1	2	4
	Deep	2	4	6
OVARY	R Superficial	1	2	4
	Deep	4	16	20
	L Superficial	1	2	4
	Deep	4	16	20

	POSTERIOR CULDESAC OBLITERATION	Partial		Complete	
		4		40	

	ADHESIONS	<1/3 Enclosure	1/3-2/3 Enclosure	>2/3 Enclosure
OVARY	R Filmy	1	2	4
	Dense	4	8	16
	L Filmy	1	2	4
	Dense	4	8	16
TUBE	R Filmy	1	2	4
	Dense	4*	8*	16
	L Filmy	1	2	4
	Dense	4*	8*	16

*If the fimbriated end of the fallopian tube is completely enclosed, change the point assignment to 16.

Denote appearance of superficial implant types as red [(R), red, red-pink. flamelike, vesicular blobs, clear vesicles], white [(W), opacifications, peritoneal defects, yellow-brown], or black [(B) black, hemosiderin deposits, blue]. Denote percent of total described as R___%, W___% and B___%. Total should equal 100%.

Additional Endometriosis: _____   Associated Pathology: _____

To Be Used with Normal Tubes and Ovaries	To Be Used with Abnormal Tubes and/or Ovaries

EXAMPLES & GUIDELINES

STAGE I (MINIMAL)	STAGE II (MILD)	STAGE III (MODERATE)

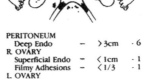

PERITONEUM
Superficial Endo – 1-3cm · 2
R. OVARY
Superficial Endo – < 1cm · 1
Filmy Adhesions – < 1/3 · 1
TOTAL POINTS 4

PERITONEUM
Deep Endo – > 3cm · 6
R. OVARY
Superficial Endo – < 1cm · 1
Filmy Adhesions – < 1/3 · 1
L. OVARY
Superficial Endo – < 1cm · 1
TOTAL POINTS 9

PERITONEUM
Deep Endo – > 3cm · 6
CULDESAC
Partial Obliteration · 4
L. OVARY
Deep Endo – 1-3cm · 16
TOTAL POINTS 26

STAGE III (MODERATE)	STAGE IV (SEVERE)	STAGE IV (SEVERE)

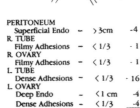
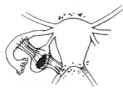
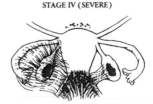

PERITONEUM
Superficial Endo – > 3cm -4
R. TUBE
Filmy Adhesions – < 1/3 · 1
R. OVARY
Filmy Adhesions – < 1/3 · 1
L. TUBE
Dense Adhesions – < 1/3 · 16
L. OVARY
Deep Endo – < 1 cm -4
Dense Adhesions – < 1/3 -4
TOTAL POINTS 30

PERITONEUM
Superficial Endo – > 3cm -4
L. OVARY
Deep Endo – 1-3cm · 32**
Dense Adhesions – < 1/3 · 8**
L. TUBE
Dense Adhesions – < 1/3 · 8**
TOTAL POINTS 52

*Point assignment changed to 16
**Point assignment doubled

PERITONEUM
Deep Endo – > 3cm · 6
CULDESAC
Complete Obliteration · 40
R. OVARY
Deep Endo – 1-3cm · 16
Dense Adhesions – < 1/3 · 4
L. TUBE
Dense Adhesions – > 2/3 · 16
L. OVARY
Deep Endo – 1-3cm · 16
Dense Adhesions – > 2/3 · 16
TOTAL POINTS 114

Determination of the stage or degree of endometrial involvement is based on a weighted point system. Distribution of points has been arbitrarily determined and may require further revision or refinement as knowledge of the disease increases.

To ensure complete evaluation, inspection of the pelvis in a clockwise or counterclockwise fashion is encouraged. Number, size and location of endometrial implants, plaques, endometriomas and/or adhesions are noted. For example, five separate 0.5cm superficial implants on the peritoneum (2.5 cm total) would be assigned 2 points. (The surface of the uterus should be considered peritoneum.) The severity of the endometriosis or adhesions should be assigned the highest score only for peritoneum, ovary, tube or culdesac. For example, a 4cm superficial and a 2cm deep implant of the peritoneum should be given a score of 6 (not 8). A 4cm deep endometrioma of the ovary associated with more than 3cm of superficial disease should be scored 20 (not 24).

In those patients with only one adnexa, points applied to disease of the remaining tube and ovary should be multiplied by two. **Points assigned may be circled and totaled. Aggregation of points indicates stage of disease (minimal, mild, moderate, or severe).

The presence of endometriosis of the bowel, urinary tract, fallopian tube, vagina, cervix, skin etc., should be documented under "additional endometriosis." Other pathology such as tubal occlusion, leiomyomata, uterine anomaly, etc., should be documented under "associated pathology." All pathology should be depicted as specifically as possible on the sketch of pelvic organs, and means of observation (laparoscopy or laparotomy) should be noted.

Property of the American Society for Reproductive Medicine 1996

For additional supply write to: American Society for Reproductive Medicine, 1209 Montgomery Highway, Birmingham, Alabama 35216

American Society for Reproductive Medicine *Revised ASRM classification: 1996*   *Fertility and Sterility®*

Appendix B

Candida albicans – symptoms of yeast infection

Clinical symptoms can be very difficult to live with:

- Thrush in the vagina and mouth, skin and nails, and athlete's foot
- Bloating, intolerance to foods, constipation, poor digestion, food allergies, abdominal pains, chemical allergies, diarrhoea
- Weak muscles, numbness, tingling and fatigue
- Loss of libido, menstrual cramps, endometriosis, mood swings, cystitis
- Loss of memory, reasoning, concentration, depression, lack of self confidence, irritability
- Nasal congestion, swelling and discomfort in joints, sensitivity to cigarette smoke and perfumes, and acne
- Headaches, migraines, blurred vision and feeling 'spaced out'
- Swollen lymph glands and recurring sore throats.

Symptoms get worse in damp and cold conditions, and sometimes after eating sugary foods. The problem with diagnosing candidiasis is that it mimics many other illnesses and many health professionals dismiss the problem. Sufferers may crave sugary or yeast-containing foods. Some doctors know it as 'gut dysfunction syndrome'.

CANDIDIASIS DIET

A high-fibre diet containing some wholegrain cereals (but not wheat), organic vegetables, some fruits, additives, hormones, and antibiotic-free meat and fish are recommended. If there is no milk allergy, then live yoghurt or a supplement containing *Lactobacillus bulgaricus* and *Streptococcus thermophilus* can be taken to repopulate the bowel.

In severe cases, no fruit should be eaten for a month and only 60g of carbohydrate at the beginning of the diet.

THESE FOODS SHOULD BE AVOIDED

- All foods containing yeast: bread, biscuits, cakes, Marmite, Yeastrel, Bisto, Oxo, Bovril, sausages, meat pies, stuffings.
- Gluten grains: wheat, rye, oats, barley for one month, then no white flour, malted or sugared cereals with added vitamins.
- All fermented liquids: alcohol, wine, vinegar, soy sauce, miso.
- Dairy produce: milk, malted milk drinks, yoghurt, buttermilk, skimmed milk.
- All fruit and juices for one month, then one piece of fruit per day or a portion of diluted juice. Fruit must always be peeled and washed. No dried fruit is allowed.
- All types of mushrooms.
- Sauces, pickles, salad dressings (especially French dressing), mayonnaise, horse-radish, tomato sauce.
- All stale vegetables – cooked or uncooked.
- All refined carbohydrates: sugars, sweets, chocolates, honey.
- Tea and coffee.
- All B vitamins, unless they are hypoallergenic and yeast-free.
- Drugs which promote the growth of yeast: oral contraceptives, corticosteroids, antibiotics, hormones.

THESE FOODS CAN BE EATEN

Breakfast Cereals, ricecakes, brown rice, millet pancakes, corn fritters, corn on the cob, sugar-free cornflakes, seeds, buckwheat pancakes, bread made from corn, millet or potato flour. After one month: Ryvita, oatcakes, eggs, bacon, grilled fish, New Zealand lamb's kidneys, homemade hamburgers, vegetables, nuts.

Lunch/Dinner Roast lamb, venison, rabbit, grilled fish, chicken, turkey, pheasant, partridge, potatoes, yams, salads, green vegetables, carrots, parsnips, peppers, pulses, onions, leeks, garlic, peeled tomatoes (after first month). Eat vegetables raw or lightly steamed. Use vegetable water for soups. Salad dressings: olive oil and lemon juice (after first month). Drinks: mineral or filtered water, herb or fruit teas, soya milk, apple juice, pineapple juice, tomato juice (after first month).

All foods must be fresh. Organic is better, if available; if not, wash and peel all fruits and vegetables.

ANTIYEAST FOODS

The following have antiyeast properties: Onion, garlic, cabbage, broccoli, Brussels sprouts, kale, watercress, mustardcress, cauliflower, turnips, cinnamon, olive oil and aloe vera juice.

ANTIFUNGAL FOODS AND SUPPLEMENTS

The conventional treatment is with Nystatin, an antiyeast medication, for six months. However, this misses the target organisms.

A positive symbiotic acid-producing bacteria such as *Lactobacillus acidophilus* (one teaspoon three times a day) should be taken. Probiotics may be used to reinoculate the bowel with bifidogenic bacteria.

Olive oil and **garlic** are known to have antiyeast properties. **Oat bran fibre** also increases the absorption of faeces, thereby removing harmful organisms from the gut.

Biotin is thought to prevent the conversion of yeast to its rhizome form.

Vitamin E (400–800IU/day), zinc (30–50mg/day) and **calcium pantothenate** (vitamin B5; 200–800mg/day) are known to aid healing of the gut mucosa.

Caprylic acid, a fatty acid derived from coconut oil, has a fungicidal action against yeast. **Caprystatin** may be taken for two months *OR*

Mycocidin, made from undecylenic acid from castor bean oil, also has a fungicidal effect.

Sorbic acid, from the berries of the mountain ash, is a fatty acid that reacts on *Candida* in the mouth and vagina.

Pau d'arco tea, from Argentina, contains lapachol, which seems to be able to produce chemicals that destroy some microorganisms. It has to be used in moderation – one cup made from one tablespoon of bark per day.

Aloe vera juice is also known to react to *Candida* cells – use two teaspoons per day in water or juice.

SUGGESTIONS FOR WEEKLY MENU PLANS

Snacks between meals: nuts, sunflower/pumpkin seeds, vegetable sticks & dips, savoury popcorn, almond butter on ricecakes, replace cow's milk with soya milk in recipes, poppadoms, cornchips, aloe vera juice in fruit juice.

	BREAKFAST	LUNCH	TEA/DINNER
1	Almond nut butter & ricecakes Herb tea	Potato & leek soup Apple Beverage	Turkey breast Potato, broccoli & carrots
2	Ewe's yoghurt with ground almonds & banana, Tea	Hummus & ricecakes Salad	Tuna Salad Jacket potato
3	Cornchips & nut butter Herb tea	Carrot & almond soup Ricecakes Apple	Chicken casserole Boiled potatoes Broccoli & carrots
4	Ricecakes & bacon Herb tea	Vegetable soup Cornchips Apple	Grilled chicken Greenbeans Sweetcorn Jacket potato
5	Potato cakes Tomato & mackerel Tea	Turkey breast Boiled potato Green beans & swede	Corn tortillas/tacos Avocado pâté Green salad Apple
6	Ewe's yoghurt with banana Herb tea	Grilled cod/haddock Potato, broccoli &carrots	Hummus & ricecakes Tomato & celery Apple
7	Ricecakes & hummus Mint tea	Potato salad Salmon salad Pear	Grilled chicken Cabbage & carrots Potato

SUGGESTIONS FOR WEEKLY MENU PLANS

Snacks between meals: nuts, sunflower/pumpkin seeds, vegetable sticks & dips, savoury popcorn, almond butter on crispbreads, replace cow's milk with soya milk in recipes, poppadoms, cornchips, aloe vera juice in fruit juice.

	BREAKFAST	LUNCH	TEA/DINNER
1	Raspberries & yoghurt Herb tea	Chicken with lemon Green salad Beverage	Mixed vegetable soup Oatcakes
2	Yoghurt & blackberries Herb tea	Cottage cheese Mixed vegetable salad	Tomato Savoury butter & ricecakes Green salad
3	Fresh peaches in yoghurt Herb tea	Broadbean, celery & Spanish onion salad Ryvita & hummus Water	Cauliflower cheese (Feta) Grilled tomato
4	Spiced apple & yoghurt Herb tea	Grilled chicken Greenbeans & carrots	Rice pilaff Stir-fried vegetables
5	Poached egg on rye toast Rooibosch tea	Corn pasta & pesto Green salad Tomato	Grilled mackerel Green salad Dates & nuts
6	Soya yoghurt & strawberries Herb tea	Brown rice casserole with leeks & nuts, mint & cucumber	Baked potato with spinach & mace Mustard & cress Sliced tomato
7	Oatmeal porridge & berries Caro	Nut roast Green salad	Mixed green salad Poached salmon

Appendix C

SYMPTOMS AND PAIN CALENDAR

Days of menstrual cycle	1	2	3	4	5	6	7	8	9	10	11	12	13	
Painkillers														
Period pain														
Menstruation														
Pelvic cramps														
Left side abdominal pain														
Right side abdominal pain														
Low abdominal pain														
Backache														
General pain														
Pain in left leg														
Pain in right leg														
Pain in stomach														
Pain in abdomen														
Pain in head														
Bowel movement pain[a]														
Urination[b]														
Sexual intercourse pain[c]														
Bloating														
Breast tenderness														
Forgetfulness														
Anxiety														
Depression														
Mood swings														
Insomnia														
Increased appetite														
Irritability														

^aB = before
A = after
F = frequency
A = after
D = during
^bP = pain
^cD = during

Menstruation
H = heavy blood loss
C = clots
L = light blood loss
B = brown blood
S = spotting
R = red blood
Bk = Black blood

List medications used
1 = Mild, normal activities
2 = Moderate, interferes with daily life
3 = Severe, unable to function

Please fill in for one month

14	15	16	17	18	19	20	21	22	23	24	25	26	27	28	29	30	31

Appendix D

Natural methods of family planning

This involves couples working as a team to plan their baby by using the fertile phase as a marker for receptivity to sperm. They may maximize their chances of conception by accurately identifying their most fertile time in each cycle. Colleen Norman at the Fertility Education Centre (see p. 394) in Cardiff has produced several booklets to give practical help with charts and information. It is an easy system to use – with colour-schemed charts and visual formulae.

This system uses a temperature chart, a vaginal mucus chart and a menstrual cycle chart.

There should be a minimum of six low temperatures before ovulation, and the first three thereafter should be high. Mucus symptoms need to be recorded from menstruation to peak for the days around ovulation.

References

References to medical journals use standard abbreviations of journal titles

CHAPTER 2

1 Gambert H R, 'Factors that control thyroid function: Environmental effects and physiological variables' in *The Thyroid Gland*, eds I E Braverman and R D Utiger, J B Lippincott, Philadelphia, pp. 347–57, 1991

2 Casper R C, *Women's Health: Hormones, Emotions and Behaviour*, Cambridge University Press, Cambridge, p. 91, 1998

3 Murray M and Pizzorno J, *Encyclopaedia of Natural Medicine*, Optima Macdonald Press, p. 388, 1995

4 Hedge G H, Colby H D and Goodman R L, Chapter 9 'Female Reproduction' in *Clinical Endocrine Physiology*, W B Saunders, Philadelphia & London, 1987

5 Love S, *Dr. Susan Love's Hormone Book*, Random House, New York, p. 173, 1997

6 Edwards R G and Brody S A, *Principles and Practice of Assisted Human Reproduction*, W B Saunders, Philadelphia & London, p. 496, 1995

7 Ibid, p. 185

8 Binkley S A, *Endocrinology*, HarperCollins College Publishers, London, p. 388, 1995

9 Edwards R G and Brody S A, *Principles and Practice of Assisted Human Reproduction*, W B Saunders, Philadelphia & London, p. 168, 1995

10 'Human Reproduction' 10: 101, 1995, quoted in Leiberman S and Bruning N, *The Real Vitamin & Mineral Book*, Avery Press, New York, p. 265, 1997 (2nd edn)

11 Ziegler E E and Filer L J, *Present Knowledge in Nutrition*, ILSI Press Washington, DC p. 174, 1996 (7th edn)

12 Fredericks C, *Guide to Women's Nutrition: Dietary Advice for Women of All Ages*, Putnam Publishing Group, New York, 1989

13 Ambrus J L, 'Estrogens and clotting factors' in *Consensus on Menopause Research*, eds P A Van Keep, R B Greenblatt and M Albeaux-Fernet, MTP Press, Lancaster, 1976

14 Katchadourian H, *The Biology of Adolescence*, W H Freeman, San Francisco, p. 18, 1997

15 Binkley S A, *Endocrinology*, HarperCollins College Publishers, London, p. 389, 1995

16 Ibid, p. 412

17 Ibid, p. 381

18 Vernon M W, IVF Center, Central Baptist Hospital, Lexington, Kentucky personal communication, 1996

19 Oliker A J and Harris A E, 'Endometriosis of the bladder in a male patient' in *J Urol*, 106: 858, 1971

20 O'Connor D T, *Endometriosis: Current Review in Obstetrics and Gynaecology 12*, Churchill Livingstone, Edinburgh, p. 20, 1987

21 Sampson J A, 'Peritoneal endometriosis due to menstrual dissemination of endometrial tissue into the peritoneal cavity' in *Am J Obstet Gynecol*, 14: 422, 1927

22 Halme J M G *et al.*, 'Retrograde menstruation in healthy women and in patients with endometriosis' in *Obstet Gynaecol*, 64 (4): 151–4, 1984

23 Vernon M W, 'Animal Models in Endometriosis Research' in *Infertility and Reproductive Medicine Clinics of North America*, W B Saunders, Philadelphia & London, p. 565, 1987

24 Meyer R, 'Uber Endometrium in der Tube, sowie uber die Hierausentstehenden wirklichen Sarcomatosa' in *Zentralbl Gynakol*, 51: 1482, 1927

25 Hurst B S and Rock J A, 'Anatomic and functional considerations in the development of a classification for endometriosis and pelvic pain and infertility' in *Proceedings of the Vth World Congress on Endometriosis*, eds H Minaguchi and O Sugimoto, Parthenon Publishing, London, 1997

26 Kolberg R, 'NEWS: Endometriosis enigma: Do the cells themselves hold the crucial clues?' in *J NIH Res*, 9: 23–5, 1997

27 Ibid

28 Vernon M W, Beard J S, Graves K and Wilson E A, 'Classification of endometriotic implants by morphological appearance and capacity to synthesize prostaglandin F' in *Fertil Steril*, 46: 801, 1986

29 Evers J L H, Dunselman G A J and Goeij A F T H, 'Endometriosis and peritoneum: Teflon or Velcro?', *Abstract at the First Nordic Congress on Endometriosis*, Stockholm, Sweden, April 2001

30 Passwater R A and Cranton E M, *Trace Elements, Hair Analysis and Nutrition*, Keats Publishing, New Canaan, p. 66, 1983

CHAPTER 3

1 Lemonick M D, 'Teens before their time' in *Time*, 30 Oct 2000, pp. 66–74

2 Trickey R, *Women, Hormones & the Menstrual Cycle*, Allen & Unwin, pp. 258–73, 1998

3 Vines G, 'Sweet but deadly' in *New Sci*, pp. 26–30, 1 Sept 2001

4 Zammit V A, 'Insulin stimulation of hepatic triacylglycerol secretion and the etiology of insulin resistance' in *J Nutr*, 131: 2074, 2001

5 Middlemann Whitney C, *The Role of Insulin Resistance in the Polycystic Ovary Syndrome*, ION dissertation publication, 1999

6 Barbieri R L, Makris A and Ryan K J, Insulin stimulates androgen accumulation in incubations of human ovarian stroma and theca. *Obstet Gynaecol*, 64 (suppl): S73–80, 1984

7 Franks S, Robinson S and Willis D S, Nutrition, insulin and polycystic ovary syndrome, *Rev Reprod*, 1: 47–53, 1996

8 Legro R S, The genetics of polycystic ovary syndrome. *Am J Med*, 98 (suppl 1a): S9–16, 1995

9 British Medical Association and The Royal Pharmaceutical Society of Great Britain, *British National Formulary*, Sept: 305, 1998

10 Velasquez E M *et al.*, 'Metformin therapy in polycystic ovary syndrome reduces hyperinsulinemia, insulin resistance, hyperandrogenemia and systolic blood pressure, while facilitating normal menses and pregnancy' in *Metabolism*, 43: 647–52, 1994

11 Dunaif A *et al.*, 'Profound peripheral insulin resistance, independent of obesity, in polycystic ovary syndrome' in *Diabetes*, 38: 1165–74, 1989

12 Steiner R A, 'Molecular motifs linking body weight, nutrition and reproduction', (Plenary session), *ASRM 57th Annual Meeting*, 23 Oct, 2001

13 Groop L A and Tuomi T, 'Non-insulin dependent diabetes mellitus – a collision between thrifty genes and an affluent society' in *Ann Med*, 29: 37–53, 1997

14 Trickey R, *Women, Hormones & the Menstrual Cycle*, Allen & Unwin, p. 267, 1998

15 Reaven G M, 'Role of insulin resistance in human disease' in *Diabetes*, 37: 1595–1607, 1998 (Banting lecture)

16 Rupp H, 'Insulin resistance, hyperinsulinaemia and cardiovascular disease, The need for novel dietary prevention strategies' in *Basic Res Cardiol*, 87: 99–105, 1992

17 Trickey R, *Women, Hormones & the Menstrual Cycle*, Allen & Unwin, p. 270, 1998

CHAPTER 4

1 Bradley D, *Hyperventilation Syndrome*, Celestial Arts Publishing, Berkeley CA, 1992

2 Willcox B, Willcox C and Suzuki H, *The Okinawa Way: How to Improve Your Health and Longevity Dramatically*, Penguin Books, p. 64, 2001

3 Kronhausen E, Kronhausen P and Demopoulos H B, *Formula for Life*, William Morrow, New York, p. 95, 1989

4 Kohlmeier L, Rehm J and Hoffmeister H, 'Lifestyles and trends in worldwide breast cancer rates' in *Ann NY Acad Sci*, 609: 259–68, 1990

5 Hawkes N, 'Margarine linked to breast cancer' in *The Times*, 5 September 1997

6 Kassis V, 'The prostaglandin system in human skin' in *Danish Med Bull*, University of Copenhagen, Department of Dermato-Venereology, pp. 320–42, 1983

7 Ibid

8 Rock J A and Hurst B S, 'Clinical significance of prostanoid concentrations in women with endometriosis' in *Current Concepts in Endometriosis*, Alan R Liss, pp. 61–80, 1990

9 Halme J K, 'Role of peritoneal inflammation in endometriosis associated with infertility' in *Endometriosis Today: Advances in Research and Practice, Proceedings of the Vth World Congress on Endometriosis*, eds X Minaguchi and O Sugimoto, Parthenon Publishing, New York & London, pp. 132–5, 1997

10 Lieberman S and Bruning N, *The Real Vitamin and Mineral Book*, Avery Publishing, p. 315, 1997 (2nd edn)

11 Covens A, Christopher P and Cusper R F, 'The effect of dietary supplementation with fish oil fatty acids on surgically induced endometriosis in the rabbit' in *Fertil Steril*, 49: 698–703, 1988

12 Taraye J P and Lauressergue H, 'Advantages of a combination of proteolytic enzymes, flavonoids and ascorbic acid in comparison with non-steroid inflammatory drugs' in *Arzneim Forsch*, 27(1): 1144–9, 1977

13 Hanck A and Weiser H, 'Analgesic and anti-inflammatory properties in vitamins' in *Int J Vit Nutr Res*, 27: 189–206, 1985

14 Cathcart R F *et al.*, 'Leg cramps and vitamin E' in *J Am Med Assoc*, 219: 216–17, 1972

15 Kammura M, 'Anti-inflammatory effects of vitamin E' in *J Vitaminol*, 18: 204–9, 1972

16 Greenwood J, 'Optimum vitamin C intake as a factor in the preservation of disc integrity' in *Med Ann DC*, 33: 274, 1964

17 Misra A L *et al.*, 'Differential effects of opiates on the incorporation of (14C) thiamine in the central nervous system of the rat' in *Experimentia*, 33: 372–4, 1977

18 Hieber H, 'Die Behandung vertebragener Schmerzen und Sensibilitatsstorungen mit Hochdosiertem Hydroxoxcobalamin' in *Med Monatsschr*, 28: 545–8, 1974

19 Muller P, *First International Symposium on Magnesium Deficit in Human Physiology*, 1971

20 Marone G *et al.*, 'Physiological concentrations of zinc inhibit the release of histamine from human basophils and lung mast cells' in *Agents Act*, 18: 103–6, 1986

21 Berqvist I A *et al.*, 'Enhancing quality of life in women and girls with endometriosis-related pain when traditional treatments have failed' in Proceedings of the Savolinna Quality of Life Workshop, Finland, p. 9, 2000

22 Mills D, 'The value of nutrition in the management of pain due to endometriosis' in *Progress in the Management of Endometriosis, Proceedings of the 4th World Congress on Endometriosis*, ed E M Coutinho, Parthenon Press, London, pp. 409–20, 1994

CHAPTER 5

1 Hasson H M, 'Incidence of endometriosis in diagnostic laparoscopy' in *J Reprod Med*, 16: 135, 1976

2 Ballweg M L, *Overcoming Endometriosis*, Congdon & Weed, New York & Chicago, p. 76, 1987

3 Ward N, 'Preconceptual care and pregnancy outcome' in *J Nutr Environ Med*, 5: 205–8, 1995

4 Harada T, Iwabe T and Terakawa N, 'Role of cytokines in endometriosis' in *Fertil Steril*, 76: 1–10, 2001

5 Hill A J, 'The immunology of implantation' in *Course 12, Immunology of Infertility and Pregnancy Loss*, 32nd Annual Postgraduate Program, ASRM Toronto, pp. 15–25, 1999

6 Vernon M W, 'Biochemical activity: differential responsiveness of endometriotic implants' in *Proceedings of the 3rd World Congress on Endometriosis*, eds I Brosens and J Donnez, 1993

7 Ylikorkala O *et al.*, 'Peritoneal fluid prostaglandin in endometriosis, tubal disorders and unexplained infertility' in *Obstet Gynaecol*, 63: 616–20, 1984

8 Drake T *et al.*, 'Peritoneal fluid thromboxane B2 and 6-ketoprostaglandin F1a in endometriosis' in *Am J Obstet Gynecol*, 140: 401–4, 1981

9 Vernon M W, 'Biochemical activity: differential responsiveness of endometriotic implants' in *Proceedings of the 3rd World Congress on Endometriosis*, eds I Brosens and J Donnez, 1993

10 Sharpe K L and Vernon M W, 'Polypeptides synthesized and released by rat endometriotic tissue differ from those of uterine endometrium in culture' in *Biol Reprod*, 48: 1334, 1993

11 Taylor R N, 'Immune aspects of endometriosis' in *Course 12, Immunology of Infertility and Pregnancy Loss*, 32nd Annual Postgraduate Program, ASRM Toronto, pp. 53–66, 1999

12 Tummon I S *et al.*, 'Occult ovulatory dysfunction in women with minimal endometriosis or unexplained infertility' in *Fertil Steril*, 50: 716, 1987

13 Donnez J and Thomas K, 'Incidence of the luteinizing unruptured follicle syndrome in fertile women and in women with endometriosis' in *Eur J Obstet Gynaecol Reprod Biol*, 14: 187, 1982

14 Koninckx P R, DeMoor P and Brosens I A, 'Diagnosis of the luteinized unruptured follicle syndrome by steroid hormone assays on peritoneal fluid' in *Br J Obstet Gynaecol*, 87: 929–34, 1980

15 Wardle P G *et al.*, 'Endometriosis and ovulatory disorder: Reduced fertilization *in vitro* compared with tubal and unexplained infertility' in *Lancet*, 2: 236, 1985

16 Binkley S A, *Endocrinology*, HarperCollins College Publications, pp. 406–10, 1995

17 Naples J D, Batt R E and Sadigh J, 'Spontaneous abortion rate in patients with endometriosis' in *Obstet Gynaecol*, 57: 509, 1986

18 Pittaway D E, Vernon C and Fayex J A, 'Spontaneous abortion in women with endometriosis' in *Fertil Steril*, 50: 711, 1988

19 Branch W, *Course 12, Immunology of Infertility and Pregnancy Loss*, ASRM Toronto, pp. 27–37, 1999

20 Barlow D H *et al.*, 'Changes in humoral immunity in endometriosis' in *The Current Status of Endometriosis: Research and Management*, eds I Brosens and J Donnez, The Proceedings of the 3rd World Congress on Endometriosis, Brussels, pp. 235–48, 1992

21 Swann K, Lai T and Parrington J, 'Life starts with a new conception' in *The Sunday Times*, 12 May 1996

22 Price W A, *Nutrition and Physical Degeneration*, Price-Pottinger Foundation, La Mesa, p. 397, 1945

23 Esther 2:8, *Good News Bible*, Collins, London, 1978

24 Genesis 30:14, *Good News Bible*, Collins, London, 1978

25 Judges 13:3–4, *Good News Bible*, Collins, London, 1978

26 Whorton M D and Milby T H, 'Recovery of testicular function among DBCP workers' in *J Occup Med*, 22: 177–9, 1980

27 'Help yourself to a healthy pregnancy', *She Magazine*, Tommy's Campaign Tesco leaflet, October 1996

28 Higgins I M, 'Nutrition and maternal health' in *Proceedings of the First Conference on Human Nutrition*, Ohio State Department of Health, Columbus, Ohio, 1971

29 Price W A, *Nutrition and Physical Degeneration*, Price-Pottenger Foundation, La Mesa, p. 397, 1945

30 Pottenger F M Jr, *Pottenger's Cats*, Price-Pottenger Foundation, La Mesa, 1983

31 McCarrison R, *Nutrition and Health*, McCarrison Society, London, 1984

32 Williams R J, *Biochemical Individuality: The Basis for the Genetotrophic Concept*, Wiley, New York, 1956

33 Wynn A H A and Wynn M, *The Case For Preconceptual Care in Men and Women*, AB Academic Publishers, Bicester, p. 84, 1991

34 Ward N, 'Preconceptual care and pregnancy outcome' in *J Nutr Environ Med*, 5: 205–8, 1995

35 Wynn A H A and Wynn M, *The Case For Preconceptual Care in Men and Women*, AB Academic Publishers, Bicester, pp. 68–70, 1991

36 Watteville H, Jurgens R and Pfalz H, 'Einfluss von Vitaminagel auf Fruschbarkeit, Schwangerschaft und Nachkommen' in *Schweiz Med Wochenschr*, 84: 875–82, 1954

37 Werbach M R, *Nutritional Influences on Illness*, Keats Publishing, p. 219, 1987

38 Russell L B and Russell W L, 'The sensitivity of different stages in oogenesis to the radiation induction of dominant lethals and other changes in the mouse' in *Progress in Radiobiology*, eds J S Mitchell, B E Holmes and C C Smith, Oliver & Boyd, Edinburgh, pp. 187–92, 1956

39 Wynn A H A and Wynn M, *The Case For Preconceptual Care in Men and Women*, AB Academic Publishers, Bicester, pp. 32–3, 1991

40 Ibid

41 Gregory J, Foster K, Tyler H and Wiseman M, *The Dietary and Nutritional Survey of British Adults*, HMSO, London, p. 29, 1990

42 Abraham S, Mira M and Llewellyn-Jones D, 'Should ovulation be induced in women recovering from an eating disorder or who are compulsive exercisers?' in *Fertil Steril*, 53: 566–8, 1990

43 Cameron J L, *The Menstrual Cycle and its Disorders*, eds K M Pirke, W Wuttke and U Schweiger, Springer Verlag, Heidelberg, pp. 66–78, 1989

44 Barr S I, Prior J C and Vigna Y M, 'Restrained eating and ovulatory disturbances: possible implications for bone health' in *Am J Clin Nutr*, 59: 92–7, 1994

45 Wynn A H A and Wynn M, 'Slimming and fertility' in *Modern Midwife*, 4 (6): 17–20, 1994

46 Kyo U C *et al.*, 'Changes in endocrine pancreatic function in short-term diet restriction' in *Nutrition*, 17: 425–9, 1991

47 Wynn A H A and Wynn M, *The Case For Preconceptual Care in Men and Women*, AB Academic Publishers, Bicester, p. 78, 1991

48 Coop I E, 'Effect of flushing on reproductive performance of ewes' in *J Agri Sci (Camb)*, 67: 305–23, 1966

49 Doyle W *et al.*, 'Maternal nutrient intake and birthweight' in *J Hum Nutr Diet*, 2: 415–22, 1989

50 Brosens I A, Koninckx P R and Corveleyn P A, 'A study of plasma progesterone, oestradiol 17β, prolactin and LH levels and the luteal phase appearance of the ovaries in patients with endometriosis and infertility' in *Br J Obstet Gynaecol*, 85: 246–50, 1978

51 Esch M W, Easter R A and Bahr J M, 'Effect of riboflavin deficiency on estrous cyclicity in pigs' in *Biol Reprod*, 25: 659–65, 1981

52 Barnes B and Bradley S G, *Planning for a Healthy Baby*, Vermilion, London, 1990

53 Doyle W *et al.*, 'Maternal nutrient intake and birth weight' in *J Hum Nutr Diet*, 2: 415–22, 1989

54 Wynn A H A and Wynn M, 'The need for nutritional assessment in the treatment of the infertile patient' in *J Nutr Med*, 1: 315–24, 1990

55 Le Fanu, J, 'Mother's Battle of the Bulge' in *The Times*, 30 March 1995

56 Smith N C, 'Detection of the foetus at risk' in *Eur J Clin Nutr*, 46 (suppl 1): S1–S5, 1992

57 Hackman E, 'Maternal birth weight and subsequent pregnancy outcome' in *J Am Med Assoc*, 250: 2016–19, 1983

58 Aherne W and Dunhill M S, 'Morphology of the human placenta' in *Br Med Bull*, 22 (1): 5–12, 1966

59 Hackman E, 'Maternal birth weight and subsequent pregnancy outcome' in *J Am Med Assoc*, 250: 2016–19, 1983

60 Doyle W *et al.*, 'The association of maternal diet and birth weight dimensions' in *J Nutr Med*, 1: 9–16, 1990

61 Committee to Study the Prevention of Low Birth Weight, *Preventing Low Birth Weight*, National Academy Press, Washington, 1985

62 Burke B S, Harding V V and Stuart H C, 'Nutrition studies during pregnancy' in *J Paediatr*, 23: 506–15, 1943

63 Wynn A H A and Wynn M, 'The need for nutritional assessment in the treatment of the infertile patient' in *J Nutr Med*, 1: 315–78, 1990

64 Bates G W, Bates S G and Whitworth N S, 'Reproductive failure in women who practise weight control' in *Fertil Steril*, 37: 373–8, 1982

65 Speroff L and Walllach E E, 'The changing face of infertility' in *Fertility*, pp. 8–23, 1987

66 Keen C L and Zidenberg-Cherr S, 'Should vitamin-mineral supplements be recommended for all women with childbearing potential?' in *Am J Clin Nutr*, 59 (suppl): 532S–9S, 1994

67 Ryan S, 'Scientists link falling sperm counts to chemicals in food' in *The Sunday Times*, 21 May 1995

68 Bentham P, 'VDU terminal sickness' in *Green Print*, 165: 27–35, 1980

69 Skakkebaek N and Keilding N, 'Changes in semen and the testes' in *BMJ*, 309: 1316–17, 1994

70 Whorton M D and Milby T H, 'Recovery of testicular function among DSCP workers' in *J Occup Med*, 22: 177–9, 1980

71 Skakkebaek N and Keilding N, 'Changes in semen and the testes' in *BMJ*, 309: 1316–17, 1994

72 Sharpe R M and Skakkebaek N, 'Are oestrogens involved in falling sperm counts and disorders of the male reproductive tract?' in *Lancet*, 341: 1392–6, 1993

73 Connor S, 'Mystery of the vanishing sperm' in *The Independent on Sunday*, 8 March 1992

74 Jeyendran R S, *Interpretation of Semen Analysis Results: A Practical Guide*, Cambridge University Press, Cambridge, pp.16–17, 2000

75 Prasad A S, 'Is infertility linked to zinc deficiency?' in *Better Nutrition Magazine*, 8: 13–62, 1982

76 Tuormaa T E, 'Adverse effects of manganese deficiency on reproduction and health' in *J Orthomol Med*, 11: 3, 1996

77 Murray M T, *Male Sexual Vitality*, Prima Publishing, Rocklin, pp. 50–6, 1994

78 Colburn T, Myers J P and Dumanoski D, *Our Stolen Future*, Little, Brown, London, 1996

79 Link A, *Chlorine, Pollution and the Parents of Tomorrow*, Women's Environmental Network, London, 1991

80 Mormann R, *Endometriosis Association 10th Anniversary Handbook*, Milwaukee 1991

81 Urlocker K, 'Surviving infertility' in *Infertility Awareness*, 9 (2): 4–5, 1993

CHAPTER 6

1 Kistner R W, 'The treatment of endometriosis by inducing pseudopregnancy with ovarian hormones: a report of 58 cases' in *Fertil Steril*, 10: 539, 1959

2 Grant E, *Sexual Chemistry*, Cedar Press, London, pp. 47, 97, 166, 237, 1994

3 Hurst B S and Schalaff W D, 'Treatment options for endometriosis: Medical therapies' in *Infertility and Reproductive Medicine Clinics of North America Vol 2*, ed D Olive, W B Saunders, Philadelphia & London, 3: 645, 1992

4 Gunning J E and Moyer D, 'The effect of medroxyprogesterone acetate on endometriosis in the human female' in *Fertil Steril*, 18: 759, 1967

5 O'Connor D, *Endometriosis*, Churchill Livingstone, Edinburgh, p. 13, 1989

6 Sensky T E and Liu D T, 'Endometriosis: associations with menorrhagia, infertility and oral contraceptives' in *Int J Gynaecol Obstet*, 17: 573–6, 1980

7 Parazzini F *et al.*, 'Oral contraceptives use and risk of endometriosis – Italian Endometriosis Study Group' in *Br J Obstet Gynaecol*, 106: 695–9, 1999

8 Kirshon B and Poindexter A N III, 'Contraception: a risk factor for endometriosis' in *Obstet Gynaecol*, 71: 829–31, 1988

9 Barbieri R L, Evans S and Kistner R W, 'Danazol in the treatment of endometriosis analysis of 100 cases with a 4-year follow-up' in *Fertil Steril*, 37: 737, 1982

10 Holt J P and Keller D, 'Danazol treatment increases serum enzymes' in *Fertil Steril*, 41: 70, 1984

11 Hodgen G D, 'General applications of GnRH agonists in gynecology past, present and future' in *Obstet Gynecol Surv*, 44: 293, 1989

12 Warnock J K and Bundner J C, 'Anxiety and mood disorders associated with gonadotrophin-releasing hormone agonist therapy' in *Psychopharmacol Bull*, 33: 311–6, 1997

13 Luciano A A and Manzi D, 'Treatment options for endometriosis: Surgical therapies' in *Infertility and Reproductive Medicine Clinics of North America Vol 2*, ed D Olive, W B Saunders, Philadephia & London, 3: 657, 1992

14 Editorial, 'Hysterectomy prevalence and death rates for cervical cancer – United States' in *MMWR*, 41(2): 17–20, 1992

15 Santow G and Bracher M, 'Correlates of hysterectomy in Australia' in *Soc Sci Med*, 34(8): 929–42, 1992

16 Vessey M P *et al.*, 'The epidemiology of hysterectomy: findings in a large cohort study' in *Br J Obstet Gynaecol*, 99(5): 402–7, 1992

17 Colgan H, *Hormonal Health: Nutritional and Hormonal Strategies for Emotional Well-Being and Intellectual Longevity*, Apple Publishing, p. 92, 1996

18 Centerwell B S, 'Premenopausal hysterectomy and cardiovascular disease' in *Am J Obstet Gynecol*, 139: 58–61, 1981

19 Shoupe D, 'Rationale for ovarian conservation in women' in *ASRM Menopausal Medicine*, 7 (3): 1–4, 1999

20 Acher J, *Bad Medicine*, Simon & Schuster, Australia, p. 191, 1995

21 Hurlbutt K, in *Overcoming Endometriosis*, ed M L Ballweg, Congdon & Weed, New York, 1987

22 Tallo C P *et al.*, 'Maternal and neonatal morbidity associated with *in vitro* fertilization' in *J Pediatr*, 127 (50): 794–800, 1995

23 Venn A *et al.*, 'Breast and ovarian cancer incidence after infertility and *in vitro* fertilization' in *Lancet*, 243: 1627–8, 1995

24 Pouly J L *et al.*, 'The place of IVF in the treatment of endometriosis-related infertility' in *Endometriosis Today. Proceedings of the Vth World Congress on Endometriosis*, eds H Minaguchi and O Sugimoto, Parthenon Publishing Group, New York & London, p. 443, 1997

25 Dmowski W P *et al.*, 'The effect of endometriosis, its stage and activity, and of auto-antibodies on IVF and embryo transfer success rates' in *Fertil Steril*, 63: 555, 1995

26 Stolwijk A M *et al.*, 'The impact of the women's age on the success of standard and donor IVF' in *Fertil Steril*, 67: 702, 1997

27 Dmowski W P *et al.*, 'The effect of endometriosis, its stage and activity, and of auto-antibodies on IVF and embryo transfer success rates' in *Fertil Steril*, 63: 555, 1995

28 Cornwell J, 'Why is this so difficult? Infertility' in the *Sunday Times Magazine*, 34–42, 11 November 1996

29 Syal R, 'Revealed: 30,000 embryos used in fertility experiments' in *The Sunday Times*, 3 May 1998

30 Davies S, 'Nutritional medicine. Has it a role in handicap prevention and the medical treatment of infertility, including assisted ovulation, IVF and GIFT?' in *J Nutr Med*, 1: 251–8, 1990

31 Whitworth N, 'IVF and sperm abnormalities' in *The Times*, 1996

32 Speroff L and Walsh E E, 'The changing face of infertility' in *Fertility*, 8–23, 1987

33 Igarashi M, 'Augmentative effects of ascorbic acid upon induction of human ovulation in clomiphene-ineffective anovulatory women' in *Int J Fertil*, 22(3): 168–75, 1977

34 Reuben C and Priestley J, *Essential Supplements for Women*, Thorsons, London, p. 190, 1991

35 British Medical Association & Royal Pharmaceutical Society of Great Britain, *British National Formulary*, 1996

36 British Medical Association & Royal Pharmaceutical Society of Great Britain, *British National Formulary*, p. 264, 1996

37 Mills D S, 'The role of nutrition in preconceptual care within a health promotion setting', *Master of Arts Degree Investigative Study*, University of Brighton, April 1996

38 British Medical Association & Royal Pharmaceutical Society of Great Britain, *British National Formulary*, 1996

39 Hawkes N, 'Why grapefruit juice and drugs don't mix' in *The Times*, 24 November 1997

40 Oakley A, *From Here to Maternity – Becoming a Mother*, Penguin, Harmondsworth, p. 283, 1981

41 Friedson E, 'Dilemmas in the doctor/patient relationship' in *A Sociology of Medical Practice*, eds C Cox and A Mead, Collier Macmillan, London, 1975

42 Gilligan C, *In a Different Voice: Psychological Theory and Women's Development*, Harvard University Press, Cambridge, Mass, 1982

43 Wastell D and Macdonald V, 'Drug salesmen face jail over gifts to GPs' in *Sunday Telegraph*, 27 July 1997

44 Bequaert Holmes H and Purdy L M, eds, *Feminist Perspectives in Medical Ethics*, Indiana University Press, Bloomington & Indianapolis, p. 100, 1992

45 Ibid, p. 72

46 Pellegrino E D and Thomasina D C, *For the Patient's Good*, Oxford University Press, New York, pp. 20–1, 1988

47 Phillips M, 'Losing our humanity at the embryo bank' in *The Sunday Times*, p. 17, 6 December 1998

48 Lauersen N H and de Swann C, *Endometriosis Answer Book*, Fawsett Columbine, New York, p. 197, 1988

49 'Too many hysterectomies in the UK' in *Lancet*, 349: 1226, 1997

50 Lilford R J, 'Hysterectomy: Will it pay the bills in 2007?' in *BMJ*, 314: 160–1, 1997

51 Lazarus K, Weinsier R L and Boker J R, 'Nutrition knowledge and practices of physicians in a family-practice residency programme: the effect of an education programme provided by physician nutrition specialists' in *Am J Clin Nutr*, 58: 319–25,1993

52 Green L W, Erikson M P and Schor E L, 'Preventive practices by physicians: behavioural determinants and potential interventions' in *Am J Prev Med*, 4: 101–7, 1988

53 Null G, *No More Allergies*, Villard Books, New York, 1992

54 Meldrum J M, 'A response to the health of the nation: a summary of the government's proposals' in *J Nutr Med*, 2: 415–21, 1991

CHAPTER 7

1 Berdanier C D, 'Nutrient-gene interactions' in *Present Knowledge in Nutrition*, eds E E Ziegler and L J Filer Jr, ILSI Press, Washington, 1996 (7th edn)

2 Williams R J, *Biochemical Individuality: The Basis for the Genetotrophic Concept*, Wiley & Sons, New York, 1956

3 Null G, *The Complete Guide to Health and Nutrition*, Arlington Books, London, p. 499, 1984

4 Ibid, p. 499

5 Quotes extracted from 'Human Reproduction' 10: 50–55, 1995, reproduced in *The Real Vitamin and Mineral Book*, S Lieberman and N Bruning, Avery Press, New York, p. 325, 1997

6 Binkley S A, *Endocrinology*, HarperCollins College Publishers, p. 384, 1995

7 Quotes extracted from 'Human Reproduction' 10: 50–55, 1995, reproduced in *The Real Vitamin and Mineral Book*, S Lieberman and N Bruning, Avery Press, New York, p. 325, 1997

8 Weil A, 'Eight weeks to optimum health' in *Spontaneous Healing*, Warner Books, p. 82, 1995

9 Null G, *The Complete Guide to Health and Nutrition*, Arlington Books, London, p. 427, 1984

10 Griswold R E, 'The health tape', from *The Love Tapes*, Ediner, Minnesota, 1988

CHAPTER 8

1 Usher R, 'The sunnier, southern side of the street' in *Time*, 12 Nov, p. 65, 2001

2 Philpott W H and Kalita D K, *Brain Allergies: The Psychonutrient Connection*, Keats Publishing, New Canaan, p. 6, 1987

3 Batdielder T, 'Depression: an anthropological perspective' in *Townsend Lett Docs*, April: 32–4, 2001

4 Holford P and Coos H, *Natural Highs*, Piatkus, London, p. 74, 2001

5 Begley S, 'Fighting addiction: How it all starts inside your brain' in *Newsweek*, 12 Feb, p. 58–60, 2001

6 Begley S, 'The brain in winter' in *Newsweek Special Issue, Winter*, pp. 139–43, 2001

7 Ibid, p. 24–9

8 Thompson R F, *The Brain: An Introduction to Neuroscience*, W. H. Freeman & Co., p. 120, 1985

9 Thompson R, *The Brain: An Introduction to Neuroscience*, W. H. Freeman & Co., p. 130, 1985

10 Lombard J and Germano C, *The Brain Wellness Plan*, Kensington Books, pp. 132–3, 1997

11 Thompson R, *The Brain: An Introduction to Neuroscience*, W. H. Freeman & Co., p. 112, 1985

12 Godfrey P *et al.*, 'Enhancement of recovery from psychiatric illness' in *Lancet*, 336: 392–5, 1990

13 Helfrich R, *Take Control of Your Health*, Duckworth Books, p. 44, 1996

14 Chaitow L, *The Healing Power of Amino Acids*, Thorsons Press, p. 38, 1989

15 Braverman E R and Pfeiffer C C, *The Healing Nutrients Within: Facts, Findings and New Research on Amino Acids*, Keats Publishing, New Canaan, pp. 120–36, 1987

16 Chaitow L, *Amino Acids in Therapy*, Thorsons, pp. 73–5, 1985

17 Helfrich R, *Take Control of Your Health*, Duckworth Books, p. 52, 1996

18 Erdmann R and Jones M, *The Amino Revolution*, Century Books p. 56, 1988

19 Chaitow L, *Amino Acids in Therapy*, Thorsons, pp. 58–61, 1985

20 Ibid, pp. 32–3

21 Ibid, p. 59

22 Helfrich R, *Take Control of Your Health*, Duckworth Books, p. 50, 1996

23 Lombard J and Germano C, *The Brain Wellness Plan*, Kensington Books, p. 28, 1997

24 Erdmann R and Jones M, *The Amino Revolution*, Century Books p. 181, 1988

25 Chaitow L, *Amino Acids in Therapy*, Thorsons, p. 58, 1985

26 MacDonald Baker S, *Detoxification & Healing*, Keats Publishing, New Canaan, pp. 8–12, 1997

27 Philpott W H and Kalita D K, *Brain Allergies: The Psychonutrient Connection*, Keats Publishing, New Canaan, pp. 7–8, 1987

28 Philpott W H and Kalita D K, *Brain Allergies: The Psychonutrient Connection*, Keats Publishing, New Canaan, pp. 3–4, 1987

29 Thompson R, *The Brain: An Introduction to Neuroscience*, W. H. Freeman & Co., p. 141, 1985

30 Snyder S H, 'Pain pathways' in *Sci Am*, 236 (3): 44–56, 1977

31 Thompson R, *The Brain: An Introduction to Neuroscience*, W. H. Freeman & Co., p. 128, 1985

32 Lombard J and Germano C, *The Brain Wellness Plan*, Kensington Books, p. 158, 1997

33 Sprongen K, 'Taming raging hormones' in *Newsweek Special Issue, Winter*, pp. 30–2, 2001

34 Yoshino S, Fujimori J and Kohda M, 'Effects of mirthful laughter on neuroendocrine and immune systems in patients with rheumatoid arthritis' in *J Rheumatol*, 234: 793–4, 1996

35 Lombard J and Germano C, *The Brain Wellness Plan*, Kensington Books, p. 196, 1997

36 Lombard J and Germano C, *The Brain Wellness Plan*, Kensington Books, pp. 199–200, 1997

37 Ibid, pp. 202–10

38 Ibid, p. 208

39 Roberts H J, *Aspartame (Nutrasweet): Is It Safe?*, The Charles Press, p. 198, 1990

40 Blaylock R L, *Excitotoxins: The Taste That Kills*, Health Press, p. 79–80, 1994

41 Lombard J and Germano C, *The Brain Wellness Plan*, Kensington Books, pp. 30–9, 1997

CHAPTER 9

1 Null G and Feldman M D, *Reverse the Ageing Process Naturally*, Villard Books, New York, 1993

2 Collins J K, O'Sullivan G and Shanahan F, 'Probiotics bacteria – interaction with the human immune system' in *Gut Flora and Health – Past, Present and Future*, The Royal Society of Medicine Press, pp. 13–14, 1996

3 Rosenburg L E, 'Inborn errors of nutrient metabolism: Garrod's lessons and legacies' in *Genetic Factors in Nutrition*, eds A Valezquez and H Bourges, pp. 61–77, 1984

4 Vernon M W, personal communication, 1997

5 Thomas E J and Rock J A, *Modern Approaches to Endometriosis*, Kluwer Academic Publishers, Lancaster, p. 14, 1991

6 Dmwoski W P, Braun D and Gebel H, 'The immune system in endometriosis' in *Modern Approaches to Endometriosis*, E J Thomas and J A Rock, Kluwer Academic Publishers, Lancaster, p. 97–108, 1991

7 Meek J, *Immune Power*, Optima Macdonald, London, pp. 33–4, 1990

8 Ibid, p. 143

9 'Sugar and immunity' in *The New York Times*, 14 July 1987, quoted in G Null and M Feldman, *Reversing the Aging Process Naturally*, Villard Books, New York, p. 24, 1993

10 Meek J, *Immune Power*, Optima Macdonald, London, p. 34, 1990

11 Ibid, p. 33

12 Barlow D H, Kennedy S H, Fernandez-Shaw S and Starkey P M, 'Changes in humoral immunity in endometriosis' in *The Current Status of Endometriosis: Research & Management*, eds I Brosens and J Donnez, Parthenon Publishing, Lancaster, pp. 235–49, 1992

13 Kirkwood E and Lewis C, *Understanding Medical Immunology*, John Wiley, Chichester, p. 26, 1994 (2nd edn)

14 Barnes B and Bradley S G, *Planning for a Healthy Baby*, Vermillion, London, p. 68, 1990

15 Null G and Feldman M D, *Reversing the Aging Process Naturally*, Villard Books, New York, pp. 90–3, 1993

16 Ibid, pp. 90–3

17 Nothnick W B, 'New insights into the treatment and classification of endometriosis', *ASRM Florida Roundtable Discussion Paper*, pp. 1–15, 2001

18 Thomas E J and Rock J A, *Modern Approaches to Endometriosis*, Kluwer Academic Publishers, Lancaster, p. 97, 1991

19 Meek J, *Immune Power*, Optima Macdonald, London, p. 139, 1990

20 Weir D M, *Immunology*, Churchill Livingstone, Edinburgh, p. 53, 1988 (6th edn)

21 Ballweg M L, 'Immunotherapy for endometriosis' in *Endometrium and Endometriosis*, Blackwell Science, Oxford, pp. 367–75, 1997

22 Halme J and Hammond M G, 'The role of growth factors in endometriosis' in *The Current Status of Endometriosis: Research & Management*, eds I Brosens and J Donnez, Parthenon Publishing, Lancaster, p. 211, 1992

23 Ibid, p. 212

24 Halme J, Hammond M G, Hulka J S, 'Retrograde menstruation in healthy women and in patients with endometriosis' in *Obstet Gynecol*, 64: 151–4, 1984

25 Halme J K, 'Role of peritoneal inflammation in endometriosis associated with infertility', *World Congress on Endometriosis*, p. 72, Yokohama, Japan, 1996

26 Evers J L H, 'The immune system in endometriosis: introduction' in *The Current Status of Endometriosis: Research and Management*, eds I Brosens and J Donnez, Proceedings of the 3rd World Congress on Endometriosis, Brussels, Parthenon Publishing, Lancaster, pp. 223–33, 1992

27 Harada T *et al.*, 'Role of cytokines in endometriosis' in *Fertil Steril*, 76: 1–10, 2001

28 Kauma S, *Course 12, Immunology for the Infertility Specialist. Immunology of Infertility and Pregnancy Loss*, ASRM meeting, Toronto, pp. 1–25, 1999

29 Haney A, Muscato J and Weinberg J, 'Peritoneal fluid cell populations in infertile patients' in *Fertil Steril*, 35: 696–8, 1981

30 Taylor R N, 'Immune aspects of endometriosis' in *Course 12, Immunology of Infertility and Pregnancy Loss*, ASRM meeting, Toronto, pp. 53–65, 1999

31 Odukoya O A, Wilson A P and Cooke I, 'The prevalence of endometrial IgG antibodies in patients with endometriosis' in *Hum Reprod*, 10 (5): 1214–19, 1992

32 Vallatton M B and Forbes A P, 'Antibodies to cytoplasm of ova' in *Lancet*, 2: 264–5, 1996

33 Braley J, *The Immuno Review*, 1 (1 & 2): 1993, (personal communication, ION Conference, 1995, London)

34 Singh A, Nery Danta Z, Stone S C, and Asch R H, 'Presence of thyroid antibodies in early reproductive failure: biochemical versus clinical pregnancies' in *Fertil Steril*, 63(2): 277–81, 1995

35 Howard S, 'Module 16: Current thinking in coeliac disease' in *Pharmacy Magazine*, CEI–CEVIII, February 1997

36 Toates F, *Stress – Conceptual and Biological Aspects*, John Wiley, Chichester, pp. 8, 65, 75–77, 83, 276, 1996

37 Null G and Feldman M D, *Reverse the Ageing Process Naturally*, Villard Books, New York, p. 59, 1993

CHAPTER 10

1 McCance X and Widdowson A, *Comparison of Foods 1939 and 1991*, 1991

2 Kendall P, 'Why fruit and veg were better for us 50 years ago', *The Daily Mail*, 5 March 2001

3 McKeown T, *The Role of Medicine: Dream, Mirage or Nemesis?* Basil Blackwell, Oxford, 1979, quoted in *The Modern Rise of Population*, Arnold, London, 1979

4 Lange T, 'The Food Programme', *BBC Radio 4 Food Choices*, 13 March 1997

5 'Ready-cooked meals account for 35 per cent of food bills' in *The Guardian*, 15 November 1994

6 Lipski E, *Digestive Wellness*, Keats Publishing, New Canaan, p. 29, 1996

7 Collins J K, O'Sullivan G and Shanahan F, 'Probiotic bacteria – interaction with the human immune system' in *International Congress and Symposium Series 219, Gut Flora and Health – Past, Present and Future*, eds A R Leeds and I R Rowland, Royal Society of Medicine Press, London, pp. 13–19, 1996

8 Chaitow L and Trenev N, *Probiotics*, Thorsons, London, 1990

9 Collins J K, O'Sullivan G and Shanahan F, 'Probiotic bacteria – interaction with the human immune system' in *International Congress and Symposium Series 219, Gut Flora and Health – Past, Present and Future*, eds A R Leeds and I R Rowland, Royal Society of Medicine Press, London, pp. 13–19, 1996

10 Ibid

11 Lipski E, *Digestive Wellness*, Keats Publishing, New Canaan, p. 227, 1996

12 Office of Population and Census Statistics, *The Dietary and Nutritional Survey of British Adults*, HMSO, London, 1991

13 Marks J, 'Current status and future prospects' in *International Congress and Symposium Series 219, Gut Flora and Health – Past, Present and Future*, eds A R Leeds and I R Rowland, Royal Society of Medicine Press, London, pp. 57–69, 1996

14 Stuttaford T, 'Medical briefing: dialysis could be hard and dangerous' in *The Times*, p. 5, 1 November 2001

15 Cannon G, *Superbug – Nature's Revenge, Why Antibiotics Can Breed Disease*, Virgin, p. 102, 1995

16 Gibson G R and Beaumont A, 'An overview of human colonic bacteriology in health and disease' in *International Congress and Symposium Series 219, Gut Flora and Health – Past, Present and Future*, eds A R Leeds and I R Rowland, Royal Society of Medicine Press, London, pp. 57, 1996

17 Schiffrin F J *et al.*, 'Immune modulations of human blood cells following the ingestion of lactic acid bacteria' in *J Dairy Sci*, 78: 491–7, 1995

18 Crayhon R, *Health Benefits of FOS (Fructo-oligosaccharides)*, Keats Publishing, New Canaan, p. 28, 1995

189 Brostoff J and Gamlin L, *The Complete Guide to Food Allergy and Intolerance*, Bloomsbury Press, London, pp. 129, 230, 1989

20 National Institutes of Health, Bethesda, Maryland, *Food Allergy and Intolerance*, 1996

21 Hollander D and Tarnawski H, 'Ageing-associated increase in intestinal absorption of macromolecules' in *Gerontology*, 31: 133–7, 1985

22 Petres T J and Bjarnason I, 'Uses and abuses of intestinal permeability measurements' in *Can J Gastroenterol*, 12 (3): 1988

23 Reichelt K L *et al.*, 'Gluten, milk proteins and autism: results of dietary intervention on behaviour and urinary peptide secretion' in *J Appl Nutr*, 42: 1–11, 1990

24 Ballweg M L, *Endometriosis Sourcebook*, Contemporary Books, Chicago, pp. 200–2, 1995

25 Feldman D, 'Steroid hormone systems found in yeast' in *Science*, August 1984

26 Edwards D A, 'Depression and *Candida*' in *J Am Med Assoc*, 253: 340, 1995

27 Rivas V and Rogers T J, 'Studies on the cellular nature of *Candida albicans*-induced suppression' in *J Immunol*, 130: 376, 1983

28 Null G, *The Complete Guide to Health and Nutrition*, Arlington Books, London, p. 129, 1984

29 Lamb K and Nichols T R, 'Endometriosis: A comparision of associated disease histories' in *Am J Prev Med*, 2 (6): 324–9, 1986

30 Null G, *No More Allergies*, Villard Books, New York, p. 3, 1992

31 Golos N and Golos-Golbritz F, *If It's Tuesday It Must Be Chicken*, Keats Publishing, New Canaan, 1979

32 Null G, *Good Food, Good Mood*, St Martin's Press, New York, p. 13, 1998

33 Cohen R, 'The health dangers of dairy products' in *Nexus*, pp. 23–8, August 1998

34 Chaitow L and Trenew N, *Probiotics*, Thorsons, London, pp. 70–1, 1990

35 Councell C E, Taha A and Ruddell W S J, 'Coeliac disease and auto-immune thyroid disease' in *Gut*, 35: 844–6, 1994

36 Lindsay R S and Toft A D, 'Hypothyroidism' in *Lancet*, 349: 413–7, 1997

37 Weetman A P, 'Hypothyroidism: screening and subclinical disease' in *BMJ*, 314: 1175, 1997

38 Singh A, Dantas Z N, Stone S C and Asch R H, 'Presence of thyroid antibodies in early reproductive failure: biochemical versus clinical pregnancies' in *Fertil Steril*, 63(2): 277–81, 1995

39   Howard S, 'Current thinking in coeliac disease' in *Pharmacy Magazine* CEI–VII, February 1997

40   Sher K S and Mayberry J F, 'Female fertility, obstetric and gynaecological history in coeliac disease. A case control study' in Sher K S, Jayanthi V, Probert C S J, Stewart C R and Mayberry J F, 'Infertility, obstetric and gynaecological problems in coeliac sprue' in *Digest Dis*, 12: 186–90, 1994

41   Councell C E, Taha A and Ruddell W S J, 'Coeliac disease and auto-immune thyroid disease' in *Gut*, 35: 844–6, 1994

42   Hemming W A, 'The entry into the brain of large molecules derived from dietary protein' in *Proc Roy Soc Lond*, 200: 175–92, 1978

43   Maki M and Collin P, 'Coeliac disease seminar' in *Lancet*, 349: 1755–9, 1997

44   Johnston S D *et al.*, 'Prevalence of coeliac disease in Northern Ireland' in *Lancet*, 349: 1370, 1997

45   Cronin C C and Shahan F, 'Insulin-dependent diabetes mellitis and coeliac disease' in *Lancet*, 349: 1096–7, 1997

46   Lark S, *Fibroid Tumors and Endometriosis: A Self-Help Book*, Celestial Arts, Berkeley, 1993

47   Fredericks C, *Guide to Women's Nutrition. Dietary Advice for Women of All Ages*, Perigree Books, New York, p. 32, 1989

48   Stock S, 'Nutrition and hormones' in *Nutr Ther Today*, 3: 4, 1995

49   Ibid

50   Cowan D W *et al.*, 'Breast cancer incidence in women with a history of progesterone deficiency' in *Am J Epidemiol*, 114: 209–17, 1981

51   Spallholz J E *et al.*, 'Immunological responses of mice fed diets supplemented with selenite selenium' in *Proc Soc Exp Biol Med*, 143: 685–9, 1973

52   Stock S, 'Nutrition and hormones' in *Nutr Ther Today*, 3: 4, 1995

53   Challem J J and Lewin R, 'Managing endometriosis through nutrition' in *Endo Assoc USA Newsletter*, 10 (4), 1989

54   Devlin T M, *Textbook of Biochemistry with Clinical Correlations*, John Wiley, pp. 570–90, 1986 (2nd edn)

55   Lemon H M *et al.*, 'Re: ethnic differences in estrogen metabolism in healthy women' in *J Nat Cancer Inst*, 89 (21): 1626–8, 1997

56   Lemon H M *et al.*, 'A method for estimating catechol estrogen metabolism from excretion of noncatechol estrogens' in *Cancer*, 68 (2): 444–50, 1991

57   Goldin B R and Gorbach S I, 'The effect of milk and lactobacillus feeding on human intestinal bacterial enzyme activity' in *Am J Clin Nutr*, 39: 756–61, 1984

58   Ockerman P A, Bachrack L, Glans S and Rassner S, 'Evening primrose oil as a treatment of premenstrual syndrome' in *Recent Adv Clin Nutr*, 2: 404–5, 1986

59   Link A, 'Fertility and the environment' in *Nutr Ther Today*, 3(3): 6–81, 1991

60   Vidal J and Cone M, 'Out for the count: do toxic chemicals reduce male fertility' in *The Guardian*, 15 February 1995

61   McLachlin J A and Arnold S F, 'Environmental estrogens' in *Am Sci*, 84: 452–61, 1997

62   Ibid

63   Rier S E *et al.*, 'Production of interleukin-6 and tumor necrosis factor-alpha by peripheral blood mononuclear cells from rhesus monkeys with endometriosis' in *J Immunol*, 150: 49a, 1992

64   Rier S *et al.*,'Serum levels of TCDD and dioxin-like chemicals in rhesus monkeys chronically exposed to dioxin: correlation of increased serum PCB levels with endometriosis' in *Toxicol Sci*, 59: 147–59, 2001

65   Poulter S, 'The suspect salmon: how healthy fish could be polluting our children's diets' in *The Daily Mail*, p. 37, 13 November 2001

66 The Women's Environmental Leaflet: 'Living with dioxins', p. 15, 1993 in Hume Hall R 'New threat to public health: organochlorines and food' in *Nutr Health*, 8: 333, 1992

67 'Prostaglandins & Leukotrienes, March 1985, 2nd International Congress on Essential Fatty Acids' quoted in Lieberman S and Bruning N, *The Real Vitamin & Mineral Book*, Avery Books, New York, p. 315, 1997 (2nd edn)

68 MacDonald Baker S, *Detoxification & Healing: The Key to Optimum Health*, Keats Publishing, New Canaan, p. 25, 1997

69 Gambert H R, 'Factors that control thyroid function: Environmental effects and physiological variables' in Braverman I E and Utiger R D, eds, *The Thyroid Gland*, J B Lippincott, Philadelphia, pp. 347–57, 1991

70 Chaitow L and Trenev N, *Probiotics*, Thorsons, London, p. 47, 1990

71 Fredericks C, *Guide to Women's Nutrition: Dietary Advice for Women of All Ages*, Putnam Publishing Group, New York, p. 36, 1989

72 Messina M, Messina V and Setchell K, *The Simple Soyabean and Your Health*, Avery Publishing, New York, p. 73, 1994

73 Ibid

74 Ministry of Agriculture, Fisheries and Food, 'Assessment on phyto-oestrogens in the human diet', *J Environ Health*, November 1997

75 Zeligs MA, 'Safer estrogen with phytonutrition' in *Townsend Lett Docs*, April: 83–8, 1999

76 Watts D L, 'Nutritional interrelationships, minerals, vitamins, endocrines' in *J Orthomol Med*, 5: 11–20, 1990

77 Gambert S R, 'Factors that control thyroid function: environmental effects and physiologic variables' in eds L E Braveman and R D Utiger, *The Thyroid Gland*, J B Lippincott, Philadelphia, pp. 347–57, 1991

78 Fredericks C, *Guide to Women's Nutrition: Dietary Advice For Women of All Ages*, Perigee Books, p. 53, 1989

79 Singh A *et al.*, 'Presence of thyroid auto-antibodies in early reproductive failure: biochemical versus clinical pregnancies' in *Fertil Steril*, 63(2): 277–81, 1995

80 Councell L and Trenew N, *Probiotics*, London, Thorsons, pp. 70–1, 1990

81 Ditcoff B A and Gerfo P L, *The Thyroid Guide*, London, HarperCollins, p. 28, 2000

82 Dees C *et al.*, 'Dietary estrogens stimulate human breast cells to enter the cell cycle' in *Environ Health Perspect*, 105(3): 1997

83 'The ice cream story' in *The Sunday Observer*, 29 May 1983

CHAPTER 11

1 Walker C and Cannon G, *The Food Scandal*, Century Publishing, London, p. 68, 1984

2 Quoted in Doll R and Peto R, *Causes of Cancer*, Oxford University Press, Oxford, 1981

3 Silverberg E, 'Cancer Statistics, 1985' in *Cancer J Clin*, 35(1): 19, 1985

4 Buss D H, 'Food patterns in the British Isles' in *Ann Nutr Metabol*, 35 (suppl): 12–21, 1991

5 Badura B and Kickbish I, *Health Promotion Research: Towards a New Social Epidemiology*, WHO Regional Publications, Copenhagen, European Series No. 37: 233, 1991

6 Lappalainen R *et al.*, 'Perceived benefits of healthy eating among a nationally representative sample of adults in the European Union' in *Eur J Clin Nutr*, 51(2): 247–57, 1997

7 Margetts B M, 'Basic issues in designing and interpreting epidemiological research' in *Design Concepts in Nutritional Epidemiology*, eds B M Margetts and M Nelson, Oxford University Press, New York, pp. 22–4, 1997

8 Nelson M M and Evans H M, 'Relation of thiamine to reproduction in the rat' in *J Nutr*, 55: 151–63, 1955

9 Brosens I A, Koninckx P R and Corveleyn P A, 'A study of plasma progesterone, oestradiol–17B, prolactin and LH levels and the luteal phase appearance of the ovaries in patients with endometriosis and infertility' in *Br J Obstet Gynaecol*, 85: 246–50, 1978

10 'Dietary reference values for food, energy and nutrients for the United Kingdom' in *HMSO Report 41*, HMSO, London, pp. 90, 94, 102, 146, 167, 1991

11 Laursen N H and De Swann C, *Endometriosis Answer Book*, Fawcett Columbine, 1988

12 Esch M W, Easter R A and Bahr J M, 'Effect of riboflavin deficiency on estrous cyclicity in pigs' in *Biol Reprod*, 25: 659–65, 1981

13 Ballweg M L, *Overcoming Endometriosis*, Congdon & Weed, 1987

14 Grant E, *Sexual Chemistry*, Cedar Press, London, 1992

15 Colgan M, *Hormonal Health*, Apple Publishing, Vancouver, 1996

16 Christianson R E, Oeshli F W and van den Berg B J, 'Caffeinated beverages and decreased fertility' in *Lancet*, 1(8634): 378, 1989

17 Goldstein F, Goldman M B and Cramer D W, 'Infertility in women and moderate alcohol use' in *Am J Publ Health*, 84(9): 1429–32, 1994

18 Cited by Hope J, 'Just a little tipple can damage your fertility' in *The Daily Mail*, 21 August 1998

19 Ellis R, 'Alcohol trebles the risk of miscarriage', in *The Mail on Sunday*, 10 February 2002

20 Van Voorhis B J *et al.*, 'The effects of smoking on ovarian function and fertility during assisted reproduction cycles' in *Obstet Gynecol*, 88(5): 785–91, 1996

21 Marks K, 'Women smokers leave daughters a deadly legacy' in *The Daily Telegraph*, 3 February 1994

22 Derbyshire D, 'Babies "poisoned" by mothers who smoke' in *The Daily Mail*, 24 August 1998

23 Passwater R A and Cranton E M, *Trace Elements, Hair Analysis and Nutrition*, Keats Publishing, New Canaan, 1983

24 Zeigler E E and Filer L J Jr, *Present Knowledge in Nutrition*, ILSI Press, Washington, p. 316, 1996 (7th edn)

25 Joo S J and Betts N M, 'Copper intakes and the consumption patterns of chocolate foods as sources of copper for individuals in the 1987–1988 nationwide food consumption survey' in *Nutr Res*, 16(1): 41–52, 1996

26 Ellis R, ' Warning: smoking cannabis can seriously damage your baby', *The Mail on Sunday*, 6 January 2002

27 Null G, *No More Allergies*, Villard Books, New York, p. 3, 1992

28 Lieberman S and Bruning N, *The Real Vitamin and Mineral Book*, Avery Books, New York, p. 315, 1997 (2nd edn)

29 Yudkin J, 'Objectives and methods in nutrition education: let's start again' in *J Hum Nutr*, 1981

CHAPTER 13

1 Gudice L C, 'Insulin-like growth factor and other endometrial modulators in endometrial development and endometriosis' in *Endometrium and Endometriosis*, eds M Diamond and K Osteen, Blackwell Science, Cambridge, pp. 24–31, 1996

2 Osteen K G, Bruner K L and Sharpe-Timms K L, 'Steroids and growth factor regulation of matrix metalloproteinase expression and endometriosis' in *Sem Reprod Endocrinol*, 14: 247–55, 1994

3 Osteen K G, Bruner K L and Eisenberg X, 'Progesterone and transforming growth factor beta co-mediate matrix metalloproteinase expression in a model of endometriosis' in *Endometriosis Today, Proceedings of the Vth World Congress on Endometriosis*, eds H Minaguchi and O Sugimoto, Parthenon Publishing, New York, 13: 210–15, 1994

4 Lessey B A *et al.*, 'Aberrant integrin expression in the endometrium of women with endometriosis' in *J Clin Endocrinol Metabol*, 79: 643–9, 1994

5 Ibid

6 Haney A F, Muscanto J J and Weinberg J B, 'Peritoneal fluid cell populations in infertility patients' in *Fertil Steril*, 25: 696–700, 1981

7 Halme J *et al.*, 'Increase activation of peritoneal macrophages in patients with endometriosis', in *Am J Obstet Gynecol*, 148: 85–90, 1983

8 Olive D L, Montoya I and Schenken R M, 'Macrophage-conditioned media enhanced endometrial stromal cell proliferation *in vitro*' in *Am J Obstet Gynecol*, 164: 953–8, 1991

9 Vega M *et al.*, 'Functional luteolysis in response to hydrogen peroxide in human luteal cells' in *J Endocrinol*, 147: 177–82, 1995

10 Nothnick W B and Vernon M W, 'Immunomodulation of endometriotic implants' in *Endometriosis Today, Proceedings of the Vth Congress on Endometriosis*, eds H Minaguchi and O Sugimoto, Parthenon Publishing, New York, 13: 107–17, 1997

11 Nothnick W *et al.*, 'New insights into the classification and treatment of endometriosis' in *Int J Gynaecol Pathol*, 20: 140–6, 2001

12 Sharpe, K L and Vernon M W, 'Polypeptides synthesized and released by endometriotic tissue differ from those of the uterine endometrium in culture' in *Biol Reprod*, 48: 1334–40, 1993

13 Knight J, 'Far from the madding cows' in *New Scientist*, 24 January 1998

14 Evers J L H *et al.*, 'Endometrium and peritoneum: Teflon or Velcro?', abstract presented at *1st Nordic Congress on Endometriosis*, Stockholm, April 2001

15 Smith S K *et al*, 'Multiple gene expression regulating angiogenesis in endometrium', abstract presented at *1st Nordic Congress on Endometriosis*, Stockholm, April 2001

16 Geirsson R T, 'Familial endometriosis', abstract presented at *1st Nordic Congress on Endometriosis*, Stockholm, April 2001

17 Zondervan K and Kennedy S, 'Risk factors for endometriosis – is prevention possible?', abstract presented at *1st Nordic Congress on Endometriosis*, Stockholm, April 2001

18 Hummelsoj L, 'Worldwide experiences of women with endometriosis', abstract presented at *1st Nordic Congress on Endometriosis*, Stockholm, April 2001

19 Symposium at the National Institutes of Health, Washington, D C, April 2000. Kevin Osteen, PhD, Director of Endometriosis Association Research Program at Vanderbilt University School of Medicine, was a key planner for the symposium. This research is highlighted in the *Endometriosis Association Newsletter*, 22 (3), 2001

20 Trempe Norcum M, 'Research recap: Designer oestrogens, anti-oestrogens, and bisphosphonates – what the new drugs can and can't do' in *Endometriosis Association Newsletter*, 19 (5–6), 1999

21 Duczman L and Ballweg M L, 'Endometriosis and cancer: what is the connection?' in *Endometriosis Association Newsletter*, 20 (3–4), 1999

22 Mills D, 'Endometriosis: possible nutritional strategies' in *Lamberts Nutr Bull*, 2: 1–12, 1992

23 O'Connor D, *Endometriosis*, Churchill Livingstone, Edinburgh, p. 145, 1989

24 Coutinho E M, 'Progress in the management of endometriosis' in *The Proceedings of the 4th World Congress on Endometriosis 28 May 1994*, Parthenon Publishing, London, p. 1, 1994

CHAPTER 14

1   MacDonald Baker S, *Detoxification & Healing*, Keats Publishing, New Canaan, p. 62–3, 1997
2   Vecchiarelli A *et al.*, 'Protective immunity induced by low-virulence *C. albicans*: cytokine production in the development of the anti-infectious state' in *Cell Immunol*, 124: 334–44, 1989
3   Ballweg M L, 'Immunotherapy for endometriosis: the science behind a promising new treatment' in *Endometrium and Endometriosis*, Blackwell Science, Oxford, pp. 367–76, 1997
4   Helfrich R, *Take Control of Your Health*, Duckworth Books, 1996

Glossary

Abdomen	Belly. The area of the body below the lungs and above the hips. Internally known as the peritoneal cavity. (*see* Peritoneal cavity)
Acute	Describes a disease of rapid onset, severe symptoms and brief duration. Acute abdomen as with ectopic pregnancy or ruptured ovarian cysts. (*see* Pain)
Adhesions	Used in medicine to describe the abnormal attachment of organs to each other by fibrous scar tissue. Caused usually by trauma to tissue from an injury or surgery. Endometriosis causes adhesion formation in the peritoneal cavity from the congealed sticky blood strands. (*see* Endometriosis *and* Peritoneal cavity)
Adipose tissue	The fat storage tissue of the body.
Aflatoxins	A poisonous substance in the spore of fungus which affects peanuts.
Allergy	A hypersensitive immune response acquired by some individuals to environmental substances. These environmental substances are called allergens, the most common of which are pollen, dust and animal dander. With foodstuffs the most common allergens are wheat, dairy and citrus fruits. (*see* Immune system)
Amenorrhoea	The absence of the menstrual period (monthly bleeding). (*see* Menstrual cycle *and* Menstrual period)
Amino acid	The fundamental chemical constituents of all proteins. The digestive tract breaks down proteins into amino acids in order for that portion to be absorbed into the bloodstream. Used as building blocks by the body to produce hormones, enzymes, prostaglandins, etc. (*see* Proteins)
Anabolic hormones	Hormones which stimulate the formation of the larger chemicals of the body from the smaller precursor chemicals. For instance, an anabolic hormone stimulates the building up of body proteins, like muscle proteins, from amino acids. Testosterone is an anabolic hormone which is formed from oils hormones) and stimulates the build-up of muscle proteins, which is why it has been used by some athletes to increase their muscle size.
Analgesic	A drug that relieves pain.
Anaemia	A condition in which the blood has a deficiency of red blood cells (RBCs) or haemoglobin, the iron-based molecule in RBCs that carries oxygen in the blood. Anaemia may be caused by deficiencies of iron, copper, B12 or B6. (*see* Red blood cells).

Anorexia nervosa	An illness common in female adolescents, in which the patients starve themselves or use other techniques, such as vomiting or taking laxatives, to induce weight loss. Motivated by a false perception of their bodies as fat. Linked to deficiencies in iron and zinc. Zinc is used by 20 enzymes in the brain and by the hypothalamus, the seat of appetite control.
Anovulation	No ovulation occurs during the menstrual cycle. (*see* Luteinizing unruptured follicle syndrome)
Antagonist	A substance such as a vitamin, mineral or hormone whose action opposes that of another substance. Thus taking zinc at the same time as iron can cut down the absorption of both. They should be taken at different times.
Antibiotics	Drugs that inhibit the growth of microorganisms. Prolonged use may disrupt gut flora and oestrogen excretion. Using probiotics after taking a course of antibiotics will replace the bifido bacteria. (*see* Probiotics)
Antibody	A Y-shaped protein produced by the immune system B lymphocytes that attacks matter that is 'alien' to the body. (*see* Immune system)
Antigens	Substances that are 'alien' to the body and which elicit an immune response when they enter the body, for example, viruses and bacteria. (*see* Immune system)
Antihistamine	A drug which inhibits the release of histamine in the body. This effect can dampen pain and allergic reaction. Some antihistamines make the user drowsy and unable to operate machinery or drive.
Antioxidants	These are comprised of vitamins, minerals and compounds found in food which can neutralize the damaging effects of free oxidizing radicals. Antioxidants prevent cells from ageing too rapidly.
ART	Assisted reproductive technology. The use of processes like IVF, GIFT and ICSI to help infertile couples conceive. (*see In vitro* fertilization, Gamete intrafallopian transfer, Intracytoplasmic sperm injection). For endometriosis the pregnancy rate is 20–35 per cent per attempt.
Ascorbic acid	*see* Vitamin C
Autoimmune disease	When the immune system wrongly attacks its own tissue and treats it as if it were 'alien' matter. A false recognition pattern seems to evolve.
Bacteria	A loosely used term that refers to microorganisms that are usually rod-shaped and are not viruses or fungi. Some bacteria, such as the bifido bacteria in our gut, are beneficial. Other types of bacteria are dangerous to health, for example, salmonella.
Bifidobacteria	These bacteria prevent the colonization of the intestine by harmful pathogenic bacteria and yeasts. They protect the integrity of the mucosal barrier which prevents harmful substances from entering the bloodstream. They also assimilate B vitamins and promote bowel movements.
Biochemistry	The chemistry of living organisms.
Bioflavonoids	Give colour to leaves and plants. Used to be called vitamin P. Strengthen capillary walls and help prevent bruising. Found in fruits and vegetables.

Blastocyst	An early stage of embryonic development that occurs at 7–8 days after fertilization. A blastocyst consists of a hollow ball of cells with a localized thickening that will develop into the embryo. (*see* Embryo *and* Zygote)
Bonds	In chemistry, the physical, magnetic, electrical and chemical forces that keep atoms attached to each other.
Bone marrow	Cells found in the centre of the long bones (such as the femur) that manufacture most of the blood cells.
Boron	Boron is an element which works very much like oestrogen to prevent loss of minerals from the bone and osteoporosis. Synergy with vitamin D and calcium. Modulates immune and inflammatory processes.
Brain	The highly developed mass of nervous tissue that forms the upper end of the central nervous system. Encased in the skull. It sends nervous ganglia throughout the body to receive and send messages. Two-thirds of the brain is made of oils. It relies on nutrients to pass messages across gaps, and the neurotransmitters are based on proteins.
Bulimia	Insatiable overeating, due to neurological causes. The hypothalamus may be at fault.
Butyric acid	Liberated in a healthy large intestine. Helps the acidophilus and bifido bacteria to stick to the gut membrane, thereby protecting it. Required as a primary source of energy for all cells on the intestinal wall, which renew themselves every three days. Aids the natural healing of the gut membrane after antifungals have been used to eradicate *Candida albicans*. Plays a supporting role in the release of immunoglobulins from the gut mucosa.
Caffeine	An alkaloid drug, obtained from coffee, chocolate, coke and tea, that has a stimulant action, particularly on the central nervous and reproductive systems.
Calcium	Metallic element essential for the normal development and functioning of the body, muscle function and constituent of bones and teeth. Its uptake is facilitated by vitamin D. Works in the immune and nervous systems.
Calorie	A unit of measure used to determine the amount of energy in foodstuffs. It is equal to the amount of energy that would be able to raise the temperature of one gram of water one degree Centigrade.
Cancer	Malignant growth of abnormal cells which may invade and spread to other parts of the body and can cause death.
Candida albicans	A genus of yeast (fungus) that is commonly found in the human gut flora. In some individuals *Candida albicans* will overwhelm the digestive and immune system. If a yeast infection develops, it can lead to food intolerances and disrupt normal hormonal regulation.
Carbohydrate	A group of compounds, including the sugars, starch and fibres (non-starch polysaccharides), that contain carbon, hydrogen and oxygen. Used by the body for energy production, but excess intake is converted to fat and stored in adipose tissue. Fibre is essential to health and should be eaten daily.
Carcinogenic	A substance or action that causes cancer, such as benzene, chemicals, pesticides.

Catabolic hormones	Hormones which stimulate the breakdown of the larger chemicals of the body to form smaller precursor chemicals. For instance, some catabolic hormones stimulate the breakdown of body proteins, like muscle proteins, into amino acids (muscle wasting). The opposite to anabolic hormones.
Cataracts	Clouding of the lens of the eye resulting in blurred vision.
Cell	The basic unit of all living organisms, which can reproduce itself exactly using the DNA blueprint at its core. A group of cells is referred to as a tissue. The body is made up of many different types of cells – nerve, immune, sperm, connective tissue, fat cells, etc.
Cell-mediated immunity	This involves free-floating white cells in the bloodstream which neutralize 'alien' invaders.
Cell membrane	The phospholipid layer which protects the cell organelles from damage, allowing substances to move in and out. Made up from oils. (*see* Cytoplasm)
Cellulose	A fibrous carbohydrate consisting of linked glucose units that cannot be digested by the human. It passes through the body unchanged, but is able to absorb water, cholesterol and oestrogens. It speeds up excretion time and helps the body rid itself of harmful toxins. The cell walls of all fruits, vegetables, cereals, nuts and seeds are made of cellulose.
Cervix	The small opening of the uterus into the vagina. (*see* Uterus *and* Vagina)
Chelate	A chemical substance which attaches in a claw-like manner to metals and can prevent the metals, especially heavy metals such as lead, mercury and cadmium, from hurting the body.
Chemotactic	Movement of a cell or organism in response to a stimulus – a chemical change.
Chemotoxins	Chemicals which have a toxic effect in the body.
Chlamydia	A virus-like bacteria which can causes damage to the reproductive system leading to infertility. Studies show 81.7 per cent of women under 25 years of age to be infected.
Cholecalciferol	*see* Vitamin D
Choriocarcinoma	Highly invasive malignant tumour that can develop from the chorion, a membrane that surrounds the fetus. Hydatioiform mole occurs when the blastocyst turns cancerous. (*see* Chorion)
Chorion	The embryonic membrane that totally surrounds the embryo and serves as a protective barrier while in uterus. (*see* Embryo)
Chromium	Needed for glucose tolerance factor along with vitamin B3. Used for fatty acid synthesis. Deficiency leads to heart disease. Normalizes blood sugar levels.
Chromosomes	Thread-like structures in the cell nucleus that carry genetic information. The human has 46 chromosomes – 23 from the father, 23 from the mother. (*see* Gene *and* DNA)
Chronic	Describes a disease of long duration, involving slow changes. (*see* Endometriosis *and* Pain)
Cis fatty acid	The natural form in which oils exist. Builds a strong cell membrane. Found only in cold-pressed oils.

Clomiphene	A synthetic non-steroidal compound used in IVF that stimulates the pituitary to produce hormones (FSH and LH) that induce follicular growth and egg development by the ovary. (*see* Follicle-stimulating hormone, Luteinizing hormone *and* Ovarian follicle)
Codeine	An analgesic derived from morphine but less potent as a painkiller and sedative, and is less toxic.
Coenzymes	Non-protein organic compounds such as vitamins and minerals that, as part of an enzyme, play an essential role in a chemical reaction. (Without sufficient supplies of the coenzyme the reaction could not take place.)
Collagen	The main supportive protein of the skin, tendons and bone. It relies on uptake of vitamins A and C, essential fatty acids and zinc for its formation.
Complementary medicine	Systems of healing which complement orthodox medicine, including homeopathy, herbal remedies, acupuncture, osteopathy, chiropractic, naturopathy, hydrotherapy and faith healing.
Conception	The process of fertilization of the egg when the egg and sperm collide and new life begins. (*see* Fertilization *and* Pronuclei)
Congenital	From birth.
Constipation	Difficult, incomplete, or infrequent evacuation of the bowels. Insufficient fibre reduces water uptake, leading to a build-up of toxins and reduced excretion of cholesterol and oestrogens. Related to some food intolerances. Wheat, bananas, cheese and eggs can trigger constipation. Vitamin C and magnesium are known to soften stools.
Coenzyme Q10	Aids the heart muscle in its uptake of oxygen. Has strong antioxidant properties which are protective to all body cells. Also works within cells in process of energy production.
Corpus luteum (CL)	The structure that forms from the follicles of the ovary after ovulation. The corpus luteum produces the hormone progesterone which supports the pregnant state. (*see* Ovary, Ovulation *and* Progesterone)
Cytoplasm	The fluid matrix inside the living cell which surround all the organelles. (*see* Cell)
Department of Health	A department of central government in the UK that supports the Secretary of State for Health in meeting his obligations which include the National Health Service, and the prevention and control of infectious diseases.
Dermatitis	Infection or irritation of the skin.
D-Gamma linolenic acid (DGLA)	An omega-6 essential fatty acid found in evening primrose oil.
Diabetes mellitus	An endocrine disease caused by insufficient insulin production by the pancreas. Blood sugars, like glucose, are not used properly by the body cells of people with diabetes mellitus. There is a new research link between high insulin levels and polycystic ovaries. (*see* Pancreas)

Diet	The mixture of foods that a person eats. A balanced diet contains adequate quantities of all the macro- and micro-nutrients. As we are all unique individuals, our needs will vary.
Diethylstilboestrol (DES)	A synthetic oestrogen used as a drug replacement for natural oestrogen. DES given to pregnant women in the 1960s to prevent abortion was found to cause abnormal development of their growing baby's reproductive tract.
Dietitian	A trained dietitian looks at a person's calorie intake and assesses which foods should be eaten if they are ill, underweight or overweight.
Dioxins	A powerful toxin used in industrial processes and as an aerial herbicide. Used in 'agent orange' during the Vietnam war. Known to damage the reproductive system due to its oestrogenic effect on body cells, and thought to be a carcinogen. Stored in body fat so care must be taken when dieting to go slowly. Powerful immunosuppressants.
D,L-Phenylalanine (DLPA)	Phenylalanine is an amino acid that occurs as two mirror images, the L and D form. The L form occurs naturally in nature, and the D form is man-made. D,L-Phenylalanine is a mixture of the L and D forms and is used for pain relief, as an appetite suppressant and works an anti-depressant.
DNA	Deoxyribonucleic acid. The scientific name for the chemical that our genes are made of. It is found in all living cells and acts as a blueprint for cell reproduction and renewal. If part of the DNA is corrupted, then cell mutations can occur. (*see* Gene *and* Chromosomes)
Dopamine	A hormone which is found in the adrenal glands and brain.
Dyspareunia	Painful or difficult sexual intercourse experienced by a woman. Can be caused in endometriosis if adhesions stick organs together, or if there are large ovarian cysts or internal inflammation.
Ectopic pregnancy	The development of a pregnancy in an area of the body other than the uterus. An ectopic pregnancy in the Fallopian tubes may lead to the death of the mother after eight weeks if it is not found and removed. A major obstetric problem.
Eczema	A non-contagious inflammation of the skin that is characterized with redness, itching and sometimes sores. May be related in some to dairy intolerances and low fatty acid intake.
Embryo	The first cells of the newborn from fertilization to about 8 weeks of development.
Embryology	The study of the growth and development of the embryo.
Endocrine system	The body's control system that involves interactions between hormones. The word endocrine means internal secretions which act as messengers. Includes the hypothalamus, hypocampus, thyroid, parathyroid, thymus, adrenal glands, ovaries, testes pituitary, pancreas, liver, and placenta.
Endocrinology	The study of the endocrine glands and the substances they secrete (hormones). (*see* Hormones)
Endogenous	Contained or produced in the body.

Endometriosis	The disease condition where endometrium develops and grows in areas and organs of the body other than where it belongs. The endometrium is normally found lining the uterus. Endometriosis may cause pain and infertility. (*see* Uterus *and* Endometrium)
Endometriotic implants	The pieces of endometrium that develop outside the womb, such as on the bowel, bladder, ovaries and appendix, in women who have endometriosis. (*see* Endometrium)
Endometrium	The inner lining of the uterus that is the surface where the blastocyst/embryo implants during pregnancy. The endometrium is the tissue that is lost during the menstrual period and it is also the source of tissue for endometriosis formation. It relies on oestrogen for its growth. (*see* Uterus *and* Endometriosis)
Endorphins	Small molecules secreted by the pituitary gland that act as a natural analgesic to control pain. They are thought to be concerned with controlling the activity of the endocrine glands. Thiamine is known to be used by endorphins.
Enzyme	An organic chemical, usually a protein, that speeds up biochemical reactions or causes the breakdown of large molecules into smaller molecules. They act as catalysts as the reaction does not change them. The cofactors used to create enzymes are vitamins and minerals. Each enzyme is very specific. They are vital for body function.
Enzyme saturation	When all cells are replete with all the nutrients which they require in order to work at their optimum level.
EPA (eicosapentaenoic acid)	An omega-3 EFA found in fish liver oils. The body metabolizes EPA to form anti-inflammatory prostaglandins and to keep blood thin. Important in prevention of heart disease, PMS and cancers.
Epididymis	The collecting tube on the side of each testis that stores sperm before ejaculation. (*see* Testes, Sertoli cell *and* Sperm)
Epithelial cells	The surface cells that usually cover the outer or innermost layers of an organ.
EPO (evening primrose oil)	Gamma-linolenic acid (GLA). The precursor to anti-inflammatory prostaglandins. A useful addition to the diet in conditions such as endometriosis, arthritis, asthma, PMS, eczema and heart disease. Stops blood becoming sticky. Should not be used by those with epilepsy or manic depression. (*see* Precursor)
Essential amino acid (EAA)	Amino acid that is essential for normal growth and development but cannot be synthesized by the body. Amino acids are the smallest part of a protein. Used, for example, for tissue renewal, enzymes and hormones.
Essential fatty acid (EFA)	A fatty acid that is essential for normal growth and development but cannot be synthesized by the body. Used in brain cells and cell membranes.
Embryo transfer (ET)	The placement of embryos into the uterus at the end of an IVF cycle. (*see* In vitro fertilization *and* Uterus)
Estrogen/ oestrogen	The female sex hormone secreted in large concentrations by the ovary and placenta. Responsible for the female secondary sex characteristics. (*see* Ovary *and* Placenta) It comprises a large family of steroid hormones that includes oestriol, oestrone, oestradiol. Small amounts are produced by the adrenal cortex, fat cells and testes.

Fallopian tubes	Two tubes attached at each corner of the uterus which stretch out towards the ovaries. They are the passageways used by eggs to meet the sperm and the place of fertilization. The newly formed embryo can then enter the uterus. Also known as the oviducts. (*see* Uterus)
Family planning	The use of contraception to limit or space out the numbers of children born to a couple. To maintain the woman's health one child every two years is felt to be optimum.
Fertility rate	The number of live births occurring in a year per 1,000 women of child-bearing age (usually 15–44 years of age).
Fertilization	The fusion of a sperm and an ovum. (*see* Sperm *and* Ova)
Fetus	Baby before birth. (*see* Pregnancy)
Flatulence	Gas that forms in the gastrointestinal (GI) tract. An excess of gas can be formed when *Bacteroides* bacteria become overgrown as the bifidobacteria are destroyed by antibiotics, the pill, HRT and stress.
Folic acid	B vitamin essential for preventing fetal abnormalities. Reduced by the pill and stress. The metabolic role of folic acid is interdependent with that of zinc and vitamin B12 (both are required by rapidly dividing cells) and a deficiency in one may lead to a deficiency in the other.
Follicle	*See* Ovarian follicle.
Follicle-stimulating hormone (FSH)	The hormone released by the anterior pituitary gland that stimulates the ovary to produce follicles and mature eggs. Released in the first 14 days of the cycle. In anovulation, FSH is deficient. (*see* Pituitary, Ova *and* Ovary)
Free radicals	Small singlet oxygen molecules that have a high capacity to react chemically with other molecules. They are highly unstable as they only have one electron and try to steal another from a normal cell membrane or its DNA. This chemical reaction can be destructive, especially to protein molecules. Also known as free oxidizing radicals (FoRs).
Fructo-oligosaccharides (FOS)	*See* Prebiotics.
Gamete	A mature sex cell; the egg of the female or the sperm of the male. Gametes are haploid, containing half the normal number of chromosomes, 23 chromosomes in an ova and 23 in a sperm, so that when they join, the embryo has a full 46. (*see* Sperm, Ova, Chromosomes *and* Gamete)
Gastrointestinal (GI)	Pertaining to the stomach and intestine; the digestive tract/system.
Gene	The basic unit of genetic material, which is found at a unique place on a chromosome. A damaged P53 gene is known to be responsible for cancer formation. (*see* Chromosome *and* DNA)
General practitioner (GP)	A doctor who is the main agent of primary care, through whom patients make first contact with medical services. The majority have had no training in nutrition.

Germ cells	The precursor cells that have the potential to develop into sperm or eggs. (*see* Precursor, Sperm *and* Ova)
Gestation	The duration of a pregnancy. (*see* Pregnancy)
GIFT (gamete intrafallopian transfer)	A form of assisted reproduction in which ova are mixed with the partner's sperm and then introduced into a Fallopian tube where fertilization takes place. (*see* Ova, Sperm *and* Fertilization)
GLA (gamma-linolenic acid)	An EFA abundant in evening primrose oil. (*see* Essential fatty acid *and* EPO)
Glycoprotein	Large protein molecules that also contain sugar (carbohydrate) molecules. (*see* Proteins)
Glucose	A simple sugar used by cells in energy production. Two teaspoons are the norm in the body's eight pints of blood. (*see* Carbohydrate)
Gonadotrophins	The hormones (LH and FSH) released from the pituitary gland which stimulate the ovaries to produce follicles and undergo the process of ovulation. (*see* Pituitary, Luteinizing hormone *and* Follicle-stimulating hormone)
Gonadotrophin-releasing hormone (GnRH)	Hormone produced in the hypothalamus that stimulates the pituitary to produce and secrete gonadotrophins. Its production is dependent on absorption of zinc and vitamin B6. (*see* Pituitary gland, Luteinizing hormone *and* Follicle-stimulating hormone)
Graafian follicle	A mature follicle on the ovary prior to ovulation, containing a large fluid-filled cavity that distends the surface of the ovary. The oocyte develops inside the follicle attached to one side. (*see* Ovarian follicle, Ovary *and* Ovulation)
Gram	A unit of weight equal to 0.035oz.
Granulosa cells	The cells that line the inside of the Graafian follicle. They produce large amounts of oestrogen and the fluid of the follicle. They also supply nutrients to the egg and, as a result of this role, are also called 'nurse cells'. (*see* Ovary, Ovarian follicle *and* Oestrogen)
Growth factor	A polypeptide (small protein) that is produced by tissue that stimulates cells to proliferate.
Gynaecologist	Doctor specializing in women's reproductive illnesses.
HCG (human chorionic gonadotrophin	Hormone produced by the placenta during pregancy, used as the basis for pregnancy test. HCG maintains the secretion of progesterone by the corpus luteum of the ovary as the secretion of pituitary LH is blocked during pregnancy. Poor placental formation will lead to poor HCG secretion and the pregnancy will not be maintained. (*see* Pregnancy *and* Placenta)
Health centre	A building owned or leased by a district health authority, that houses personnel or services from one or several sections of the National Health Service.
Health education	Persuasive methods used to encourage people to adopt lifestyles that the educators believe will improve health, and to reject habits regarded as harmful to health. Disease prevention.

Health promotion	A programme of surveillance planned on a community basis to maintain the best possible health and quality of life of the members of that community, both collectively and individually.
Histamine	A chemical that can cause blood vessels to dilate. It is secreted at the site of a wound and is one of the major factors that cause the wound to become red. It is also secreted by the immune system during an immune response to antigens. Involved in anaphelactic shock. Vitamin C is antihistamine. (*see* Immune system *and* Antigens)
Holistic	Viewing the body as a whole unit which works together when considering matters of health and healing. Prevention being better than cure.
Homeostasis	The tendency of the body to always strive to maintain a stable or uniform state.
Hormones	The body's chemical messengers that are secreted by the endocrine glands.
Hormone receptors	Special proteins on or in cells to which hormones attach. Attachment (binding) of the hormone to the receptor will cause the endocrine effect of the hormone. Can be disrupted by exogenous hormones. (*see* Endocrinology *and* Hormones)
Hormone replacement therapy (HRT)	The administration of oestrogen and progesterone to replace these hormones in women who have no ovarian function due to menopause or surgery. Natural menopause should not be a problem if a woman is well nourished. (*see* Menopause, Oestrogen, Progesterone *and* Ovary)
Hyperventilation	Rapid deep breathing. Lowers the carbon dioxide in the blood and can lead to unconsciousness, dizziness and 'spaced-out' feelings. Low oxygen supply to cells causes malfunction.
Hypoglycaemia	Low glucose sugar in the blood. This can lead to irritability, weakness, fatigue, excessive sweating. The body relies on insulin and glucose tolerance factor (B3 and chromium-based) to control blood sugar levels. (*see* Diabetes mellitus)
Hypothalamus	Part of the base of the brain that is connected to the pituitary gland. Secretes hormones that control the production and secretion of the pituitary hormones. The seat of appetite control. Also controls body temperature. Integrates hormone control and nervous system activity. (*see* Pituitary gland)
Hypothyroid	A condition where the thyroid secretes insufficient amounts of thyroid hormones T3, T4, which affect TSH from the pituitary. Causes constipation, skin coarseness, sluggishness, lethargy, dull brain, loss of outer third of eyebrows. (*see* Thyroid)
Hysterectomy	Surgical removal of the uterus. Should only be essential if diseased. Removal of the uterus has been seen to shorten life by five years, and lead to strokes and heart disease. (*see* Uterus)
Humoral immunity	The fluid and hormonal (humors) system of the body. The immune system depends upon antibodies produced by B lymphocytes circulating via the bloodstream.
Iatrogenic condition	A condition that results from medical treatment, as either an unforeseen or inevitable side effect, such as hair loss with chemotherapy, gut flora disruption with antibiotics.

Intracytoplasmic sperm injection (ICSI)	The injection of a single sperm directly into an ova, done by an endocrinologist. The resulting zygote is then transferred back into the woman's uterus. (*see* Ova *and* Sperm)
Immune	Having a natural resistance to harmful substances.
Immune system	The defence system of the body that helps fight off infections from bacteria, viruses and other 'alien' substances.
Immunoglobins	Immune cells are produced by B lymphocytes, which form antibodies against 'alien' bacterial protein material.
Infant mortality rate (IMR)	The number of deaths of infants under one year of age per 1,000 live births in a given year.
Infertility	Inability of a couple to induce conception after 12–18 months of unprotected sexual intercourse.
Inflammation	The body's response to injury, which may be acute or chronic. It is associated with a local increase in temperature and the activation of the immune system. Histamines are released. (*see* Immune system)
Integrins	The 'adhesive' material which enables one cell to 'stick' to another in order to form the structure of the body. Forms the connective tissue collagen.
Interferon	Produced by macrophages and T lymphocytes. Protects cells from damage by shutting down the mitochondria, the energy production site, to stop the virus from reproducing. Needs choline, manganese and vitamin C. Our ability to produce interferon is damaged by pesticides.
Interleukins	Regulating chemicals secreted by the white blood cells (leukocytes). Interleukin-2 stimulates T lymphocytes and is used in the treatment of cancer. (*see* White blood cells)
In vitro fertilization (IVF)	The fertilization of the egg outside the body, usually in a dish in a specially designed incubator.
Iron	A metallic element essential to the process of respiration and therefore life. It stimulates immunity, boosts physical performance and allows blood to carry oxygen to cells for energy production.
Lactation	The production and release of milk from the breast. (*see* Prolactin *and* Pituitary gland)
Laparoscope	A fibreoptic surgical instrument that can be inserted through a small incision in the belly button to view the contents of the peritoneal cavity.
Laparoscopy	A surgical procedure for the examination of the peritoneal cavity using a laparoscope. Also called 'belly-button' surgery.
Laparotomy	A surgical procedure for the examination of the peritoneal cavity using a longer incision in the abdominal wall (belly).
Leaky gut	Where the gut membrane has been eroded or breached, and toxins can enter the bloodstream and set up intolerances and toxic feelings. Autointoxification.
Leukotrienes	A subgroup of series two prostaglandins (PG2). They increase inflammation and blood-clotting. Responsible for bronchial constriction (as in asthma) and inflammatory processes.

Lindane	A powerful insecticide which has oestrogenic properties. Found in chocolate and milk, and linked to breast cancer.
Linoleic acid	An omega-6 polyunsaturated cis fatty acid. We cannot make this and depend upon good oils in foods. Found in vegetable oils such as sunflower and safflower oils.
Linolenic acid (LA)	An omega-3 cis fatty acid. We cannot make this and depend upon food intake. The alpha form is found in fish oils and linseed. (*see* EFA)
Lipids	Water-insoluble substances which have a greasy feel. They include neutral fats, fatty acids, steroids and waxes.
Luteinizing hormone (LH)	Hormone produced by the pituitary which stimulates ovulation and the corpus luteum to produce progesterone. Released from day 14 to day 28 in the normal cycle. (*see* Pituitary gland *and* Progesterone).
Luteinizing unruptured follicle syndrome (LUFS)	The condition where a woman appears to have a normal menstrual cycle, but the egg does not ovulate (pop) out of the ovarian follicle. (*see* Anovulation)
Lymph	A transparent to yellow-coloured liquid found in lymphatic vessels. It carries lymphocytes and bathes tissues. (*see* Lymphatic system)
Lymph glands	Structures found in the lymphatic system that filter the lymph and are part of the immune system. Found in the neck, groin, armpit. They prevent 'aliens' from entering the bloodstream. (*see* Immune system)
Lymphatic system	A system of tubes (lymph vessels) that drain lymph from various organs and return the lymph to the blood. Part of the immune system. (*see* Immune system *and* Tonsils)
Lymphocyte	A type of white blood cell that originates from the lymph glands.
Lysosome	A particle inside cells which helps break down 'alien' invaders.
Lysozyme	Contained by T-cells. This is a deadly enzyme which kills germs and our own cells once released by these immune cells. Vitamin C provides some protection, 'mopping up' any excess.
Macrophage	A wandering cell that is found in tissue and blood that can phagocytize (eat) bacteria and other 'alien' matter that makes its way into the body. (*see* Phagocytize, White blood cells *and* Immune system)
Magnesium	A white metallic element that is an essential nutrient. Magnesium deficiency can lead to impaired nerve and muscle function. Marginal magnesium deficiency is becoming common. It causes loss of appetite, nausea, diarrhoea, confusion, muscle tremors and spasms, lack of coordination. Useful with PMS and abdominal cramps.
Malabsorption	When the intestines are malfunctioning and nutrients from foods are not absorbed effectively into the bloodstream. It can be due to coeliac problems when gluten damages the villi, or if the gut mucosa is damaged by drugs or constant stress. It may be corrected by slippery elm, butyric acid and NAG.
Medical	Of or relating to medicine; the diagnosis, treatment and prevention of disease.
Medicine	The science or practice of the diagnosis, treatment and prevention of disease.

Melatonin	A hormone secreted by the pineal gland in the brain. Excess melatonin hampers fertility and raises the levels of prolactin. Modern life causes imbalances in light and dark cycles which affect melatonin production. Zinc is vital in this process as is natural daylight. Exposure to electromagnetic fields reduces melatonin levels. Blocks oestrogen from binding to oestrogen receptors of cells, as in breast cancer cells (*see* Pineal gland)
Menarche	Start of menstrual cycles. Usually from the age of 12 to 17. (*see* Menstrual cycle *and* Menstrual period)
Menopause	The end of the monthly menstrual cycle that results from the use of all the eggs of the ovary. Usually starts between 44 and 55 years of age and takes 7 years to occur naturally. (*see* HRT, Ova *and* Menstrual cycle)
Menstrual cycle	The reproductive cycle of women that lasts for about one month. Controlled by the hormones of the pituitary, ovary and uterus. During the menstrual cycle, the endometrium of the uterus thickens in preparation for pregnancy. If pregnancy does not occur, the endometrium is sloughed off as the menstrual period (flow), and the cycle is repeated. (*see* Uterus, Pituitary gland, Ovary *and* Endometrium)
Menstrual period	That part of the menstrual cycle that is associated with the flow of blood out of the vagina. Also referred to as 'menstruation' or 'menstrual bleeding'. Should be pain-free and symptomless in healthy individuals. The nutrients B6, zinc, chromium, magnesium and vitamin C are known to play a role. (*see* Menstrual cycle)
Metabolism	The biochemical reactions of the body that are involved in the maintenance of life. The thyroid gland and hypothalamus are related to the metabolic rate at which foods are burnt to provide energy. Iodine and selenium are important for this process.
Microgram	One-millionth part of a gram.
Milligram	One-thousandth part of a gram.
Miscarriage	The tragic premature loss of a fetus due to natural causes.
Mitochondria	A small organelle found inside all cells that makes the energy of the cell. Exercise promotes the formation of more mitochondria.
Morula	An early embryo with approximately 16–200 cells. (*see* Embryo)
Mutagen	A substance which can cause changes in the DNA of cells of the body. (*see* DNA *and* Gene)
Mutation	A change in form, structure or characteristics of an organism due to alterations in the DNA of the nucleus. (*see* DNA *and* Gene)
Myometrium	The thick muscle layer of the uterus. It contracts during the birthing process to expel the baby. Menstrual cramps are the pain signals transmitted to the brain during myometrial contractions. In PMS these cramps can be alleviated by use of magnesium supplements. (*see* Uterus)

NAG	*N* acetyl glucosamine is an integral part of the 'glue' which holds cells together, especially the mucous membranes lining the intestines (*see* Integrins). It helps normal intestinal mucosa growth and helps to protect it from acids, enzymes and organisms. It is an amino sugar which occurs naturally in a healthy body.
Naturopathy	A system of medicine that relies upon the use of only natural substances for the treatment of disease.
Neural tube defects (NTD)	Defects of the nervous system, such as spina bifida. Attributed to deficiencies in folic acid and zinc.
Neurotransmitters	The chemicals produced at the end of a nerve that transmit to the next nerve or muscle, or produce an excitatory signal within the brain. They inhibit or excite a response. Serotonin, acetylcholine and the catecholamines depend upon tryptophan, choline and tyrosine, respectively.
Neutrophil	A type of white blood cell found in the blood that is part of the immune system. (*see* Immune system)
Nicotinic acid (niacin, nicotinamide)	Vitamin B3, which aids lowering of blood cholesterol and is protective against heart disease. Reduces high blood pressure.
Nutrients (niacin)	Food substances that are nourishing and which are the supply of materials for body metabolism. Vitamins, minerals and fatty acids are micronutrients, and fats, carbohydrates and proteins are macronutrients.
Nutritionist	A trained nutritionist or nutrition consultant assesses a person's illness and works with that person to correct individual body biochemistry imbalances and improve nutrient intake from the diet. Tests can be done to assess, for example, vitamin and mineral levels, and gut fermentation.
Obstetrician	A doctor who specializes in pregnancy and childbirth.
Oedema	Swelling, retention of fluid in spaces between cells. Oedema is spelled edema in the USA.
Oestrogen	The female sex hormone secreted in large concentrations by the ovary and placenta. Responsible for the female secondary sex characteristics. (Oestrogen is spelled estrogen in the USA.) Also produced in the adrenal glands, fat cells and testes.
Oocyte	Same as ova. (*see* Ovary *and* Ova)
Oophorectomy	Surgical removal of the ovary. (*see* Ovary)
Oral contraceptive	Orally administered drugs derived from ovarian steroids which interfere with the reproductive process and induce infertility. They disrupt blood chemistry causing vitamin A and copper levels to be raised, while lowering levels of B vitamins and zinc.
Organelles	The structures within each cell which allow the cell to function.
Organochlorines	Organic compounds containing chlorine, including chloroform, DDT, dioxins and other pesticides.
Ova and ovum	The unfertilized egg produced in the ovary. Ovum is singular (one egg) and ova more than one. (*see* Ovary)

Ovarian cysts	A fluid-filled sac, one or more of which can develop in the ovary. Most are non-malignant, but they can reach a very large size and cause gross swelling and pain. In endometriosis, chocolate cysts filled with stale dark-brown blood are common. With polycystic ovaries, many follicular cysts develop. High copper levels are related to cyst formation. The pill increases blood copper levels.
Ovarian follicle	The cyst-like structure that forms on the ovary during the menstrual cycle and which contains the developing egg and granulosa cells. (*see* Ovary, Ova *and* Granulosa cells)
Ovary	Paired almond-shaped organs lying in the pelvis that produce hormones (oestrogen and progesterone) and eggs. (*see* Oestrogen, Progesterone *and* Ova)
Ovulation	The process of expulsion of the egg from the ovarian follicle to the Fallopian tube. Occurs around day 14 or 15 of a normal cycle. (*See* Ova, Ovary *and* Fallopian tube)
Oxytocin	A protein-derived hormone secreted by the posterior pituitary that stimulates uterine contractions during the birthing process and the release of milk from the breast.
Pain	Suffering, distress of body or mind. Usually caused by disease or injury, but can be emotional pain from trauma.
Pancreas	The gland that is located under the liver that functions as both an endocrine and exocrine gland. As an endocrine gland, the pancreas secretes insulin and glucogon to control the concentration of blood sugar and, as an exocrine gland, the pancreas secretes digestive enzymes into the intestine (*see* Diabetes mellitus *and* Endocrine system).
Pelvic inflammatory disease (PID)	A general infection in the peritoneal cavity that can be caused by a variety of bacteria that gain entrance into the peritoneal cavity through the female reproductive tract from poor hygiene or infected male sperm. The disease is associated with flu-like symptoms and adhesions, leading to infertility. (*see* Peritoneal cavity, Chlamydia *and* Adhesions)
Peristalsis	Rhythmic muscular contraction in the intestines which pushes food through the digestive system. The process is involuntary. Bifidobacteria and fibre encourage peristalsis.
Peritoneal cavity	The lower abdomen (belly) which contains the reproductive tract, bladder, kidneys and adrenals, small and large intestine, liver, pancreas and stomach.
Peritoneal fluid	The fluid found in the peritoneal cavity. (*see* Peritoneal cavity)
Petechia	A small red to purplish-red area on the surface of the skin or an organ that is caused by small broken blood vessels.
Petechial implants	Endometriotic implants that are red and have the appearance of a petechia. These are the most active implants and cause the most inflammation and pain. May be producing their own oestrogens.
Peyer's patches	Clusters of cells found on the small intestine that are involved in the immune system. They act as testing stations for 'alien' food particles such as bacteria, parasites or chemicals.

Phagocytize	The ability to ingest (eat) microorganisms or other foreign matter. The process whereby white blood cells ingest microorganisms. (*see* Macrophage, Immune system *and* White blood cells)
Phytochemicals	Substances found in plants, and not in animals, which have an effect upon body biochemistry.
Phytoestrogens	Oestrogens present in plants. Isoflavones, lignans and coumestans are structurally similar to oestradiol. They have an oestrogen-modulating effect. Lower binding activity than endogenous oestrogens. Found in soya, wheat, citrus, seeds, pulses and grains.
Phthalates	Phthalic acid diesters are organic chemicals used in industry as plasticizers. They are found in low levels in foods which are wrapped in plastics. Some researchers feel that these levels are high enough to have profound effects on reducing human fertility. Oestrogenic in action.
Pineal gland	Gland found in the middle of the brain that secretes the hormone melatonin. Controls the seasonal changes in the reproductive system and hair growth in seasonal animals (such as sheep and horses). (*see* Melatonin)
Pituitary gland	Endocrine gland at the base of the brain that secretes a variety of hormones, many of which affect other endocrine glands. The major hormones of the pituitary that affect the reproductive system are follicle-stimulating hormone (FSH), luteinizing hormone (LH) and prolactin. The pituitary is divided into the anterior (front) and posterior (back) pituitary. Known to use vitamin B6 and zinc.
Placebo	An inactive substance or other pretend 'medicine' administered to a patient usually to compare its effects with those of a real drug or treatment, but which may help to relieve a condition because of the patient's belief that it will cure him/her. 'Works' by psychosomatic suggestion.
Placenta	The tissue that connects the developing fetus to the uterus of the mother. This organ has to develop over the space of one month, so nutrient intake is crucial to its healthy formation. (*see* Fetus)
Platelets	Blood cells that are important in blood clot formation. If they become too sticky, they cause heart disease problems. Vitamins C and E, garlic and root ginger thin the blood. Vitamin K is necessary for blood to clot. Sugar causes blood to become sticky.
PMS/PMT	Premenstrual syndrome/premenstrual tension. The build-up of symptoms before a period is due. May be related to faulty nutrition or malabsorption of nutrients. Responds to the use of B-complex, B6, magnesium, zinc, chromium, vitamins C and E, and essential fatty acids.
Polychlorinated biphenyls (PCBs)	Toxic chemicals commonly used in electrical components and industrial processes. Thought to be damaging to the reproductive system. Stored in body fat, so care must be taken when dieting to go slowly.
Pouch of Douglas	The blind pouch that makes the bottom of the peritoneal cavity. It lies between the vagina and colon, and below the ovaries. Also called the 'cul-de-sac' area of the peritoneal cavity. It is a prime site for endometriotic implants. (*see* Peritoneal cavity)

Precursor	One that precedes another.
Pregnancy	The condition of having a developing embryo or fetus in the body for nine months' gestation. (*see* Embryo *and* Fetus)
Premarin	Conjugated oestrogens obtained from the urine of pregnant mares used for HRT. (*see* Oestrogen)
Premenstrual	A few days before a menstrual period. PMS symptoms such as bloating, irritability, headaches and anxiety that often build up from day14 to day 28 of the cycle. (*see* Menstrual period)
Prebiotics	Fructo-oligosaccharides that encourage growth of bifidobacteria in the gut flora. 15mg per day is optimum.
Probiotics	Replenish the bifidobacteria which inhabit a healthy gut. The growth of these friendly bacteria encourages oestrogen clearance. If they are not present in healthy quantities, the oestrogen is reactivated and sent back into circulation to cause havoc. Also support immunoglobins.
Progesterone	Female steroid sex hormone which prepares the endometrium of the uterus for pregnancy and is required for the maintenance of pregnancy. Secreted by the corpus luteum in the ovary once conception has taken place to prepare the womb lining and placenta. Maintains the pregnancy and prevents release of further eggs from the ovary. (*see* Ovary *and* Corpus luteum)
Prolactin	Pituitary hormone which stimulates milk synthesis. It also stimulates the production of progesterone by the corpus luteum of the ovary. Excess melatonin causes an increase in prolactin, which lowers zinc and prostaglandins. (*see* Pituitary gland *and* Lactation)
Pronuclei	The two nuclei that form in the egg after fertilization. One nucleus contains the genes of the egg (mother) and the other nucleus contains the genes of the sperm (father).
Prostaglandin (PG)	A lipid hormone found in many cells of the body. Some are proinflammatory while others are anti-inflammatory.
Proteins	A group of complex organic nitrogen-containing compounds found throughout the body. They are composed of sequential strands of amino acids and are used for body building and repair, hormones and enzyme production.
Pseudo	Superficial resemblance, false.
Pyridoxine	Vitamin B6. Required by more than 60 enzymes, and essential for DNA and protein synthesis. It influences the nervous and reproductive systems, and plays a vital role in immunity and avoidance of PMS symptoms. Aids infertility along with zinc.
Quercetin	A flavonoid which acts as an antioxidant. Helps prevent water retention and leaking capillaries. Acts as a phytoestrogen and helps the body to convert oestradiol to oestriol – the safe form of oestrogen.
Red blood cells	The major cell type found in the blood. Its main function is to transport oxygen throughout the body. Also called erythrocytes.

Retrograde	To move backwards. Endometriosis may be a result of retrograde menstruation – that is, menstrual flow into the peritoneal cavity via the Fallopian tubes instead of into the vagina.
Riboflavin	Vitamin B2, part of the body's antioxidant mechanism. Needed for correct thyroid function. Used alongside vitamin B5 in the reproductive system.
Scurvy	A disease condition that develops as a result of vitamin C deficiency. People with scurvy have anaemia, weakness, spongy gums and a tendency to bleed. (*see* Anaemia)
Selenium	A non-metallic element resembling sulphur. Small amounts of selenium are required for normal metabolism. Major antioxidant. Needed for thyroid function alongside iodine. Significant in sperm motility.
Seminal fluid	The fluid in the ejaculate that contains sperm. High levels of zinc in each ejaculation, 1.5mg. (*see* Sperm *and* Testes)
Serotonin	A neurohormone produced in large amounts in the pineal gland of the brain. It is also found in other tissues of the body, including blood platelets and intestinal walls. It is believed to play a role in inflammation. Features in the process of sleep, prevention of depression, anxiety and mood disorders.
Sertoli cell	The cells of the testes that surround the developing sperm. They supply nutrients to the developing sperm and secrete fluids that help push the sperm out of the testes and into the epididymis. (*see* Sperm, Testes *and* Epididymis)
Sex steroids	Lipid-soluble steroid hormones involved in the reproductive process. They include oestrogen, progesterone and testosterone. Good quality cis fatty acids are essential for their formation. (*see* Steroids, Oestrogen, Progesterone *and* Testosterone)
SIDS	Sudden infant death syndrome.
Slippery elm	Herb which soothes irritated tissues, especially mucous membranes such as those in the digestive tract.
Sperm	The male reproductive cell produced in the testes and which contains the genes of the father. The head and tail of the sperm depend upon zinc. (*see* Testes *and* Seminal fluid)
Spermatogenesis	Formation of sperm in the testes. (*see* Sperm *and* Testes)
Spermatozoa	Same as sperm.
Steroids	A group of lipid-soluble biochemical substances which chemically resemble cholesterol. Cholesterol is the precursor of all steroid hormones. Vitamin D is also closely involved. The atoms of steroids are arranged in four rings. The major steroid-producing organs of the body include the ovary, testis, adrenal gland and placenta.
Stilboestrol	Synthetic non-steroidal oestrogen, known as DES (diethylstilboestrol) in the USA. Causes cancer. (*see* DES)
Stillbirth	When an infant is dead at birth.
Superoxide dismutase (SOD)	A highly reactive enzyme that neutralizes free oxidized radicals (FoRs). (*see* Free radicals)

Synergy Symbiotic relationship	Working together for the good of each other. When two organisms work together for the benefit of both organisms.
T cells	A type of cell that helps the immune system. Also known as T-helper cells, which switch the immune system on, and T-suppressor cells which switch the immune system off. (*see* Immune system)
Teratogen	A substance, agent or process that induces the formation of developmental abnormalities in a fetus such as excess vitamin A, alcohol, thalidomide and measles. (*see* Fetus)
Teratogenesis	The process leading to developmental abnormalities in the fetus.
Testes	The paired organs located in the scrotum under the penis. The site of production of sperm and testosterone. (*see* Sperm *and* Testosterone)
Testosterone	Major masculinizing hormone produced in large amounts by the male testes. Dependent upon vitamin E and zinc for its manufacture.
Thymus	A ductless gland that is found under the breastbone. Doubles in size by puberty and shrinks thereafter. Functional tissue is replaced by fatty tissue. Involved with the early development of the immune system, and is the main production site for T lymphocytes (white blood cells associated with antibody production), which migrate from bone marrow to mature in the thymus. Zinc-dependent organ. (*see* Immune system)
Thyroid	The endocrine gland that controls the overall level of metabolism in the body. It is located in the neck and secretes the hormone thyroxine. For temperaure regulation. (*see* Metabolism, TSH *and* Thyroxine)
Thyroid-stimulating hormone (TSH)	The hormone secreted by the pituitary that stimulates the thyroid gland to produce thyroxine. (*see* Thyroid *and* Thyroxine)
Thyroxine	The major hormone secreted by the thyroid. Thyroxine regulates general metabolism. Iodine-dependent. Requires riboflavin, vitamin B2, selenium, tyrosine and vitamin E for its formation. Antagonistic with oestrogen. If oestrogen is too high, thyroxine will be low and vice versa. (*see* Thyroid)
Tocopherol	*see* Vitamin E.
Tonsil	A small almond-shaped mass on the back of the mouth that is composed mostly of lymphoid tissue. It is believed to be a source of the white blood cells that phagocytize (eat) the bacteria that enter the mouth and nose. (*see* Lymphatic system, Phagocytize *and* White blood cells)
Transit time	In reference to the digestive system, transit time is the time that foodstuffs spend in the gastrointestinal tract from the time of ingestion to defecation. Should be 12–24 hours.(*see* Gastrointestinal)
Uterus	The organ of the reproductive system where pregnancy occurs. Also called the womb. It is a muscular organ that is about the size of a small fist, with an inner lining of mucus-like tissue called the endometrium. Magnesium aids relaxation of uterine muscles. (*see* Endometrium)

Vagina	The lower part of the female reproductive tract that connects the cervix of the uterus to the exterior. (*see* Uterus *and* Cervix)
Villi	Finger-like projections in membranes of the gut which can be damaged by gluten grains in susceptible people. The villi increases the surface area for nutrients to be absorbed, so their damage leads to malabsorption.
Vitamins	A general term for a group of unrelated biochemical substances that occur in food in small amounts and are required for normal metabolic functioning of the body. They may be either water-soluble or fat-soluble substances.
Vitamin A	A vitamin found primarily in fish-liver oils, and some yellow and dark-green vegetables, functioning in normal cell growth and development. Deficiency causes roughening and hardening of the skin, night-blindness and deterioration of mucous membranes in the lung. Found in two forms: retinol (animal) and beta-carotene (plant-based). Excess amounts of vitamin A retinol are toxic.
Vitamin B1	Thiamine. Deficiency can cause learning defects.
Vitamin B2	Riboflavin. Deficiency can cause limb defects.
Vitamin B3	Nicotinamide or niacin. Deficiencies can cause harelip or cleft palate.
Vitamin B5	Pantothenic acid. The anti-allergy vitamin. Needed for reproduction. Aids memory.
Vitamin B6	Pyridoxine. Most commonly deficient especially in those who take the pill, HRT or other sex hormones because of their abnormal amine metabolism. Lowered by the pill. Deficiency can cause depression, urinary tract cancer or dermatitis. Precursor of progesterone.
Vitamin B12	Cyanocobalamin. Often deficient in smokers or vegetarians. Only found in animal produce.
Vitamin B-complex (other)	Water-soluble vitamins found primarily in yeast, liver, eggs, and certain vegetables. Taking too much of one B vitamin can cause shortages of the others. Lowered by the pill. Also produced in the small intestine by bifidobacteria.
	Folic acid. Lowered by the pill, HRT and fertility stimulants. Taking the pill causes localized folate deficiency of the cervix, which may trigger cervical cancer. Extra required during pregnancy. Deficiency can cause anaemia and spina bifida. Aspirin, anaesthetic gas and sulphasalazine interfere with folate absorption. Has oestrogenic properties. (*see* Anaemia *and* HRT)
	Choline. Important in the synthesis of phosphatidylcholine (lecithin) and other phospholipids, DNA and RNA. Insecticides inactivate choline enzymes, thus preventing the uptake of manganese in plants, which is then linked to a fall in manganese absorption. Choline and inositol are important for liver enzyme function, and aid the breakdown of oestrogens so that they can be excreted safely by the body.
	Inositol. Aids choline in oestrogen degradation in the liver. Involved in the synthesis of phospholipids, so is essential for the digestion and absorption of fats and their uptake by cells.

Biotin. Not a true vitamin as it is made by the bifidobacteria in the gut. Prevents overgrowth of yeast in the intestines. Biotin deficiency resembles Alzheimer's disease. Drugs like antibiotics cause a deficiency.

Vitamin C	Ascorbic acid. Water-soluble vitamin present in citrus fruits, rosehip powder and chilli peppers. Lowered by pill hormones, smoking and tetracyclines. Antiviral, antibacterial, antihistamine. Smokers are deficient as each cigarette burns up 25mg of vitamin C.
Vitamin D	Fat-soluble vitamin that is produced in response to skin exposure to the sun. Also found in fish oils. Deficiencies in vitamin D cause rickets. A precursor of cholesterol and thought to be a hormone in its own right. Deficiency may cause problems in hormone formation.
Vitamin E	Fat-soluble vitamin that belongs to the tocopherol family and found in wheatgerm oil, cereals and egg yolk. Rats fed a vitamin E-deficient diet have fertility problems. Important in preventing sticky platelets and blood clots.
Vitamin K	A fat-soluble vitamin. Has two forms: phytomenadione (plant origin) and menaquinone (animal origin). Required for normal blood-clot formation. Found in alfalfa, spinach, cabbage, fishmeal and egg yolk.
Vulvadynia	Vulval pain, the kind that is often referred to vulvadynia, may be caused by endometriosis in the surrounding tissues. Symptoms include feeling as if the vulva is constantly inflamed but in different areas; a sudden prickly feeling like horrible pins-and-needles; at times, a burning itching but with absolutely no discharge; and very painful pinching/searing to the point that you may not be able to open the legs or sit down normally, alongside the usual endometriosis pain on intercourse. It may be confused with symptoms of cystitis. A change of diet and nutritional supplements, as well as specialist treatment with a negligible dose of amitriptyline (normally given as an anti-depressant in higher doses, but used here to dampen the nerve endings), will make a difference in terms of pain. A special 'virginal' speculum can be used for examination. Amielle trainers may be used as gently as possible to ease symptoms in the area.
White blood cells	Free-floating cells found in the blood that help the immune system. Also called leukocytes. (*see* T cells *and* Macrophage)
Womb	*see* Uterus.
Xeno-oestrogens	Oestrogens from outside the body. These are oestrogens which are metabolized in the body from synthetic man-made chemicals. They disrupt normal hormone profiles. Body fat stores these chemicals and releases them as weight is lost. High exposure to these pesticidal chemicals can disrupt oestrogen levels and may be related to endometriosis.
Zinc	Metal cofactor necessary for the correct functioning of reproduction and the immune system. Lowered by the pill. Available in oysters and red meat. (*see* Sperm *and* Vitamin B6)
Zygote	The newly fertilized ovum before cleavage begins. (*see* Fertilization)

Recommended reading

Endometriosis

Ballweg, Mary Lou, *The Endometriosis Sourcebook*, The Endometriosis Association/Contemporary Books, 1995

Hawkridge, Caroline, *Living with Endometriosis*, Vermilion, London, 1996

Henderson, Lorraine, Robyn Riley and Ros Wood, *Explaining Endometriosis*, Allen & Unwin, Sydney, 1991

Wittgenstein, Kate, *Living with Endometriosis*, Addison Wesley Longman, Harlow, 1987

Fertility

Barnes, Belinda and Suzanne G. Bradley, *Planning for a Healthy Baby*, Vermilion, London, 1994

Bradley, Susan Gail with Nicholas Bennett, *Preparation for Pregnancy*, Argyll, 1995

Leese, Henry, *Human Reproduction and in vitro Fertilization*, Macmillan Education, London, 1989

Wynn, Margaret and Arthur, *The Case for Preconceptual Care in Men and Women*, A B Academic Publishers, Bicester, 1991

Digestion and absorption

Brostoff, Dr Jonathan and Linda Gamlin, *The Complete Guide to Food Allergy and Intolerance*, Bloomsbury, London, 1989 (reissued in 1998)

Chaitow, Leon and Natasha Trenev, *Probiotics*, Thorsons, London, 1990

Connoly, Pat, Crook, William and Trum Hunter, Beatrice, *The Candida Albicans Yeast-Free Cookbook*, McGraw-Hill Trade, 2000

Lipski, Elizabeth, *Digestive Wellness*, Keats Publishing, New Canaan, 1996

MacDonald Baker, Sidney, *Detoxification & Healing*, Keats Publishing, New Canaan, 1997

Murray, Michael and Joseph Pizzorno, *Encyclopaedia of Natural Medicine*, Optima MacDonald, London, 1990

Trattler, Ross, *Better Health Through Natural Healing*, Health, 1987

Foods, vitamins, minerals and essential oils

Carper, Jean, *The Food Pharmacy*, Simon & Schuster, London, 1990
—*Food, Your Miracle Medicine*, Simon & Schuster, London, 1995

Chaitow, Leon, *The Stone Age Diet*, Optima MacDonald, London, 1988

Cherry Hills, Hilda, *Good Food, Milk Free, Grain Free*, Keats Publishing, New Canaan, 1980

Coffey, Lynette, *Wheatless Cooking*, Ten Speed Press, California, 1984

Cousins, Barbara, *Cooking Without*, Moorside Natural Healing Clinic, 1989

Cox, Peter and Peggy Brusseau, *Secret Ingredients*, Bantam Books, London, 1997

Erasmus, Udo, *Fats that Heal, Fats that Kill*, Alive Books, Burnaby BC, 1996

Graham, Judy, *Evening Primrose Oil*, Thorsons, London, 1993

Hendler, Dr Sheldon Saul, *The Doctor's Vitamin and Mineral Encyclopaedia*, Arrow Books, London, 1991

Lieberman, Shari and Nancy Bruning, *The Real Vitamin and Mineral Book*, 2nd edition, Avery Press, New York, 1997
Null, Gary, *The Complete Guide to Sensible Eating*, 4 Walls 8 Window, New York, 1990
—*The '90s Healthy Body Book*, Health Communications, Florida, 1994
Null, Gary with Dr Martin Feldman, *Good Food, Good Mood*, St Martin's Press, New York, 1988

Environmental issues
Buist, Robert, *Food Chemical Sensitivity*, Prish, Dorset, 1986
Cadbury D, *The Feminisation of Nature: Our Future at Risk*, Hamish Hamilton, London, 1997
Colburn, Theo, John Peterson and Dianne Dumanoski, *Our Stolen Future*, Little Brown, London, 1996
Humphreys J, *The Great Food Gamble*, Coronet, 2002
Millstone, Erik, *Food Additives*, Penguin, Harmondsworth, 1986
Mumby, Dr Keith, *Complete Guide to Food Allergies*, Thorsons, London, 1993
Philpott, William H and Dwight K Kalita, *Brain Allergies*, Keats Publishing, New Canaan, 1987
Van Straten, Michael and Barbara Griggs, *Superfoods*, Dorling Kindersley, London, 1990
Virtue, Doreen, *Constant Craving*, Hay House, Carlstad, CA, 1996
Wunderlich Jr, Ray C, *Sugar and Your Health*, Good Health Publications, Florida, 1982

Medical ethics
Bequaert Holmes, Helen and Laura M Purdy, *Feminist Perspectives in Medical Ethics*, Indiana University Press, Bloomington & Indianapolis, 1992
Miles, Agnes, *Women, Health and Medicine*, Open University Press, Buckingham, 1991

Pain management
Sadler, Jan, *Natural Pain Relief*, Element Books, Shaftesbury, 1997
Lipton, Dr Sampson, *Conquering Pain*, Methuen, London, 1994

Miscellaneous
Anderson, Greg, *50 Essential Things to Do When the Doctor Says It's Cancer*, Plume, New York, 1993
Carter, Jean and Michael, *Sweet Grapes: How to stop being infertile and start living again*, Perspective Press
Colgan, Dr Michael, *Hormonal Health*, Apple Publishing, Vancouver, 1996
Fredericks, Carlton, *Guide to Women's Nutrition*, Putnam Publishing Group, New York, 1989
Grant, Dr Ellen, *Sexual Chemistry*, Cedar Press, London, 1994
Jones, J, *The Unofficial Guide to Smart Nutrition*, IDG Books, New York, 2000
Kenton, Leslie, *Ageless Ageing*, Arrow Books, London, 1987
Kübler-Ross, Elizabeth, *On Death and Dying*, Tavistock/Routledge, London, 1970
Langer, Stephen E and James F Scheer, *Solved the Riddle of Illness*, Keats Publishing, New Canaan, 1984
Meek, Jennifer, *Immune Power: Health and the Immune System*, Optima Macdonald, 1990
Null, Gary and Martin Feldman, *Reverse the Ageing Process Naturally*, Villard Books, New York, 1996
Pizzorno, Joseph, *Total Wellness*, Prima Publishing, Rocklin, CA, 1996
Reynolds, Simon, *Become Happy in Eight Minutes*, Plume Penguin, Harmondsworth, Middlesex, 1996
Worwood, V A, *Endometriosis and Aromatherapy* (booklet), The Earth Garden Clinic, 2 Fairview Parade, Romford, Essex RM7 7HH

Useful addresses

ACUPUNCTURE

Council for Acupuncture, 38 Mount Pleasant, London WC1X 0AP

The American Association of Acupuncture and Oriental Medicine, P O Box 162340, Sacramento, CA 95816, USA. Tel: 916 443 4770. www.aaaomonline.org

AROMATHERAPY

The International Federation of Professional Aromatherapists (IFPA), 82 Ashby Road, Hinckley, Leicestershire LE10 1SN. Tel: 01455 637987. Email: admin@ifparoma.org. www.ifparoma.org

The American Alliance of Aromatherapy (AAoA), P O Box 309, Depoe Bay, OR 97341, USA

National Association for Holistic Aromatherapy, 3327 W. Indian Trail Road PMB 144, Spokane, WA 99208, USA. Tel: (509) 325 3419. Email: info@naha.org. www.naha.org

CANCER

Macmillan Cancer Support, 89 Albert Embankment, London SE1 7UQ. Cancerline: 0808 808 2020 (9am–10pm, Monday–Friday). Email: cancerline@macmillan.org.uk. www.macmillan.org.uk

Women's National Cancer Control Campaign (WNCC), Suna House, 128–130 Curtain Road, London EC2A 3AR. Helpline: 020 7729 2229. Email: info@wnccc.org.uk. www.wnccc.org.uk

CHIROPRACTIC

The British Chiropractic Association, 59 Castle Street, Reading, Berkshire RG1 7SN. Tel: 0118 950 5950 (9am–5pm, Monday–Friday).

www.chiropractic-uk.co.uk

Anglo-European College of Chiropractic, 13–15 Parkwood Road, Bournemouth BH5 2DF. Tel: 01202 436200. Email: aecc@aecc.ac.uk. www.aeccc.ac.uk

The American Chiropractic Association (ACA), 1701 Clarendon Boulevard, Arlington, VA 22209, USA. Tel: (703) 276 8800. Email: memberinfo@acatoday.org. www.amerchiro.org

The International Chiropractors Association, 1110 N. Glebe Road, Suite 650, Arlington, VA 22201, USA. Tel: 1 800 423 4690. Email: chiro@chiropractic.org. www.chiropractic.org

Chiropractic Association (Singapore), c/o 19 Tanglin Road #04–17, Tanglin Shopping Centre, Singapore 247909. Tel: (65) 6738 9142. Email: rawdc@chiropractic-care.com.sg. www.chiropractic.org.sg

Chiropractors Association of Australia, PO Box 335, Penrith, New South Wales 2751, Australia. Tel: (02) 4731 8011. Email: nhq@caa.asn.au. www.chiropractors.asn.au

New Zealand Chiropractors' Association (NZCA), P O Box 46 127, Herne Bay, Auckland, New Zealand. Tel: 64 9 360 2089. Email: info@chiropractic.org.nz. www.chiropractic.org.nz

COUNSELLING

British Association for Counselling and Psychotherapy, BACP House, 15 St John's Business Park, Lutterworth, Leicestershire LE17 4HB. Email: bacp@bacp.co.uk. www.bacp.co.uk

ENDOMETRIOSIS GROUPS

Argentina

Endometriosis Group Argentina, Av. Santa Fe

1675 2 Piso Dito A CP 1060, Capital Federal, Buenos Aires, Argentina. Tel/fax: 54 11 4815 4802. Email: endoasist@yahoo.com. www.endometriosisgroup.com.ar

Australia

Endometriosis Association (Queensland) Inc., P O Box 39, Red Hill, Queensland 4059, Australia. www.qendo.org.au

Austria

Osterreichische Endometriose Vereinigung, Martha-Frühwirt-Zenturn, Obere Augartenstrasse 26-28, 1020 Wien, Austria. Tel: 676 4447344, Email: office@endometriose-wien.at. www.endometriose-wien.at

Belgium

Endometriose Stichting, Postbus 34, 3630 Maasmechelen, Belgium. Email: info@endometriose.be. www.endometriose.be

Brazil

ABEND (Associação Brasileira de Endometriose), Rua Claro de Camargo Sobrinho 89, Vila Pouso Alegre Barueri, SP Cep 06402-050, Brazil. Tel: 11 4198 8228. Email: abend@abend.org.br. www.abend.org.br

Denmark

Endometriose Foreningen, Kvorupvej 1, Åsted, DK-6800 Varde, Denmark. Tel: 2172 4300. Email: info@endo.dk. www.endo.dk

Finland

Endometrioosiyhdistys Finland, PL 142, 00531 Helsinki, Finland. Tel/fax: 0 50 380 6715. Email: endo@endometrioosiyhdistys.fi. www.endometrioosiyhdistys.fi

France

EndoFrance, 17 allée des Eguerêts, F-95280 Jouy le Moutier, France. Email: contact@endofrance.org. www.endofrance.org

Germany

Endometriose-Vereinigung Deutschland e.V., Bernhard-Göring-Strasse 152, 04277 Leipzig, Germany. Tel: 341 3 06 53 04 (9am–12pm Monday–Thursday, 1–6pm Thursday). Email: info@endometriose-vereinigung.de. www.endometriose-vereinigung.de

Hungary

Nok az endometriózisért alapitvány, Kapy utca 43, H-1025 Budapest, Hungary. Tel: 30 970 5613. Email: info@endometriozis.hu. www.endometriozis.hu

India

Endometriosis Society India, 6A & 6F Neelamber, 28B Shakespeare Sarani, Kolkata 700 017, India. Tel: 2240 4463/33 2865 0364. Email: mail@endosocindia.org. www.endosocindia.org

Ireland

Endometriosis Association of Ireland, Carmichael Centre, North Brunswick Street, Dublin 7, Ireland. Tel: 1 873 5702. Email: info@endo.ie. www.endo.ie

Italy

Associazione Italiana Endometriosi Onlus (AIE), Casella Postale 114, I-20014 Nerviano (MI), Italy. Tel/fax: 0331 589800. Email: info@endoassoc.it. www.endoassoc.it

Associazione Progetto Endometriosi Onlus (APE) Casella Postale 315, I-42100 Reggio Emilia, Italy. Email: info@apeonlus.info. www.apeonlus.info

Japan

Japan Endometriosis Association (JEMA), 1-20-2-301, Nippombashi Chuo-ku, Osaka, Japan. Email: info-2@jemanet.org. www.jemanet.org

Malta

Endo Support (Malta). Tel: 7906 8840. Email:endosupport@gmail.com

Mexico

Associación de Endometriosis Capitulo Mexicano. Tel: 55 51 490468. Email: mexendometriosis@yahoo.com.mx. www.mexendometriosis.com

The Netherlands

Endometriose Stichting, Antwoordnummer 1789, 2000 VC Haarlem, The Netherlands. Tel: 72 581 5320 (7–10pm Monday, 9am–12pm Wednesday). Email: info@endometriose.nl. www.endometriose.nl

New Zealand

New Zealand Endometriosis Foundation Inc., PO Box 1673, Christchurch, New Zealand.

Tel: 3 379 7959. Support Line: 0800 733277 (New Zealand callers only). Email: nzendo@xtra.co.nz. www.nzendo.co.nz

Norway

Endometrioseforeningen, Postboks 2101, 1760 Halden, Norway. Tel: 452 15 555. Email: post@endometriose.no. www.endometriose.no

Portugal

Associação Portuguesa de Endometriose, Rua Laura Alves 12-1, 1050-138 Lisboa, Portugal. Tel: 96 236 8720. www.aspoendo.org

Puerto Rico

Endometriosis de Puerto Rico, Department of Microbiology, Ponce School of Medicine, PO BOX 7004, Ponce 00731, Puerto Rico. Tel: 840 2575 ext. 2206. Email: idhaliz@endopuertorico.com. www.endopuertorico.com

Singapore

Endometriosis Association (Singapore), c/o Mount Alvernia Hospital, 820 Thomson Road, Singapore 574623. Tel: 63476640 (office hours only). Email: info@endometriosis.org.sg. www.endometriosis.org.sg

Spain

Asociacion de Endometriosis España (AEE), Calle Mayor 29, E-17455 Caldes de Malavella, Spain. Email: info@endoinfo.org. www.endoinfo.org

South Africa

Endometriosis Society of South Africa, 7 Crescent Drive, Westcliff, 2193 Johannesburg, South Africa. Tel: 011 646 0449

Sweden

Svenska Endometriosföreningen, Box 14087, S-167 14 Bromma, Sweden. Email: info@endometriosforeningen.se. www.endometriosforeningen.se

Föreningen EndoLiv, Neglingev 45, S-133 34 Saltsjöbaden, Sweden. Email: info@endoliv.se. www.endoliv.se

Switzerland

Selbsthilfegruppe Endometriose Zürich, Email: info@endo-shg.ch. www.endo-shg.ch

EndoSuisse, Rue des Moulins 5, 1562 Corcelles près Payerne, Switzerland. Tel: 079 445 8315.

Email: endosuisse@endosuisse.ch. www.endosuisse.ch

Uganda

Joyce Fertility Support Centre, 32 Windsor Crescent, Kololo (off Babiiha Avenue), P O Box 28095, Kampala, Uganda. Tel: 041 345366. Email: joycefertility@hotmail.com. www.joycefertility.com

United Kingdom

National Endometriosis Society, 50 Westminster Palace Gardens, Artillery Row, London SW1P 1RL. Tel: 020 7222 2780. Free Helpline: 0808 808 2221. Email: enquiries@endometriosis-uk.org. www.endo.org.uk

Endometriosis SHE Trust UK, 14 Moorland Way, Lincoln, LN6 7JW. Tel/fax: 0870 7743665. Email: shetrust@shetrust.org.uk. www.shetrust.org.uk

The Endometriosis and Fertility Clinic, The Hale Clinic, 7 Park Crescent, London W1B 1PF. Tel: 020 7631 0156 (bookings). Email: info@haleclinic.com; dian@endometriosis.co.uk. www.haleclinic.com; www.endometriosis.co.uk

United States

Endometriosis Association, 8585 N 75th Place, Milwaukee, WI 53223, USA. Tel: 414 355 2200. Email: endo@endometriosisassn.org. www.endometriosisassn.org

Endo Research Center, International Headquarters, 630 Ibis Drive, Delray Beach, FL 33444, USA. Tel: 561 274 7442. www.endocenter.org

ENVIRONMENTAL MEDICINE

Healthy House, The Old Co-op, Lower Street, Ruscombe, Stroud, Gloucestershire GL6 6BU. Tel: 01453 752216; 0845 450 5950. Email: info@healthyhouse.co.uk. www.healthyhouse.co.uk

Environmental Air Systems, Martin Wells, Sandyhill Cottage, Sandy Lane, Rushmore, Tilford, Farnham, Surrey GU10 2ET

Hyperactive Children's Support Group, 71 Whyke Lane, Chichester, West Sussex PO19

7PD. Email: hacsg@hacsg.org.uk.
www.hacsg.org.uk

Pesticide Exposure Group of Sufferers (PEGS), 4 Lloyds House, Regent Terrace, Cambridge CB2 1AA

Society for Environmental Therapy, Mrs H Davidson, 521 Foxhall Road, Ipswich IP3 8LW

Environmental Action, 1525 New Hampshire Avenue NW, Washington DC 20036, USA

Greenpeace USA, 702 11th Street NW, Washington DC 20001, USA. Tel: 202 462 1177. Email: info@wdc.greenpeace.org. www.greenpeace.org/usa

Friends of the Earth, 1717 Massachusetts Avenue NW, Suite 600, Washington DC 20003, USA. Tel: 877 843 8687. Email: foe@foe.org. www.foe.org

Beyond Pesticides (National Coalition Against the Misuse of Pesticides), 701 East Street SE, Suite 200, Washington DC 20003, USA. Tel: 202 543 5450. Email: info@beyondpesticides.org. www.beyondpesticides.org

Citizens for a Better Environment, 152 W. Wisconsin Avenue, Suite 510, Milwaukee, WI 53203, USA. Tel: 414 271 7280. Email: cbewleigc.@apc.org. www.wsh.org/cbe

FERTILITY

The Endometriosis and Fertility Clinic, The Hale Clinic, 7 Park Crescent, London W1B 1PF. Tel: 020 7631 0156 (bookings). Email: info@haleclinic.com; dian@endometriosis.co.uk. www.haleclinic.com; www.endometriosis.co.uk

Natural Family Planning, Mrs Colleen Norman, 218 Heathwood Road, Heath, Cardiff, South Wales. Cardiff 493120 (am only)

Infertility Network UK, Charter House, 43 St Leonards Road, Bexhill-on-Sea, East Sussex TN40 1JA. Tel: 08701 188088. www.infertility.networkuk.com

Foresight (Association for the Promotion of Pre-conceptual Care), 178 Hawthorn Road, West Bognor, West Sussex PO21 2UY. www.foresight-preconception.org.uk

Resolve, 8405 Greenboro Drive, Suite 800, Mclean, VA 22102-5120. Tel: 703 556 7172. www.resolve.org

National Childbirth Trust, Alexandra House, Oldham Terrace, Acton, London W3 6NH. Enquiry line: 0870 444 8707 (9am–5pm Monday–Thursday, 9am–4pm Friday). Email: enquiries@nct.org.uk. www.nct.org.uk

National Infertility Exchange Network, P O Box 204, East Meadow, NY 11554, USA. Tel: 516 794 5772. Email: info@nine-infertility.org. www.nine-infertility.org

HEALING

Breath Fellowship, Chilston Mead, Pembury Road, Tunbridge Wells, Kent

Crowhurst Christian Healing Centre, The Old Rectory, Forewood Lane, Crowhurst, Battle, East Sussex, TN33 9AD. Tel: 01424 830204. Email: info@btconnect.com. www.crowhursthealing.co.uk

HEALTHY EATING

The Endometriosis and Fertility Clinic, The Hale Clinic, 7 Park Crescent, London W1B 1PF. Tel: 020 7631 0156 (bookings). Email: info@haleclinic.com; dian@endometriosis.co.uk. www.haleclinic.com; www.endometriosis.co.uk

Institute of Optimum Nutrition (ION), Avalon House, 72 Lower Mortlake Road, Richmond, Surrey TW9 2JY. Tel: 020 8614 7800. www.ion.ac.uk

Allergy Care Catalogue, Pollards Yard, Wood Street, Taunton, Somerset TA1 1UP. (For unusual foods)

Lifestyle Healthcare, Centenary Business Park, Henley-on-Thames, Oxfordshire RG9 1DS. Tel: 01491 570000. Email: sales@gfdiet.com. www:gfdiet.com. (Freshly-baked, home delivered gluten-free foods)

Organic Growers Association, Aeron Park, Llangietho, Dyfed, Wales.

Organic Information, P O Box 1503, Poole, Dorset BH14 8YE. Tel: 01202 715130.

Soil Association, South Plaza, Marlborough

Street, Bristol, BS1 3NX. Tel: 0117 314 5000. Email: info@soilassociation.org. www.soilassociation.org

Food Commission, 94 White Lion Street, London N1 9PF. Tel: 020 7837 1141. Email: enquiries@foodcomm.org.uk. www.foodcomm.org.uk

Freshwater Filters, Carlton House, Aylmer Road, Leytonstone E11 3AD. Tel: 0208 558 7495. Email: mail@freshwaterfilters.com. www.freshwaterfilters.com

Friends of the Earth, 26–28 Underwood Street, London N1 7JQ. Tel: 020 7490 1555. www.foe.co.uk

Good Gardeners Association, 4 Lisle Place, Churcham, Gloucestershire GL2 8AD. Tel: 01453 520322. Email: office@goodgardeners.org.uk. www.goodgardeners.org.uk

Center for Science in the Public Interest, 1875 Connecticut Avenue NW, Suite 300, Washington DC 20009, USA. Tel: 202 332 9110. Email: cspi@cspinet.org. www.cspinet.org

Garden Organic (Henry Doubleday Research Association), Garden Organic Ryton, Coventry, Warwickshire CV8 3LG. Tel: 024 7630 3517. Email: enquiry@gardenorganic.org.uk. www.gardenorganic.org.uk

Wholefood, 24 Paddington Street, London W1M 4DR. (For organic food and books)

Vegetarian Society of the UK, Parkdale, Dunham Road, Altrincham, Cheshire WA14 4QG. Tel: 0161 925 2000. www.vegsoc.org

Vegan Society, Donald Watson House, 21 Hylton Street, Hockley, Birmingham B18 6HJ. Tel: 0121 523 1730. Email: info@vegansociety.com. www.vegansociety.com

North American Vegetarian Society, PO Box 72, Dolgeville, NY 13329, USA. Tel: 518 568 7970. Email: navs@telenet.net. www.navs-online.org

American Vegan Society, 56 Dinshan Lane, P O Box 369, Malaga, NJ 08328, USA. www.americanvegan.org

The Natural Medicine Society, Regency House, 97–107 Hagley Road, Edgbaston, Birmingham B16

The Centre for Complementary and Integrated Medicine, 51 Bedford Place, Southampton SO15 2DT. Tel: 023 8033 4752. www.complemed.co.uk

FACT (Food Additives Campaign Team), 25 Horsell Road, London N5 1XL

Greenpeace, Canonbury Villas, London N1 2PN. Tel: 020 7865 8100. Email: info@uk.greenpeace.org. www.greenpeace.org.uk

Wholelife, 89 5th Avenue, Suite 600, New York, NY 10003, USA

American College of Health Science, 6600-D Burleson Road, Austin, TX 78744

HERBALISM

National Institute of Medical Herbalists, Elm House, 54 Mary Arches Street, Exeter EX4 3BA. Tel: 01392 426022. Email: nimh@ukexeter.freeserve.co.uk. www.nimh.org

New Vitality, Hugh Sinclair Unit of Human Nutrition, School of Chemistry, Food Biosciences and Pharmacy, The University of Reading, PO Box 226, Whiteknights, Reading RG6 6AP. Tel: 01323 484 353. www.newvitality.org.uk

North American Herbalists Guild, PO Box 1683, Sequel, California 95073, USA

The American Herb Association, P O Box 673, Nevada City, CA 95959, USA. www.ahaherb.com

National Herbalists Association of Australia, P O Box 45, Concord West, New South Wales 2138, Australia. Tel: 02 8765 0071. www.nhaa.org.au

Canadian Holistic Medical Association, 491 Eglington Avenue West, Apt 407, Toronto, Ontario M5N 1A8, Canada. Tel: 416 485 3071

HOMEOPATHY

Royal London Homeopathic Hospital, 60 Great Ormond Street, London, WC1N 3HR.

Tel: 0845 1555 000. www.uclh.nhs.uk

Hahnemann Society, Hahnemann House, 2 Powis Place, Great Ormond Street, London WC1N 3HT

Society of Homeopaths, 11 Brookfield, Duncan Close, Moulton Park, Northampton NN3 6WL. Tel: 0845 450 6611. www.homeopathy-soh.org

American Foundation for Homeopathy, 1508 S. Garfield, Alhambra, CA 91801, USA

British Institute of Homeopathy, Endeavour House, 80 High Street, Egham, Surrey TW20 9HE. Tel: 01784 473800. Email: info@britinsthom.com. www.britinsthom.com

British Homeopathic Association, Hahnemann House, 29 Park Street, West Luton LU1 3BE. Tel: 0870 444 3950. www.trusthomeopathy.org

National Center for Homeopathy, 801 N Fairfax Street, Suite 306, Alexander, VA 22314, USA. Tel: 703 5487790. www.nationalcenterforhomeopathy.org

International Foundation for Homeopathy, 2366 East Lake Avenue E, Suite 30, Seattle, WA 98102, USA. Tel: 206 324-8230

Australian Institute of Homeopathy, 21 Bulah Close, Berdwra Heights, New South Wales 2082, Australia

HYDROTHERAPY

UK College of Hydrotherapy, 515 Hagley Road, Birmingham, B66 4AX. Tel: 021 429 9191

Aquatic Exercise Association, PO Box 1609, Nokomis, FL 3427, USA. Tel: 813 486 8600. www.aeawave.com

The American Board of Hydrotherapy, 16842 Von Karman Avenue, Suite 475, Irvine, CA 92714, USA

HYPNOSIS

British Society of Experimental and Clinical Hypnosis, 28 Dale Park Gardens, Cookridge, Leeds LS16 7PT. Tel: 07000 560309. www.bscah.com

The Society for Clinical and Experimental Hypnosis, Massachusetts School of Professional Psychology, 21 Rivermoor Street, Boston, MA 02132, USA. Tel: 617 469 1981. Email: sceh@mspp.edu. www.sceh.usk

New World Music, Harmony House, Hillside Road East, Bungay, Suffolk NR35 1RX. Tel: 01986 891600. www.newworld.music.com. For tapes on relaxation, pain, sleep, health by Robert E Griswold. From the series The Love Tapes, Electronic Music Research Inc

IMMUNE AND ALLERGY EFFECTS

HCG Society for Primary Immune Deficiencies, 74 Beverley Road, Whyteleaf, Surrey CR3 ODX. Tel: 020 8666 7405

Action Against Allergy, P O Box 278, Twickenham TW1 4QQ. Tel: 020 8892 2711. Email: aaa@actionagainstallergy.freeserve.co.uk. www.actionagainstallergy.co.uk

National Society for Research into Allergy, 2 Armadale Close, Hollycroft, Hinckley, Leicestershire LE10 0SZ. Tel: 01455 250715. Email: eunicerose@talktalk.net. www.nsra.mymindset.co.uk

Allergy Care Catalogue, Pollards Yard, Wood Street, Taunton, Somerset TA1 1UP. (For unusual foods)

British Society for Allergy, Environmental and Nutritional Medicine, P O Box 7, Knighton, Powys LD & 2WF. Tel: 01547 550380. Email: info@ecomed.org.uk. www.ecomed.org.uk

ME Action Campaign, 3rd Floor, Canningford House, 38 Victoria Street, Bristol BS1 6BY. Tel: 0845 123 2314. Email: admin@afme.org.uk. www.afme.org.uk

Chronic Fatigue Syndrome Foundation, P O Box 220398, Charlotte, NC 28222-0398, USA. Tel: 704 362 2343

American Liver Foundation, 75 Maiden Lane, Suite 603, New York NY 10038, USA. Tel: 212 668 1000. www.liverfoundation.org

Intestinal Disease Foundation, Inc., 1323 Forbes Ave, Suite 200, Pittsburgh, PA 15219. Tel: 412 261 5888

Candida Research Information Foundation, P O Box 2719, Castro Valley, CA 94546. Tel: 415 582 2179

Gluten Intolerance Group, 31213 124th Avenue SE, Auburn, WA 98092 3667, USA. Tel: 253 833 6655. www.gluten.net

INFORMATION

Nutrition Library, 56 London Road, Hailsham, BN27 3DD. Tel/fax: 01323 846888. Email: Dsm50@pavilion.co.uk. (Email title 'nutrition data request'. £10.00 per printout of nutrition data requested)

MAIL ORDER SUPPLEMENTS

The Nutri Centre, 7 Park Crescent, London W1N 3HE. Tel: 0207 436 5122. Email: enq@nutricentre.com. www.nutricentre.com. (Mail order bookshop on site)

Higher Nature, Burwash Common, East Sussex TN19 7LX. Tel: 01435 883484. Email: info@higher-nature.co.uk. www.higher-nature.co.uk

Health Plus Ltd, Dolphin House, 27 Cradle Hill Industrial Estate, Seaford, East Sussex, BN25 3JE. Tel: 01323 872277. www.healthplus.co.uk

Biocare, Lakeside, 180 Lifford Lane, Kings Norton, Birmingham B30 3NU. Tel: 0121 433 3727. Email: sales@biocare.co.uk. www.biocare.co.uk

Helios Homeopathic Pharmacy, 87–89 Camden Road, Tunbridge Wells, Kent TN1 2QR. Tel: 01892 537254. www.helios.co.uk

Anglo-German Homeopathic Centre, 11 Atlay Street, Westfields, Hereford HR4 9PF.

Specialist Herbal Supplies, Portslade Hall, 18 Station Road, Postslade BN41 1GB. Tel: 0800 774 4494. Email: sales@shs100.com. www.shs100.com

Nature's Best, Century Place, Tunbridge Wells, Kent TN2 3EQ. Tel: 01892 552175. www.naturesbest.co.uk

Nutricology, Inc., 2300 North Loop Road, Alameda, CA 94502, USA. Tel: 800 545 9960. www.nutricology.com

Homeopathic Education Services, 2124 Kittredge Street, Berkeley, CA 94704, USA. Tel: 510 649 0294. www.homeopathic.com

Professional Botanicals, PO Box 9822, Ogden, UT 94409, USA. Tel: 877 745 0850. www.professionalbotanicals.com

Metagenics, 100 Avenue La Pata, San Clemente, CA 92673, USA. Tel: 800 692 9400. www.metagenics.com

MASSAGE

The London College of Massage, 16 Bramley Court, Wickham Street, Kent DA16 3DG. Tel: 020 3259 0000. Email: training@londoncollegeofmassage.co.uk. www.londoncollegeofmassage.co.uk

The Northern Institute of Massage, 14-16 St Mary's Place, Bury, Greater Manchester BL9 0DZ. Tel: 0161 797 1800. Email: information@nim.co.uk. www.nim.co.uk

Massage Association, 820 Davis Street, Suite 100, Evanston, IL 60201, USA

NATUROPATHY

British College of Naturopathy and Osteopathy, Lief House, 120–122 Finchley Road, London NW3 5HR. Tel: 020 7435 6464. www.bcno.ac.uk

General Council and Register of Naturopaths, Goswell House, 2 Goswell Road, Street BA16 0JG. Tel: 08780 456984. www.naturopathy.org.uk

American Association of Naturopathic Physicians, 4435 Wisconsin Avenue NW, Suite 403, Washington DC 20016. Tel: 866 538 2267. www.naturopathic.org

Canadian Naturopathic Association, Suite 205, 1234 17th Avenue SW, P O Box 3143, Station C, Calgary, Alberta, Canada. Tel: 413 244 4487

Australian Natural Therapists Association (ANTA), Suite 1, MBA House, Trades Place, Maroochydore, Queensland 4558. Tel: 1800 817 577. www.anta.com.au

NUTRITIONAL TESTING

Biolab Medical Unit, The Stone House, 9 Weymouth Street, London W1N 3FF. Tel: 020 7636 5959. Email: info@biolab.co.uk. www.biolab.co.uk

British Society for Allergy, Environmental and

Nutritional Medicine, P O Box 7, Knighton LD7 1WT. Tel: 01547 550378. Email: info@ecomed.org,uk. www.ecomed.org.uk

McCarrison Society, c/o Institute of Brain Chemistry and Human Nutrition, London Metropolitan University, North London Campus, 166–222 Holloway Road, London N7 8DB. Tel: 020 7133 2440. Email: info@mccarrisonsociety.org.uk. www.mccarrisonsociety.org.uk

The Doctors Laboratory Plc, 58 Wimpole Street, London W1M 7DE. Tel: 020 7480 4800

Diagnostech, The Cottage, Lakeside Centre, 180 Lifford Lane, Kings Norton, Birmingham B30 3NT. Tel: 0121 458 3407

Great Smokies Diagnostic Laboratory, 63 Zillcoa Street, Ashville 28801-1074, North Carolina, USA. European link: Health Interlink Ltd, Interlink House, Unit B, Asfordby Business Park, Welby, Melton Mowbray, Leicestershire LE14 3JL. Tel: 01664 810011. Email: info@health-interlink.com. www.health-interlink.com

Trace Elements Inc., 4501 Sunbelt Drive, Addison, Texas 75001. Tel: 800 824 2314. www.traceelements.com. (Hair mineral analysis)

PAIN

Input Programme, St Thomas' Hospital, Lambeth Palace Road, London SE1 7EH. Tel: 020 7188 7188. www.guysandstthomas.nhs.uk. (For the relief of chronic pain)

BackCare, 16 Elmtree Road, Teddington, Middlesex TW11 8ST. Helpline: 0845 130 2704. Email: website@backcare.org.uk. www.backcare.org.uk

American Chronic Pain Association, P O Box 850, Rocklin, CA 95677, USA. Tel: 1 800 533 3231. www.theacpa.org

PMS

National Association for Premenstrual Syndrome, 41 Old Street, East Peckham, Kent TN12 5AP. Tel: 0879 777 2178. www.pms.org.uk

OSTEOPOROSIS

National Osteoporosis Society, Camerton, Bath, Avon, BA2 OPJ. Tel: 0845 130 3076. Email: info@nos.org.uk. www.nos.org.uk

REFLEXOLOGY

The British Reflexology Association, Monks Orchard, Whitbourne, Worcester WR6 5RB. Tel: 01886 821207. Email: bra@britreflex.co.uk. www.bra@britreflex.co.uk

The International School of Reflexology, P O Box 12642, St Petersburgh, FL 33733, USA

SURGERY

The Hysterectomy Association, The Gables, Acreman Close, Cerne Abbas, Dorset DT2 7JU. Tel: 0871 7811141. Email: info@hysterectomy-association.org.uk. www.hysterectomy-association.org.uk

Hysterectomy Support Network, 3 Lymne Close, Green St Green, Orpington, Kent BR6 6BS. Tel: 0181 856 3881

Medical Self Care, Box 717, Inverness, CA 94937, USA. Tel: (415) 663 8462

Family Health Service, Medical Records Assessment: contact your local branch

The Patients Association, P O Box 935, Harrow, Middlesex HA1 3YJ. Tel: 0845 608 4455. Email: mailbox@patientsassociation.com. www.patientsassociation.com

Medical Information Bureau, Consumer Infomation Office, P O Box 105, Essex Station, Boston, MA 02112, USA. Tel: 866 692 6901. Email: infoline@mib.com. www.mib.com

SYSTEMIC KINESIOLOGY

Academy of Systemic Kinesiology, 39 Browns Road, Surbiton, Surrey KT5 8ST

WOMEN'S HEALTH

Women's Environmental Network, P O Box 30626, London E1 1TZ. Tel: 020 7481 9004. Email: info@wen.org.uk. www.wen.org.uk

National Women's Health Network, 514 10th Street NW, Suite 400, Washington DC 20004, USA. Tel: 202 347 1140. Email: nwhn@nwhn.org. www.nwhn.org

Jean Hailes Foundation for Women's Health, P O Box 1108, Clayton, South Victoria 3169, Australia. Tel: 03 9562 7555. Email: clinic@jeanhailes.org.au. www.endometriosis.org.au

The Endometriosis and Fertility Clinic, The Hale Clinic, 7 Park Crescent, London W1B 1PF. Tel: 020 7631 0156 (bookings). Email: info@haleclinic.com; dian@endometriosis.co.uk. www.haleclinic.com; www.endometriosis.co.uk

The Cystitis and Overactive Bladder Foundation, 76 High Street, Stony Stratford, Bucks MK11 1AH. Tel: 01908 569169. Email: info@cobfoundation.org. www.cobfoundation.org

Pelvic Inflammatory Disease Support Group, c/o Womens Health, London EC1. Tel: 020 7251 6580

Pelvic Pain Support Network, P O Box 6559, Poole, Dorset DH12 9DP. Email: info@pelvicpain.org.uk. www.pelvicpain.org.uk

Post Natal Depression Support Group, 66 Glencester Road, Bishopston, Bristol BS7 8BH. Tel: 01272 232 360

Stillbirth and Neonatal Death Society (SANDS), 28 Portland Place, Argyle House, London W1N 4DE. Tel: 0207 436 5881.

Email: helpline@uk-sands.org. www.uk-sands.org

Support for Termination after Abnormalities (SAFTA), 29 Soho Square, London W1V 6JB

Mooncup Ltd, Dolphin House, 40 Arundel Place, Brighton BN2 1GD. Tel: 01273 673845. info@mooncup.co.uk. www.mooncup.co.uk

Vulval Health Awareness. Tel: 07765 947599. Email: info@vhac.org. www.vhac.org

YOGA

Yoga Biomedical Trust, 90-92 Pentonville Road, London N1 9HS. Tel: 020 7689 3040. www.yogatherapy.org

The American Yoga Association, P O Box 19986, FL 34236, USA. Email: info@americanyogaassociation.org. www.americanyogaassociation.org

OTHER USEFUL ADDRESSES

www.endometriosis.co.uk
www.makingbabies.com
www.obgyn.net
www.foodlaw.rdg.ac.uk/additive.html
www.bantransfats.com
www.worldhunger.org/articles/global/ray.html
www.hsph.harvard.edu/reviews/transfats.html
www.purdeyenvironment.com
www.healthfocus.net/function/htm

Internet cafes and many libraries have facilities for you to use a computer to surf the Internet

Index